EMPTY SLEEVES

Empty Sleeves

Amputation in the Civil War South

BRIAN CRAIG MILLER

The University of Georgia Press   *Athens and London*

Portions of the introduction and chapter 2 were originally published in
Lawrence Kreiser and Randal Allred, eds., *The Civil War in Popular Culture:
Memory and Meaning* (Lexington: University Press of Kentucky, 2014), 25–44.
Portions of the introduction were originally published online, *New York Times*
Opinionator Blog, *Disunion*, December 20, 2013.

Set in Berthold Baskerville by Graphic Composition, Inc., Bogart, Georgia.

Most University of Georgia Press titles are
available from popular e-book vendors.

Printed digitally

Library of Congress Cataloging-in-Publication Data

Miller, Brian Craig.
    Empty sleeves : amputation in the Civil War South / Brian Craig Miller.
        xvi, 257 pages : illustrations ; 23 cm.
        Includes bibliographical references (pages 227–246) and index.
    ISBN 978-0-8203-4331-0 (hardcover : alkaline paper) – ISBN 978-0-8203-4332-7
(paperback : alkaline paper) – ISBN 978-0-8203-4333-4 (ebook) 1. United States–
History–Civil War, 1861–1865–Medical care. 2. Amputation–Social aspects–Southern
States–History–19th century. 3. Surgery, Military–Southern States–History–19th century.
4. United States–History–Civil War, 1861–1865–Veterans. 5. Disabled veterans–
Southern States–Social conditions–19th century. 6. Amputees–Southern States–Social
conditions–19th century. 7. Masculinity–Social aspects–Southern States–History–
19th century. 8. United States–History–Civil War, 1861–1865–Social aspects.
9. Confederate States of America–Social conditions. 10. Southern States–Social
conditions–19th century. I. Title.
    E625.M55 2015
    973.7'75–dc23

                                                                    2014023161

British Library Cataloging-in-Publication Data available

FOR NICHOLAS

CONTENTS

ILLUSTRATIONS

TABLES

ACKNOWLEDGMENTS

The genesis of this book emerged in the spring of 2003, when I was taking a graduate seminar in Reconstruction at the University of Mississippi. My professor, Nancy Bercaw, encouraged me to explore amputation in the aftermath of the Civil War within a gender framework. Her insights, encouragements, and careful readings of early drafts of my main arguments have been invaluable, and I owe a great deal of debt to her.

I am continually humbled by the proficiency, exuberant assistance, and diligent patience of archivists and librarians across the country. I am grateful to the following archival and library staffs, who made hundreds of lonely hours in the archives a pleasurable and productive experience: the Virginia Historical Society, the Library of Congress, the National Archives, the University of Texas at Austin, the Texas Land Grant Office, the Mississippi Department of Archives and History, the Louisiana State Archives, Manuscripts and Special Collections at Perkins Library at Duke University, the Southern Historical Collection at the University of North Carolina at Chapel Hill, the Arkansas State History Commission, the University of Arkansas Special Collections, the Florida State Archives, the South Caroliniana Library, the South Carolina Department of Archives and History, the South Carolina Historical Society, the University of Georgia, Emory University, the Atlanta History Center, the Georgia Archives, Missouri State Archives, the University of Kentucky, Kentucky Department for Libraries and Archives, Kentucky Historical Society, Auburn University, the University of Alabama at Tuscaloosa, and the Alabama Department of Archives and History.

In addition, at several research locations, staff members and archivists eagerly embraced my project and went the extra mile to hunt for obscure sources. I am humbled by the following individuals who made the research for a book like this possible: John Coski and Teresa Roane at the Museum of the Confederacy; Lorri Eggleston and Terry Reimer at the National Museum of Civil War Medicine in Frederick, Maryland; Eric Boyle at the U.S. Army Medical Museum; Jean Carefoot at the Texas State Archives; Jennifer Ford at the University of Mississippi; Lee Miller, Sean Benjamin, and Eira Tansey at the Manuscripts and Special Collections at Tulane University; Siva Blake at the Historic New Orleans Collection; Tara Laver, Gabe Harrell, and Germaine Bienvenieu at LSU in Baton Rouge; Darla Brock at the Tennessee State Library and Archives; Darrell Meadows and Jennifer Duplaga at the Kentucky Historical Society; Jason Stratman at the Missouri History Museum; Tamoul "Tee" Quakhaan at the Free Library in Philadelphia; Jeanie Braun and Kristine Kruger at the Margaret Herrick Library connected to the Academy of Motion Picture Arts and Sciences, and Mike Flannery and the ever diligent Peggy Balch at UAB.

Researching around the South requires extensive financial resources, and thus I am indebted for the financial support that came in the form of research fellowships at the Kentucky Historical Society and the Reynolds Historical Fellowship at the University of Alabama at Birmingham Medical School. I am also grateful to Emporia State University for a summer research grant that allowed me to research across five states.

The supportive and diligent hands of the staff at the University of Georgia Press have nurtured this book. I am grateful to Derek Krissoff for taking an initial interest in my work and to Beth Snead for her tireless efforts. Mick Gusinde-Duffy has offered endless support since his arrival at UGA Press, and I look forward to a lengthy working relationship with him in the future. Additional thanks go to Joseph Dahm for an excellent copyedit and John Joerschke and Beth Snead for their assistance through production. I also greatly appreciate the carefully constructed reader reports I received from a few anonymous readers, who supported the project and pushed me to take this book to surprising places. I am forever indebted to them for their expertise, kindness, and intellectual vigor.

I am especially grateful to the people who have offered encouragement on the manuscript as it developed, from conference papers to chapters that appeared in edited collections. I would like to thank Wendy Venet, George Rable, Laura Edwards, Mike Flannery, Shauna Devine, William Blair, John Boles, Louis Masur, Conevery Bolton Valencius, and Christopher Phillips for their helpful comments on various sections of the manuscript and encouragement to keep working. Very special thanks go to Steve Berry, who organized an outstanding symposium of Civil War weirdos that gathered together in the fall of 2009. I am so very proud that Steve not only graced this work with his brilliance and editorial diligence but has also enriched my life as a dear friend. At that symposium, I met Amy

Murrell Taylor, who read each and every word of this book and offered spot-on suggestions and endless encouragement. The lasting friendships forged in Athens have significantly shaped my work and my life, and I am grateful to Anya Jabour, Steve Nash, Michael DeGruccio, Andy Slap, and Dan Sutherland, who all offered source materials, suggestions, and unending encouragement. My life has been enriched by my friendship with Kathryn Meier. Her gracious nature and inquisitive mind have enriched my own thinking of suffering in the Civil War. Thanks to Joan Cashin for always emailing me the random amputees she stumbled upon on a daily basis. I am also grateful to Pete Carmichael, who sent me amputees and became one of my very first Civil War pals. I thank him today as he is embarking upon a difficult journey: one that I know he will succeed at. In addition, the incomparable Diane Miller Sommerville offered so much assistance to nurture me as an author. I cannot thank her enough for her patience, her encouragement, her support, and her willingness to share so many sources. LeeAnn Whites, a thoughtful scholar and splendid conversationalist, provided endless encouragement and many hearty meals during my travels through Missouri. Her work has profoundly affected how I think about the Civil War, and her friendship has made each day as a Civil War scholar a better one. Megan Kate Nelson, a marvelous email pen pal and an even better friend, shared her own work on amputees, as well as many hours of talking about life and limbs. Finally, I thank Lesley Gordon for her friendship and her support of my career. If it takes a village of historians to raise and nurture a manuscript, I am honored to have the above-mentioned scholars in my village. No village idiot here, other than myself if I have made errors throughout the book.

A note of extreme gratitude goes to friends and colleagues who continue to make each of my days a better one: Greg Schneider, Darla Mallein, John Neff, Mike Gray, Barb Gannon, Minoa Uffelman, Paul Beazley, Alice Hull-Lachassee, Brian Van Norman, Terry Bax (who let me use his house to write), Courtney Roy (who let me use her home in D.C.), and Matt Stanley (who provided some material culture for me to peruse). A note of special gratitude to those who molded my life, especially my brother, Brent, my sister, Brooke, and my parents, Craig and Linda. I am proud to be the son that you raised and the historian that you nurtured through our Civil War family vacations.

I am also thankful that I went for a run with Nick on a sunny afternoon along the trolley trail in March 2009. Since that fateful afternoon, a turning point in my life, I have been blessed by your sense of humor and your many great virtues, of which patience and understanding allow me to be not only a better educator, researcher, and writer but also a better man. I always tell my students that they need to do what they love and have someone to love while doing it. I am extraordinarily blessed to have both facets in my own life. You are truly my today and I cannot imagine my tomorrow without you.

EMPTY SLEEVES

Empty Sleeves in Civil War History and Memory

As the guns fell silent and the smoke cleared from the battlefield at Shiloh on April 7, 1862, Union captain John W. Tuttle scoured the torn landscape in search of wounded comrades. Tuttle found several damaged Union and Confederate soldiers "painfully" dragging themselves through the "deep black mud." The officer assisted the men to an area of the battlefield being used as a field hospital, where "the most shocking and sickening sight of the day or any other day during the war met our view. It was two or three wagon loads of amputated hands, arms, feet, and legs thrown in a heap." Tuttle had trained himself to react nonchalantly when encountering "dead and mangled bodies on the field." But he had failed to prepare himself for this "naked and ghastly mass of human flesh," which haunted him the rest of his life.[1]

The wartime images of amputation, mangled limbs, and bloody stumps remain vital to our understanding of the unprecedented level of suffering wrought by the Civil War. The darker side of the conflict often piques curiosity but remains difficult for many Americans to grasp. We like to think of our Civil War in terms of noble officers and honorable soldiers engaged in grand charges across open terrain. We like to only believe that the battles fought and won eventually secured the triumph of freedom and emancipation. Yet freedom and reunion came at a heavy price. Over the course of four years, hundreds of thousands of Americans fell dead in pristine pastures, beneath towering oaks, and along the banks of trickling streams and mighty rivers. The projectiles of war wounded hundreds of thousands more, creating a generation of men suffering from festering wounds and nagging injuries and struggling following the removal of their hands, feet, fingers, toes, arms, or legs by a medical surgeon.

The specter of empty sleeves and bloodthirsty surgeons haunts us still, in some cases literally. On a recent Haunted History tour of New Orleans, a guide stopped a group of tourists in front of the Hotel Provincial, located on Chartres Street in the heart of the French Quarter. The picturesque hotel, boasting free Wi-Fi and a daily continental breakfast, previously served as the location of a Civil War hospital. Apparently, as guests dine on cheese Danish and attempt to get a restful night's sleep, the ghost of a Civil War surgeon, still wearing his blood-splattered apron, roams the halls. Pints of blood materialize in the bathroom sinks, and a few spectral patients still wander the hotel halls.[2]

Amputation scenes are easier to come by at the cinema. Indeed, in Hollywood war movies a dismemberment scene is de rigueur. Our popular perception of Civil War hospitals and amputation emerged in 1939, embodied by the nursing services of Scarlett O'Hara in the epic film *Gone with the Wind*. O'Hara works tirelessly as a volunteer at Peachtree Military Hospital in Atlanta. As the artillery shells of Union general William T. Sherman's guns rattle the hospital, Scarlett and Dr. Meade walk by a Confederate soldier with an injured leg. Despite a lack of chloroform, Meade quickly condemns the leg to amputation. As the distraught Confederate screams out in pain, Scarlett, ordered to assist in the operation, approaches the table with great curiosity and trepidation. The camera remains squarely on her face, revealing a look of horror and disgust as she witnesses an amputation without any anesthetic. Scarlett departs the hospital, emphatically telling an orderly who has relayed a message that the physician needs her: "Let him wait. I'm going home. I've done enough. I don't want any more men dying and screaming. I don't want anymore." In the carriage ride back to her temporary home, the dashing Rhett Butler asks Scarlett if she has grown tired of seeing "men chopped up."[3]

Amputations appear in most Civil War films. In *Dances with Wolves*, Lieutenant John Dunbar (portrayed by Kevin Costner) musters enough courage to escape amputation and ride toward enemy lines in an apparent suicide mission. Even in *Ride with the Devil*'s depiction of irregular warfare, bushwhacker Jack Bull Chiles loses an arm during an impromptu amputation. In the 1959 film *The Horse Soldiers*, after members of the Union

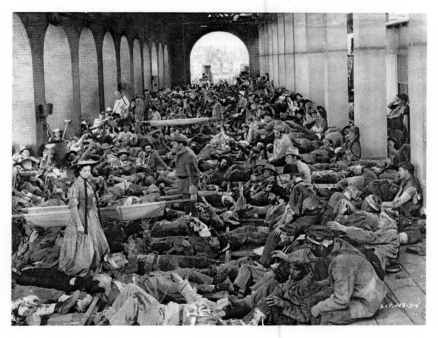

Figure 1. Scarlett O'Hara (Vivien Leigh) moves among the wounded in Atlanta in this moving scene from *Gone with the Wind*. Courtesy of the core collection, production files of the Margaret Herrick Library, Academy of Motion Pictures Arts and Sciences.

cavalry ride into Newton Station, Colonel John Marlowe (John Wayne) and Major Kendall (William Holden) interact with a Confederate prisoner named Colonel Johnny Miles. As Colonel Marlowe argues about whether or not Confederate property can be considered contraband, Major Kendall interrupts the conversation, having recognized the Confederate prisoner from their time fighting Indians together before the war. Kendall also notices that his former comrade lost his right arm: "Sorry about the arm, John. When did that happen?" "I want neither your solicitude nor to recall our association," responds the defiant Confederate, Colonel Miles, who then looks at Colonel Marlowe and asks, "Have I your permission to retire, sir?" Marlowe casually orders some men to take the Confederate prisoner to his holding cell. As Marlowe and Kendall watch Colonel Miles recede into the background, Kendall remarks, "I can't figure a man like Miles giving up that easy. He's West Point. Tough as nails." "Maybe losing that arm took a lot out of him," responds Marlowe. Kendall quickly rejoins, "The man I knew could lose both arms and still kick you to death."[4]

Even in the most recent Civil War film, Steven Spielberg's *Lincoln*, the horrific nature of Civil War medicine makes its inevitable appearance. Lincoln is embarked on a carriage ride with his son Robert through the streets of Washington. As father and son debate Robert's desire to enlist in the war effort, the carriage parks in front of a military hospital. Robert refuses to follow his father into the hospital, as he knows that his father plans to use a hospital filled with Union amputees as a way to dissuade him from military service. As Robert passes by the hospital door, a bloody wheelbarrow races by. Robert follows it to the top of a hill, where black workers reveal its contents: severed hands, feet, arms, and legs. The workers then dump the fresh appendages into a pit filled with festering and decrepit limbs. The image disturbs Robert, and also sent gasps through sold-out crowds in theaters across the country.[5]

However crude, Hollywood's attempts to recognize and depict the suffering inflicted by war and amputation have often surpassed historians' own. Only recently have historians begun to view their subjects through the lens of suffering. For most of the twentieth century the Civil War tended to be digested as a set of casualty figures (recently revised upward to potentially 850,000) that awed us without being actually awful. Over the past few years, however, Civil War history has taken a darker turn. Some social and cultural historians have explored the impact of Civil War death on politics and culture. Environmental historians have started to examine how the destruction of war altered portions of the American landscape. Medical historians have focused on sickness and disease, paying particular attention to the impact of illness on the body of Civil War soldiers and civilians. Even given this dark turn, however, the consequences of amputation on Civil War soldiers and civilians, both during and after the war, have remained largely unexplored.[6]

The scope of the phenomenon alone justifies attention. Thousands of soldiers returned home missing a limb and created a permanent class of disabled and dependent men. Such veterans faced bouts of chronic pain, immobility, and the gawks and stares of citizens who viewed the missing appendages as a macabre spectacle. Disabled men were thrown back upon their spouses and families to assist them in dealing with the everyday physical and emotional rigors of life. Damaged veterans also remained dependent on society's willingness to concede that amputation and the altering of the white male body had shattered traditional gender roles, as injured men no longer appeared or functioned as they had prior to the war. Amputated men were also dependent on government programs, whether at the federal level for Union veterans or the state level for Confederate veterans, to fashion prosthetic limbs and extend pension payments. The destruction of slavery, the perseverance of the Union, and the triumph of liberty, freedom, and equality all ensured that the sacrifices of north-ern men would be recognized, memorialized, and cherished for genera-tions beyond the battlefield. Disabled southern soldiers faced a different cultural climate. Their sacrifices, at least to Union victors, seemed the fair wages of error; federal financial assistance was withheld, and amputated Confederates were left scarred, disillusioned, and defeated. To face these challenges, Confederate amputees relied solely on themselves, their com-munities, and eventually their (often dysfunctional) state governments.[7]

Prior to the Civil War, southern men asserted their manhood through mastery and control of women and children, slaves, their land, and their households, as well as through their horses, guns, friends, and feats of strength. Other men defined their manhood through honor, an externally validated sense of self-worth that men then internalized. Such worth was demonstrated to the general public through dressing and acting like a proper man, eating and socializing as a man should, and exhibiting the proper set of emotions, facial expressions, manners, and behaviors. Men, in short, were to *embody* their own patriarchal power; they were to be ro-bust and strong, and to set their claims to honor before their peers, in acts and rituals as diverse as dueling, drinking, and electioneering. Even men without slaves or property identified themselves first *as men* and as "mas-ters of small worlds."[8]

In such a world, the white male physique was the defining marker of manhood. The female body, perceived as frail, remained dependent on the strong masculine body for survival. Virtually every southerner, for in-stance, knew the parable of the oak and the vine, in which the vine asks the oak to "bend your trunk so that you may be a support to me." "My support," replies the mighty oak, "is naturally yours, and you may rely on my strength to bear you up, but I am too large and too solid to bend. Put your arms around me, my pretty vine, and I will manfully support and cherish you [and] while I thus hold you up, you will ornament my trunk."

Thus tutored, southerners viewed aristocratic white women as actually "*incapable* of performing labor," according to one historian. Black bodies too were almost by their nature "disabled." Yes, they might be mulishly strong, but they were not steady; they were no oaks. And owning to their forced labor, black bodies routinely broke down, or they were "broken," by the whip, the lash, or other devices that left permanent scars. At the same time, slaves mutilated their own bodies as a form of resistance, to slow down work patterns or prevent them from performing a specific duty while enslaved. At daguerreotype parlors, museums, and traveling shows, Americans upheld the beauty of the healthy white body and bore witness to the deviant bodies of often racialized freaks. They gawked in horror at dwarves, for instance, and at fat ladies, conjoined twins, and individuals born without any arms or legs. For years prior to the Civil War, damaged and disabled bodies had been relegated to the slave cabins and freak show tents all across the American south.[9]

Prior to the Civil War, a man who sacrificed an arm or a leg in battle lost more than an appendage. While white southern men may have accepted amputation as a reasonable medical course of action, their society was fairly unforgiving, and the presence of an empty sleeve in the antebellum era often forced physically damaged men to work harder to resecure their manhood. Thomas William Ward, a veteran of the War for Independence in Texas, lost his leg at San Antonio in 1836. Four years later, he contributed to a cannon salute in Austin, Texas, to celebrate the fourth anniversary of Texas independence. However, the cannon exploded and shattered Ward's right arm, prompting a second amputation. Although he recovered, the double amputee was now both a sympathetic figure and something of a freak. With a shattered male physique, Ward remained dependent on government appointments in order to earn a living, including an appointment as Texas land commissioner and consul to Panama. Sam Houston, who appointed Ward to the consul position, felt an enormous amount of sympathy, writing, "I had recommended him for his present position, because, he was mutilated, and I pitied him."[10]

Pity is thin gruel. Unlike the thousands of amputees created by the Civil War, Ward struggled almost alone, as he variously contemplated suicide and lashed out in anger at his political rivals. He eventually married Susan Bean, in hopes that the loving marriage would heal his battered identity. Instead, the relationship turned sour and evaporated, and in his mismanaged rage Ward lashed out at his wife, who later vented about her estranged husband in public, remarking how she had "sacrificed herself by marrying a man with one leg and one arm." Finally Ward secured a prosthetic limb that both added to his personal comfort and masked his apparent disability. The artificial device diminished the number of people who viewed him as a "cripple" or an object of derision. Although Ward surrounded himself with men and women who recognized his missing limbs as markers of bravery, sacrifice, and manhood, the general public had not been educated in how to think and feel, and they viewed him as a disfigured oddity. Military heroism may have shaped his manhood among those in his inner circle, but it could not trump societal perceptions of the shattered male physique.[11]

As southern white men marched off to war in 1861, their military service cemented their masculine status. Men endured a kind of hypermasculinization, historian Clyde Griffen has argued, in "actual ordeals which combined murderous male conflict with male camaraderie" and created the "central event of this generation's lives." Believing they fought for an honorable cause, soldiers proved their manhood by taking up arms to protect a wife, a child, or a homestead from invading Yankees. They stood shoulder to shoulder with other men and proved their manly worth in battle before an audience of their peers who recognized and validated the honorable performance. Members of the community and the individual families of the soldiers certainly recognized the art of soldiering as an honorable profession and a clear marker for manhood. Southern soldiers marched off optimistic of securing a victory that would prove they were simply better men than their northern counterparts. They used the war to "aggressively defend their manhood," historian LeeAnn Whites argued. After all, Johnny Reb believed he held a distinct advantage over Billy Yank because southern men rode horses, shot guns, and defended their homeland in the decades prior to 1860, solidifying their own internal self-worth. This is not to say that northern men did not define their manhood through similar venues. Southern men simply believed they held the advantage and looked forward to using the war to prove their superior manhood in battle.[12]

Soldiers on both sides foresaw a quick and majestic war that would secure individual and collective rationales for heading into combat. The reality of the Civil War shattered romantic notions of warfare, as men found their will and nerve routinely tested. Some men did become inured to the constant drilling, grueling marches, and gruesome scenes; they passed the war's test of manhood, though often at staggering cost. Others failed the examination altogether and, consumed with fear, ran away. Still others found their will to fight broken by letters from loved ones calling for a speedy return home to fulfill their manly duty to the health and welfare of wives and children.

But the wounded faced a different set of masculine challenges. They were broken, physically and often psychologically. At the moment of their wounding, and in the early days of treatment, they were often separated from comrades, among strangers. Thousands found their fates in the hands of surgeons or physicians, who, of necessity, made quick decisions about how to preserve life, with less thought to the quality of the life they preserved. As historian Stephen Berry noted, "Regardless of its source or severity, though, a wound was one's own. No man had another exactly like it. The moment a soldier got hit, he and his wound were alone in the world, and they would walk the road to recovery alone too."[13]

Soldiers returned to their families with scrapes, scars, and festering wounds. In many cases, southern soldiers could either mask their scars of war or proudly display them. After all, as historian Jennifer Travis noted, a wound carried "some degree of honor." Yet, southern society before the war had few precedents for upholding such markers of manhood, especially among upper-class men who had placed a premium on a pristine, manly physical appearance. Confederate amputees could not mask their physical sacrifices and returned to a society that would now partially embrace and partially shun its incomplete and damaged "heroes."[14]

The outcome of a war fundamentally shapes how a society views its veterans and their physical and mental sacrifices. The triumphant northern veterans returned return home to cheering crowds and joyous parades that trained their society to immediately recognize their red badges of courage. The same cannot be said for southern men, who returned defeated. Their failure in war fundamentally altered perceptions of manhood, as southern men lost not only the war but also "the right to construct their sense of manhood exactly as they pleased," as LeeAnn Whites noted. Would society still recognize their physical sacrifices as worthy of respect, love, and admiration? Would a loving spouse look at an amputated husband with affection or horror? Would a potential business client find admiration in an amputee or recoil in horror? Could these damaged white bodies still control and inspire fear in black people, particularly in the postemancipation era? Was the empty sleeve simply too much to bear for both the veteran and their society? Could white southerners find a way to redefine manhood that incorporated the physically scarred veteran?[15]

As southern amputees returned home, they faced a host of psychological burdens, including "a loss of self-esteem, loss of completeness of the body image, loss of respect for one's appearance and functional ability, and inability to relate to oneself, one's spouse, and one's family, friends, and employer in a normal manner," according to one physician. Some men turned to a prosthetic limb to help fill the empty sleeve and mask the disability. Even with a mechanical substitute, however, veterans faced enormous psychological challenges, as they struggled to cope with new limitations and new kinds of dependency. Individuals who encountered an amputee on a daily basis were encouraged to offer support, rather than recoil in disgust, in order to accelerate a smooth transition back to society.[16]

No wonder many Confederate men worried about how their amputations and wounds would be judged by family, friends, and society. As historian Megan Kate Nelson has argued, "As the ruins of men dispersed throughout the country, their fragmented bodies became sites of debate about both wartime and post-war masculinity." It is reasonable to assume that white southerners would view the actions of their soldiers as honorable. But, viewing the sometimes grotesque results of those actions, southern society had to reassess and reconfigure their understanding of honor and the male physiognomy. After all, as one physician noted, "the amputee internalizes society's attitude." Southern white men and women had to incorporate the imperfect southern male body within their traditional notions of manhood and did so by recognizing damaged veterans as "heroes" within the construction of a Lost Cause mythology.[17]

The challenges amputees posed to southern society were not merely visual and symbolic. Amputated men exhibited a profound level of dependency, which had traditionally been seen as a marker of childhood, femininity, or enslavement. Wounded soldiers depended on surgeons to make a proper medical recommendation; on women to provide continued medical care, emotional support, and often basic functioning; on employers to cheerfully accept diminished capacity without seeming to stoop to charity or pity; and on the state to provide prosthetics, validation, and, ultimately, a

pension. The process by which this new level of white male dependency—
on other men, on women, on employers, and on the state—became soci-
etally and culturally accepted (however ambivalently) was, I argue, a critical facet in the remaking of white manhood in the postbellum South.[18]

The empty sleeve became an iconic symbol in the aftermath of the
Civil War. High-profile amputees, like Richard Ewell and John Bell Hood,
came to embody Confederate sacrifice and Confederate "incompleteness."
They wore the story of the war on their bodies: true, something important
had been lost, but still they stood erect and unbowed. Beneath these high-
profile cases, however, and even within them, lurked a greater sense of
desperation. Before the war, patriarchy had been embodied by the white
male physique and figure. Slaves might break down physically. Women
might break down emotionally. But men did not break. As the war progressed, men lost body parts and prewar notions of dependency and disability no longer applied, as the strong body fell victim to the power of
shot and shell. After the war, the many challenges to southern notions
of masculinity, including defeat and emancipation, were exacerbated for
amputees. As they limped home to their families and communities, amputated men remained dependent on their spouses, peers, and communities
to reconstruct their manhood in the midst of new challenges brought on
by disability. Historians have posited that women "reconstructed" southern masculinity, but this grossly underestimates how grievous a beating
these men's bodies had taken. Rather, these men ended up on the sidelines in Lost Cause memory, finding limited help for their disabilities, as
benevolent groups could not financially deal with so many veterans and
state governments initially remained hesitant to create an entirely new
class of dependents. Only after years had passed, and many of the war's
amputees had faded into history, did the states conclude that they had no
choice but to step in to help make men whole, or at least not an embarrassment to themselves.

The lack of documented evidence pertaining to amputation in the Confederacy presents historians with a daunting task to uncover the experiences of southern amputees. No concrete figures are available as to how
many Confederate amputees existed and survived the war. The *Official
Records* of the war contain numerous detailed casualty reports that list the
number of amputees, but they usually pertain to Union soldiers. Hospital
records in the Confederacy also fail to offer reliable figures on amputees.

This is partly because, in the early years of the war, without a bureaucratic system of medical record keeping, amputation cases went largely unrecorded. As Confederate doctor J. T. Gilmore explained, "The almost total absence of organization in the medical department at that period sufficiently explains why no mention is made in the official reports of many important operations performed in the early part of the war." Later in the war, surgeons did remark on the nature of surgeries, including amputation, because medical paperwork had been regularized and included spaces for comments about specific amputations and operations. Unfortunately, the Confederacy destroyed many of these viable medical records upon the evacuation of Richmond in 1865. As Joseph Jones remarked, "The destruction of a large portion of the records in the Surgeon General's office in Richmond was a serious . . . loss to the medical department." Destroyed, dilapidated, and unorganized medical records prevent historians from ever knowing how many amputations took place in the Confederacy during the Civil War.[19]

Limited documentation in the South is not the only hurdle historians have faced when tackling the medical ramifications of the Civil War. Further obscuring a reliable figure on the number of Confederate amputations are numerous erroneous and fabricated accounts pertaining to amputation. One incident recalled by W. L. Henderson exemplifies the kind of false accounts that ended up in the medical records. Henderson recalled having witnessed the amputation of a soldier in Memphis in March 1862, by Dr. E. S. Fenner. Henderson remembered seeing the patient four months later in perfect health after having lost his leg at the hip, a rare procedure that had an extremely high mortality rate. Dr. C. H. Mastin, the inspector of hospitals, denied any knowledge of Fenner performing the unusual operation and spoke to Fenner in 1865, who revealed that he had never participated in the amputation. Henderson fabricated the report because early in the war, with hip amputations being so dangerous and rare, medical professionals desired any examples of an early successful amputation to use as a model for future surgeries. Henderson's false report provided early inspiration and hope to other surgeons, only to be dashed by the cold, hard facts.[20]

Another methodological challenge to the history of Civil War amputations is the scarcity of detailed accounts by the surgeons who performed the operations or the amputees themselves. While many surgeons corresponded with their wives, they avoided discussing the graphic details of amputation, which might have shocked or sickened their spouses. The hospital records, once standardized, afforded limited space to talk significantly about the amputation beyond what was performed and the prescribed treatment during the recovery period. Literate Confederate soldiers, who profoundly chronicled the minutia of their daily lives, failed to leave us the same extent of detail in regard to the loss of a limb. Several soldiers mentioned their amputation in a letter or a diary entry, but few men wrote exhaustively about what their empty sleeve meant to them as a soldier or a southern man. At the same time, southern masculinity precluded an open dialogue from men about their feelings, as any emotional turmoil was expected to remain hidden. For those who actually mentioned their amputations in wartime correspondence, the mail ended when the firing stopped. Memoirs occasionally filled in some gaps, but only a small minority took up authoring as a hobby or profession in the postwar years. Amputees faded back into the fold of society and reappeared only at veterans' events or in newspaper anecdotes. Damaged men also faced decreased visibility in society due to limited life expectancy, especially for those who faced significant trauma to their body. Pension applications provided such an arena for expression, but the men worried more about proving they had lost a limb than describing what it all meant.

Empty Sleeves is the first full-scale study to examine what losing a limb meant to Confederate surgeons, soldiers, women, and society in general. Despite the limitations on source materials, extensive research has brought together insights gleaned from surgical and medical manuals, hospital records, surgeon reports, letters, diary and journal entries pertaining to amputation, legislative records, pension files and applications, newspaper reports, and numerous anecdotes about what it meant to lose a limb. The book combines political, medical, military, social, cultural, and gender history to create a first look at how disability studies might help us better understand the postwar South.

Yet this book focuses solely on amputees – men who lost arms, legs, fingers, toes, hands, or feet and men who underwent surgery to remove damaged bone, thus resulting in a shortened limb. Thousands of men returned home with different kinds of wounds: nagging gunshot injuries that resulted in early obituaries; losses of hearing, sight, memory, and even basic personality; gruesome head and facial injuries including crushed and missing jawbones and shattered teeth; sexual dysfunction and GI disorders; and wrecked health deriving not merely from battlefield wounds but from four years of poor diet, fatigue, chronic dysentery, and exposure to camp diseases. *Empty Sleeves*, then, is only the beginning of what must become a detailed investigation of how southern society absorbed the massive medical trauma of the Civil War.[21]

Chapter 1 tackles the medical dimensions of amputation through the eyes of the men who altered the male body: the Civil War surgeons. When Confederate soldiers suffered gunshot wounds, they largely depended on their surgeons to provide appropriate medical care and skillful amputations. Unfortunately, popular culture (and even some historians) has portrayed Civil War surgeons as butchers, incompetents, or men too overwhelmed to provide decent care. A survey of medical sources, including accounts from doctors, hospital records, and a wealth of surgical manuals, however, reveals a different portrait. To be sure Confederate surgeons were overwhelmed with patients, especially early in the war, when they faced supply and staff shortages and had to make massive adjustments to their expectations of care. But adjust they did. The war's first year jolted the surgical community, but surgeons quickly learned from early mistakes and became quite adept at saving both patients and limbs. Although some men undoubtedly did amputate rashly, the vast majority of Confederate surgeons were not saw-happy. Rather, they evolved as the war progressed, used caution with amputation, and produced far fewer amputees than the historical literature has suggested. Surgeons knew their own manhood and reputation was at stake each day they arrived at a field hospital. Thus, they tended to consult with their colleagues and numerous surgical and medical manuals that presented extensive arguments about when to amputate and when to put down the scalpel and saw. In short, despite often gritty circumstances, surgical professionalization was actually advanced by the war, even on the Confederate side.

Chapter 2 is also set in the hospital tent but turns the lens on the patients who either rejected or accepted amputation. As soldiers and officers alike entered the wards, their thoughts drifted toward family, religion, survival, fellow comrades in arms, and their postwar livelihood. Some soldiers succumbed to death, knowing they had died honorably from battle. Others, sometime violently, resisted amputation in order to maintain their complete male physique or to get back to the field of battle as quickly as possible. For the vast majority of Confederate soldiers and officers who accepted amputation, their long adjustment was marked by an array of emotional reactions, from humor and sorrow to anger and disillusionment. Generally soldiers recovered better where they found themselves surrounded by other amputated men who could create a supportive environment for their adjustment to their empty sleeve. Fellow amputees also assisted a soldier in dealing with the lengthy road of rehabilitation, the use of a prosthetic limb, and readjustment to postwar society.

The lives of the South's physically shattered white men cannot be explored without also exploring women, who were largely responsible for the men's postsurgical care before and after their homecoming and were integral to the construction and reconstruction of southern manhood after the war. Chapter 3 explores how amputated men remained dependent on southern white women in profound ways. As nurses, women were often the first faces patients saw during their recovery, and although the women saw nursing as their patriotic duty, the sheer dreadfulness of their duties left deep impressions. After the war, some women were forced to persist in permanent nursing roles, caring for their own broken family members. They also formed benevolent societies that shaped the culture and discourse regarding male disability. In addition, southern white women participated in private and even public debates over whether they should marry an amputated man. The Civil War upended notions of dependency, as amputated men remained dependent on willing women to care for their crippled bodies and maintain both their health and welfare, including their "unpunctured vanity," as Margaret Mitchell noted in *Gone with the Wind*. Whatever their societies' perceptions, however, southern white women displayed a wide range of reactions to their new duties and to amputated men as potential suitors.

The final two chapters explore male dependency on fellow citizens and state governments. Chapter 4 chronicles the return of Confederate amputees to their homesteads and the numerous challenges their disabilities created for themselves and their wider society. Where northern amputees entered a more centralized bureaucracy, southern amputees relied on a looser network of in-home care, civilian organizations, veteran-friendly employers, and benevolent societies. As a whole, the South's culture seemed deeply ambivalent about amputated men, with reactions, individual and official, that ranged from apathy to empathy. Benevolent societies did make headway in teaching southerners, especially the young, how to regard amputated men when encountering them in public life. Even with the assistance of benevolent groups and their fellow citizens, amputated men struggled to find meaningful employment and sometimes basic sustenance, as economic opportunities dissipated, and they ended up begging on street corners all across the southern landscape.

The final chapter examines how the destitute condition of many Confederate amputees finally forced the state governments to institute a series of social welfare programs to permanently care for their needs. The U.S. government constructed an aggressive prosthetics and pension program to exclusively care for Union veterans. In the South, veterans remained dependent on financially strapped state governments. Despite dilapidated budgets, however, the former states of the Confederacy worked to eventually extend limited benefits to wounded veterans, including artificial limbs, land grants, and educational vouchers that provided tools for amputated men to remain self-sufficient or dependent on themselves and their families for their economic vitality. Such benefits were hotly debated, and some former Confederate states became enmeshed in extensive political controversy over how (and how much) to care for their broken "heroes." Unionist sentiment, constitutional issues, and the sense that Confederate men were essentially traitors trumped legislative efforts to provide pensions and prosthetics in Maryland, Texas, Arkansas, and Kentucky. Other states debated whether they should issue "Yankee limbs" manufactured by northern companies or establish their own manufacturing facilities to produce prosthetics. Only decades later, after southern states had been redeemed and amputated men faded from society, did legislatures construct a means of sustenance for the truly disabled in the form of a pension. It took most states decades to realize they had to acknowledge that Confederate veterans must become dependent wards of the state in order to survive. Such contentious debates not only shed light on the underreported quest to care for amputated veterans but also highlight the rocky and uneven road to reconciliation in the shadow of the Civil War.

The American Civil War produced an entire generation of wounded, disfigured, and disillusioned men who returned to a world they no longer recognized. Many survived to lead meaningful lives even as they coped with the new realities of emancipation, destruction, and defeat. But their sheer number and peculiar circumstances made them impossible for the culture to ignore. White manhood, which had been the very antithesis of disability and dependency in the antebellum years, now had to make room for a new category of men who were partial, needy, damaged, and broken down. Much has been written about how American culture adjusted to the sheer amount of death meted out by the Civil War. But less has been written about those who did not quite die, who died in part and returned to bear living witness through their ravaged bodies to the steep cost of war.

ONE

The Surgeons

Gray Anatomy

The soldier is already dreaming of glory and renown, and, therefore,
eagerly grasps the theories of war; but military tactics necessarily leave
out of the question the ghastly field, its wounded, and the bed of suffering.
There the province of the physician begins, and on the field of battle
itself, his knowledge, and skill are put to the severest test.
–Dr. Moritz Schuppert, *Treatise on Gun-Shot Wounds*

Surgeons, be ready to give the best attention to our wounded; for doubt
not, many a manly form shall bleed pure patriotism, ere another sunset!
–Rev. J. T. Clarke, *Prepare for Battle*

How many lives were lost through ignorance, want of experience, want
of skill, want of suitable appliances will, of course, never be known.
–F. E. Daniel, M.D., *Recollections of a Rebel Surgeon*

Years after the close of hostilities, a surgeon remembered, in stunning detail, each specific moment of the amputation of a Confederate soldier in
Atlanta. The doctor recalled, "I see a strong man stretched prone on the
table. I see the aproned surgeons, stern of visage, kind and gentle of heart;
I see the gleam of a long life; I see the warm life blood spur out as it cleaves
the quivering white flesh." The doctor still heard the sound of the saw as
it grated through "the bleeding bone" and could envision that "ghastly
wound, gaping gory; its flabby flaps weeping crimson tears." As the "thirsty
sponge" drank the bloody tears of the wound, the empty chasm quickly
"dried" and the surgeon stitched the wound and placed a roller bandage
"around the stump." The patient next traveled to a cot beneath an oak tree
where he found an attentive nurse sitting by his side, sweeping away the
flies that tried to cohabitate with his newly forged stump.[1]

This chapter explores the lives of surgeons in the Confederacy and
their role in altering the image of the southern white male body during
the Civil War. At the start of the conflict, a miniscule number of surgeons

found themselves overwhelmed by limited supplies, a lack of training, and a plethora of patients. As a result, some doctors did perform ill-advised operations and produced an immense amount of suffering, chronic pain, and unnecessary death. But in underappreciated ways surgeons adapted as the war progressed. Despite persistent negative connotations as butchers, many surgeons received extensive training in a profession that gradually learned how to remove limbs only when medically necessary. Soon after the war started, surgeons had access to medical manuals that provided step-by-step instructions on how to deal with patients who had sustained even the most daunting injuries, and they tended to amputate only as a last resort, resulting in far fewer amputees than is usually suspected. Surgeons, as men, appeared to identify sympathetically with patients who were desperate to retain their manhood and, on numerous occasions, shunned amputation.

As we have seen, the inevitable hospital scene in numerous Hollywood films has shaped our impressions of Civil War surgeons as men who called for their next patient, swiped the saw or scalpel across a blood-stained apron, hacked and sawed away at an appendage of human flesh, then tossed the limb and called for their next victim. While films have a powerful ability to shape popular perception, historians have unfortunately added to the myth of the saw-happy surgeon. One historian, for instance, has called medical professionals "one of the Civil War's most dismal failures" for their apparent addiction to amputation; another has wondered if "wounded soldiers often would have been better off without any treatment—even with a lead ball remaining in them, with its potential toxic effects." One prominent Civil War historian has argued that Civil War surgeons "knew of few ways except amputation to stop gangrene" and has further noted that surgeons ended up divided between the radicals, who were only "probably right" in their belief that amputation "saved more lives than it threatened," and the conservatives, who tried to save a limb. Another historian has claimed that medical personnel "operated in ignorance, and continued to make the same mistakes throughout the war, which often led to unnecessary suffering and death." Others have criticized the overworked medical personnel as they "carelessly threw body parts everywhere." Finally, one prominent historian has claimed in a recent narrative that "surgeons and doctors who were on hand were liable to make matters worse" as they established a hospital that resembled "nothing so much as a butcher's shop on market-day." Indeed, in many of the grand narratives of the Civil War era, medical personnel are universally lumped together and swiftly condemned as an inept and careless group who deserve blame for the war's horrific level of casualties.[2]

To be sure, there are some medical historians who have viewed surgeons in a more flattering light. H. H. Cunningham has argued, for instance, that scenes of butchery have been exaggerated, lamenting that "the most outrageous statements find credulous listeners." Given the war-related shortages of proper instruments among Confederate surgeons, Cunningham has praised the medical officers for their ingenuity and skill that overcame supply deficiencies. Another medical historian has reminded historians of the primitive state of medical care in the nineteenth century and its successful evolution throughout the Civil War. Amputation, he claims, was "the most successful major operative procedure of the time." Two other medical historians have come forward with similar arguments, praising surgeons for their "ingenuity, careful attention to detail, and humane interest in wounded soldiers." Alfred Jay Bollet, in a recent article, notes that while negative characterizations about surgeons appeared in the newspapers in the early years of the war, no one has unpacked the significance of their disappearance in the later years. Surgeons were no longer written up in the press, Bollet concludes, because "competence" does not make headlines. Unfortunately, it is those early impressions that have wormed their way into most of the recent grand narratives written about the Civil War.[3]

Many surgeons, who defined their manhood by their medical reputation, would have been surprised by history's negative characterization, especially as contemporary sources challenge both the arguments of prominent historians and the popular negative stigma. Jonathan Letterman, a surgeon with the Union Army of the Potomac, remembered in 1866 that surgeons, especially at Antietam, practiced "conservative surgery" and should have amputated more often than they did. William Keen, one of the leading surgeons in the United States during the war, remembered, "The popular opinion that the surgeons did a large amount of unnecessary amputation may have been justified in a few cases, but, taking the army as a whole, I have no hesitation in saying that far more lives were lost from refusal to amputate than by amputation."[4]

The negative reputation of a Civil War surgeon eager to cut without sufficient sympathy or knowledge emanated from the very ghastliness of the act of amputation itself. We cannot deny the horrific nature of removing a limb. For thousands of soldiers, a battlefield injury prompted their very first visit to a doctor, a surgeon, or a hospital. Almost none had witnessed an amputation or a surgeon perform any sort of operation. Then there was the nature of the wounds. Lead- and shrapnel-crushed bones, shredded flesh, damaged blood vessels and vital organs produced a natural reaction to pain: cries, moans, screams, and groans. Without any prior exposure to such an environment, damaged soldiers quite naturally panicked and concluded that anyone who *could* do such things must be a monster. The process of amputation, we must remember, produced a high level of trauma not just to patients but to other observers as well. The recollections of sights and sounds associated with amputation often appear most vivid among those who were merely witnesses.

The sheer potential horror of the hospital experience prompted hundreds of soldiers and civilians to view the field hospital as ghoulish ground. A private soldier recalled his very first visit to a Civil War hospital as "the most painful thing of all." "It resembles a butcher's shamble," he claimed, "with maimed and bloody men lying on all sides—some with their arms off; some with their legs off; some awaiting their time, while the doctors, with upturned cuffs and bloody hands, are flourishing their knives and saws." The doctors stood among "piles of bloody-looking limbs" with dead bodies still lying "on the dissecting table." He called it simply a "ghastly picture." Charles Hutson, shot in the face at First Manassas, witnessed a crowded hospital scene in Charlottesville, Virginia, "with groaning men, some undergoing the agonies of amputation." Following the Battle of Seven Pines, William R. Gorman, a member of the Fourth North Carolina, felt somehow that Mother Nature herself should be weeping. "Nature smiles sweetly and the birds sing as enchantingly as though no deeds of blood and carnage had been perpetrated near this now peaceful spot," he noted. Gorman felt compelled to go to the local field hospital to "alleviate the horrible suffering" and saw a horrific scene: "piled in heaps lay [the] amputated arms and legs" stacked "like cord-wood," and the "piercing cries" of patients broke through the chloroform and "the stillness of night" until "the very corpses trembled."[5]

There is a reason the pile of amputated limbs makes it into every Hollywood movie: it made such a deep impression on everyone who saw it at

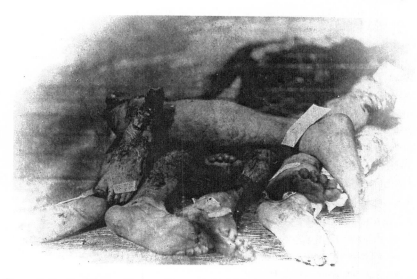

Figure 2. A pile of severed legs and feet at a Civil War hospital. Courtesy of Contributed Photographs Collection, Otis Historical Archives, National Museum of Health and Medicine.

the time. One soldier from Louisiana saw a huge box filled to the brim with hands, arms, and feet. He noted that the box "was so full that two horrible and bloody feet protruded out of the top." Richard Henry Brooks, a member of the Fifty-First Georgia, casually commented in a letter to his wife on November 3, 1862, "The doctors cut off somebody's leg, arm, hand, or foot or some other part nearly every day here [Lynchburg, Va.]." One southern woman, who found her home commandeered as a hospital, remarked, "Then came the amputating surgeon to finish what the bullet had failed to do. Arms and legs lay in a promiscuous heap on our back piazza." Kate Cumming recalled that surgeons routinely at a hospital in Corinth, Mississippi, had "amputated limbs thrown into the yard," where they remained after an operation.[6]

Obviously the very sight of a pile of limbs left a powerful and lasting impression on Confederate soldiers trying to make sense of the unprecedented level of carnage and destruction after a battle. Virginian artillerist Edmund Samuel Duffey witnessed lifeless limbs next to their former occupants all around the Second Manassas battlefield. Confederate soldier Berry Benson recalled during the Seven Days Campaign around Richmond in June 1862: "Before leaving the hospital, I went in the garden and was shocked to see lying about it, hands and arms and legs that had been amputated—a dreadful sight." Following the battle at Perryville, Kentucky, a pile of legs and arms "rose like a pyramid to the floor of the second story gallery," according to one soldier. Lieutenant Colonel William Owen, who served in the artillery with the Confederacy during the war, described hearing the "screams and groans" of men undergoing amputation and seeing piles of arms and legs, an image that he never forgot. He concluded, "No longer do the rush, roar and boom of the shot and shell, and the volleys of musketry bring fire to the soldier's eye and make his blood tingle through his veins in glorious excitement; but now the saw and knife prove that all is not glory."[7]

In addition to the sights and sounds of amputation, soldiers and civilians also smelled the aftermath of numerous field operations. Field hospitals, particularly the piles of corpses and rotting limbs, created a stench that engulfed nearby homes and areas. In Little Rock, Arkansas, one citizen noted the "nauseous aura overhanging" the city, especially as temperatures warmed and "just about everybody had the smell of putrification in his nostrils." Men, women, and children across the city "suffered the shock of unsightly mangled bodies." One civilian remembered, "Amputated arms, legs, as well as bodies, of the dead were buried as expeditiously as possible. But the odor of festering sores and of death could be detected whenever anyone went near any of the improvised hospitals."[8]

Time and again, as soldiers, civilians, and nurses described amputation, the word "butcher" cropped up in letters and diaries as a descriptor for surgeons. The label, according to one historian, originates in the soldiers' frame of reference: butchering back home. Most soldiers were farmers and had ample experience breaking down pigs, deer, cows, chickens, and other forms of livestock and game. Even Abraham Lincoln was comfortable enough with butchering to use it as a metaphor for Grant's grand five-army campaign of 1864: "Those not skinning can hold a leg." Thus, when soldiers saw the surgeon operating, they connected his performance to their own experiences dismembering an animal back home. Civilians and soldiers conveying their impressions of the first surgery they had probably ever seen would naturally adopt this metaphor. (And it is not necessarily as insulting as it might seem; butchering, in that day and age especially, was understood as a skill requiring a great deal of precision.) Even so, in referring to surgeons as butchers, Confederate soldiers butted up against the budding professionalism, not to mention the masculine honor, of medical men who were not keen on highlighting such comparisons. A butcher takes lives; a doctor preserves them.[9]

To be sure, errors were made, and some were quite costly. In one instance, a botched amputation resulted in a bone protruding from a leg; the patient could not bear the excruciating pain from any pressure on the limb. While fighting in Georgia in 1862, one Confederate soldier shuddered when he reflected on the image of a "surgeon sharpening his instruments and whetting his saw to take [from] them those necessary member[s] of our body that God has given us for our indispensable use." Theodore Livingston, a clerk at the Fairgrounds Hospital in Atlanta, noted in 1863 that he would rather "take Yankee lead in the head" than be the subject of a "young swell head" doctor to perform experiments on during an operation. One Alabama soldier criticized the reputation of all medical professionals when he observed, "I believe the Doctors kill more than they cure. Doctors ain't got half sense."[10]

Occasionally, soldiers might be enlisted to assist in amputations, an assignment few relished, which provided an opportunity for them to assess the state of amputation within Civil War medicine. One private, J. W. Gibson, fervently believed that doctors made "many useless amputations." His impression did not change when he was forced to hold the head of a Union soldier about to undergo amputation while chloroform was administered. Then Gibson dropped the head of the patient, due to "how they cut and slashed," and thought he could give the Union man a chance to "wake up and fight." Gibson informed the doctors that he did not enlist in order to be an accomplice to so much useless butchery. The doctors "laughed at me and said they would soon teach me to be a surgeon."[11]

The negative impressions of surgeons also stems from the overwhelming challenges Confederate medical personnel faced, especially in the early years of the war. The Confederacy suffered from a severe shortage of surgeons readily available to perform medical procedures, averaging about one surgeon for every 312 enlisted soldiers. Officially, the Confederate Medical Department consisted of 1,242 surgeons and 1,994 assistant surgeons. Yet the Union medical corps dwarfed its Confederate counterpart, eventually employing more than 11,000 doctors. The already limited number of Confederate medical personnel actually declined during the heat of battle, as some assistant surgeons headed off to fight. In one case, it led to the death of a soldier who had his thigh crushed in battle and bled to death before the surgeon returned. Few men who served as surgeons during the Civil War had performed military surgery during the Mexican or Crimean War. Although many physicians across the South used a scalpel before the Civil War, they treated few gunshot wounds and performed few if any amputations. And Confederate armies covered large swaths of territory, exacerbating the shortage by spreading thin the available medical personnel. Devastating waves of casualties at major battles that commenced in isolated areas further strained the small pool of skilled physicians.[12]

Confederate surgeons faced more than insufficient numbers. Technological developments in weaponry in the mid-nineteenth century yielded devastating bodily injuries that required more amputations than had been necessary during previous American military engagements. The soft lead minié ball, combined with Napoleonic tactics, created a surgeon's nightmare. Bullets shattered and crushed bones, splintering joints and necessitating, according to physician J. Julian Chisolm, "more frequently amputations and resections." Another Confederate surgeon, Deering Roberts, directly blamed ammunition for causing so many Civil War amputations. "The shattering, splintering, and splitting of a long bone," he said, "by the impact of the minié or Enfield ball were, in many instances, both remarkable and frightful, and early experience taught surgeons that amputation was the only means of saving life." Roberts believed that southern surgeons properly viewed amputation as a "conservative" approach that saved lives.[13]

In cases where physicians opted not to amputate, the slow-moving lead projectiles drove bits of clothing and dirt into wounds, producing later infections that necessitated amputation. Confederate soldiers also faced a "bullet bomb," which exploded upon contact with the bone due to an explosive material in the hollow portion of the bullet. "The consequence is a most ghastly wound," noted one Richmond editorialist. Artillery shells also tended to produce a great deal of ragged spinning shrapnel that amputated men before surgeons ever got to them. One artist depiction of the engagement at Fort Henry in February 1862 revealed two Confederate soldiers shattered by artillery fragments, each missing arms as a result of the bombardment.[14]

Inevitably, long marches and sudden engagements made it impossible for field hospitals to have adequate time to prepare for the onslaught of wounded. James B. Roden, of the Seventh Louisiana, remarked that at Spotsylvania, the operating table consisted of "a barn door on two trestles." Rev. Samuel A. Agnew, after the Battle of Tishimingo Creek in 1864, witnessed wounded men "lying on pallets" awaiting amputation at a local church. When other temporary hospitals appeared, they did not have enough medical personnel available, which meant that regular soldiers were often assisting in a variety of amputations. After the Battle of New Hope Church in 1864, surgeons were so shorthanded that they drafted a chaplain to assist.[15]

As large battles climaxed on the front lines, chaos swirled in the rear, as hundreds of patients flooded temporary hospitals to receive immediate medical attention. The main surgical manual employed by the Confederate Army was published by J. Julian Chisolm in 1862. The manual provided extensive guidance on what surgeons needed to do to save a damaged limb. This guidance had been bought dear as it was the challenges faced by the first wave of medical personnel that provided Chisolm with the information he used to codify best practices. And, given the shortages faced by the Confederacy, the output of surgical manuals and pamphlets throughout the war seems quite robust. Some of the new literature even provided extensive full-color illustrations and step-by-step details in order to guide the inexperienced surgeon through his medical baptism of fire. The theories and practices laid out in the manual actually did have an impact, and by 1862 there was a fair degree of standardization of medical practices across the Confederacy. Certainly there is overwhelming evidence that surgeons by and large cared about their patients and their reputations, as men as well as professionals, and studied the literature in order to understand some of the potentially difficult cases they were likely to see throughout the war. The standardization of medical practices as chronicled in the manuals eventually produced a class of reputable Confederate surgeons who exercised caution and skill, and there was a decline in the number of amputations in the later years of the war.[16]

Such standardization applied to the books themselves, and several surgical and instructional handbooks remained in print and underwent regular revision throughout the Civil War. Samuel D. Gross, who authored a manual on military surgery in 1861, argued that every regiment needed a

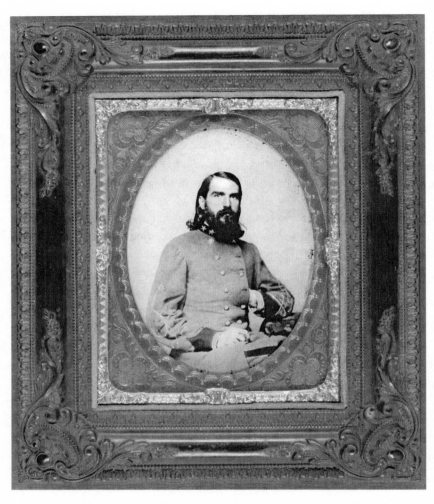

Figure 3. Col. J. J. Chisolm, Confederate surgeon and author of *A Manual of Military Surgery for the Use of Surgeons in the Confederate States Army.* Courtesy of the Library of Congress.

man capable of acting as a physician and surgeon. "He must have been educated in the modern schools; be of undoubted courage, prompt to act, willing to assume responsibility, human and sympathizing, urbane and courteous in his manners; in short, a medical gentleman." Surgeons, he continued, needed to be ready to act as a "medical philosopher" who did not dither like the "white-gloved gentry" physicians who had served in the Mexican War. This new generation of military physicians particularly needed to follow a specific set of dictates when it came to amputation. All of the prevailing medical texts urged caution. As one manual succinctly stated, "The directions here given are somewhat precise and detailed, because the success of an amputation, both as regards the life of the patient and the quality of the stump, will more often be secured by the strict observance of these simple suggestions." Consensus among medical authorities on the need to exercise restraint likely had the effect of universalizing, to a degree, a more cautionary approach to the removal of a limb.[17]

Surgical manuals also dictated that a surgeon should not begin an operation until all the tools had been placed in front of him and his assistants stood ready to perform the procedure. Tools included an amputating knife, the Catlin, or double-edged knife, amputating saws (both small and regular), and bone nippers (metal pliers with strong blades). Amputation kits and instruments remained in high demand throughout the course of the war. Given the lack of medical instruments at times, surgeons were occasionally forced to use whatever tools they could find. One surgeon recalled having "performed an amputation with a pocket knife and a common saw" during the war. Dr. George Washington Peddy, a surgeon with the Fifty-Sixth Georgia, noted in a letter to his wife in 1862, "I am offered ninety dollars just for my case of amputating and trephining instruments. They only cost me thirty-five dollars."[18]

Once the patient arrived, a Confederate surgeon assessed as best he could the nature of the wound, though the chaotic nature of the battlefield often required speed. At a time before knowledge of antisepsis, fingers seemed the most versatile and sensitive tools for probing wounds and finding bullets. Physicians learned that specific instances recommended the immediate removal of a limb, especially in cases where major nerves or blood vessels had been shredded or the crushed limb was still attached to the body. Where artillery shells had blown the appendage away, the surgeon would have to effectively reamputate to create a cleaner wound, and it was expected that such an operation should commence immediately. In addition, doctors had to weigh the likelihood that a limb saved today would ultimately kill the patient with sepsis or a bleed-out tomorrow. In such cases, amputation was the safest course.[19]

How could a surgeon make an accurate decision in the course of a few seconds? Surgeons endured a stressful environment within the battlefield hospital and faced a daunting task: a bounty of patients needing immediate care. In order to work quickly, surgeons divided patients between primary and secondary amputation cases. A primary amputation, defined as resulting from a "direct injury," usually took place either immediately after the wound occurred or shortly after the patient recovered from shock. A secondary amputation usually took place after the initial twenty-four or thirty-six hours, when initial inflammation subsided. Data from military operations noted a significantly lower mortality rate with amputations that took place immediately. As one surgeon stated simply, "Primary Amputations are far more successful than Secondary" because the sooner the amputation took place, the more likely the patient would survive.[20]

Some specific injuries received abundant coverage in the surgical manuals, and thus surgeons had plenty of information on whether and how to remove the limb. When it came to gunshot wounds to the knee joint, for instance, medical consensus dictated amputation as the only successful mode of treatment. Hunter McGuire viewed several cases of knee gunshot wounds where amputation was not done and the wound did not heal. "Whenever the surgeon persisted in his effort to save the limb, the patient died," he said. Surgeon J. W. Thompson also viewed primary amputation as the only reasonable course of action when dealing with the knee. T. G. Richardson failed to see "a single recovery without amputation from unmistakable gunshot wound of the knee joint."[21]

Again, counter to stereotypes, Civil War surgeons were well aware of anesthetics. Confederate surgeons typically administered chloroform at the beginning of an operation. Prior to the Civil War, the *Boston Medical and Surgical Journal* had published an extensive debate about the appropriate use of chloroform. After a woman died during a medical procedure from an overdose of the anesthesia, medical experts in her wrongful death trial lectured the public against the regular use of chloroform, denounced as a "dangerous anesthetic agent." The journal advocated on behalf of sulfuric ether over chloroform due to its safety, efficiency, and low cost and the fact that direct inhalation of ether did not cause death. Chloroform certainly may have killed thousands before the Civil War, and it did take the lives of some Confederate soldiers. One Kentucky soldier named Hodges, for instance, lost his leg and then his life when he "never rallied from the effects of the chloroform."[22]

Some European and Confederate physicians echoed the published concerns and refused to use chemical anesthesia. One English surgeon who served in the Crimean conflict detested the use of chloroform and instead relished "the lusty bawling of the wounded from the mart of the knife, as a powerful stimulant which has roused many a sinking man from his apathetic state." During the American Civil War, one patient endured an amputation by singing "The Bonnie Blue Flag" rather than inhaling a dose of chloroform. Another soldier from the Fourth Kentucky had most of his right arm blown away in battle, then casually walked back to the surgeon and presented his arm, dangling by a small piece of skin. The surgeon removed the arm without administering any chloroform. A member of a South Carolina artillery battalion underwent an amputation without any chloroform, and his screams could be heard up to a quarter mile away.[23]

If a surgeon did not want to use chloroform, he did have a few other options. A physician could offer a local anesthetic, usually a shot of morphine injected directly under the skin, which rapidly blunted the potential for feeling pain. Patients could also consume whiskey or other forms of alcohol to dull their senses and sensibilities. William Lindsay Brandon, a member of the Twenty-First Mississippi, shattered his ankle at Malvern Hill in 1862, the wound quickly filling his boot with blood and bone fragments. Since they had no chloroform, surgeons removed the foot after Brandon sucked down some whiskey. Although the amputation proved a success, the stump bulged with pus and blood. Doctors routinely drained the stump, an extremely painful procedure that Brandon withstood with the aid of a few shots of cognac.[24]

Although few Confederate surgeons refused to administer chloroform, most used it routinely and advocated for it fiercely. "Whenever operations are to be performed in military surgery," J. Julian Chisolm noted, "chloroform should be administered. It is a remedy which the surgeon should never be without." He called the effects of the miracle anesthesia "wonderful." Another Confederate surgeon warned, "Do not operate until your patient is fully under the influence of chloroform, until the period of anesthesia, of complete insensibility, is reached." Hunter Holmes McGuire proudly estimated that chloroform had been used twenty-eight thousand times on Confederate patients without causing any fatalities. Felix Formento, working in a hospital in Louisiana, recalled routinely using chloroform, and a surgeon stationed at Winder Hospital in Richmond stated, "In every case of operation in this division, chloroform has been used and with invariable good effect." Another Confederate surgeon suggested that chloroform was, if anything, overused, in an "almost reckless manner in which it was given to every patient put on the table." Like McGuire, though, he took comfort in the fact that the hospital did not have any major accidents with the chemical, nor did any patient perish from a chloroform overdose.[25]

Prescribing chloroform was one thing; having an ample supply was another. The Confederacy was particularly subject to shortages, including of anesthesia. Hearing their comrades screaming on the operating tables, soldiers often assumed that the surgeon had deliberately withheld chloroform, confirming the butcher stereotype, when in reality there was nothing to withhold. John Robson, a member of the Fifty-Second Virginia, recalled that Confederate medical patients routinely faced a lack of medicine, including chloroform. Another physician recalled after the war, "The Confederate surgeons were handicapped in many ways. We were short on chloroform, and had to use it as economically as possible—we had none to waste." Usually only supply issues, rather than a warped sense of compassion or a poor understanding of medicine, hampered surgeons from administering chloroform to a man about to undergo amputation. And Confederate cavalry raids, such as one committed by Thomas Jackson's cavalry on May 24, 1862, specifically sought out large stores of chloroform and carried back as much as possible.[26]

In order to get the patient to a point of "complete insensibility," the Confederate surgical manuals agreed on a few essential precautions to ensure both maximum effectiveness and the safety of the patient. In turn, Confederate medical personnel routinely followed the advice of the manuals, as cases of death by chloroform rarely appear in the medical records. Hospital workers, after placing the patient in a recumbent position, jettisoned any belts, swords, and tight clothing that might constrict breathing. The surgical assistant folded a piece of cloth in the shape of a cone and inserted a sponge soaked in chloroform. Patients received a dose of chloroform in a well-ventilated area, as the assistant placed the cloth a few inches from the mouth or nose. The first breath of the patient contained more air than chloroform. With each successive breath, the chloroform source moved closer and closer to the mouth and nose. Then the patient breathed loudly, a clear signal that the chloroform had taken affect – and the surgeon could begin the operation. In the event that an amputation lasted longer than expected and the effects of the anesthesia began to fade, the medical assistant reapplied the chloroform. In many instances, the surgeon also administered a tad of whiskey or brandy to calm the nerves of the patient and keep his pulse strong.[27]

With the anesthesia administered, Confederate surgeons usually waited five minutes before beginning the procedure. The location of the cutting directly affected the probability of survival. Surgeons played a game of inches. Amputations of lower extremities (hands, feet, lower legs, and arms) produced a higher survival rate than those closer to the trunk. Hence, for instance, amputations were urged for compound fractures of the lower but not upper portions of the femur. This had not always been the case, but at the first Battle of Manassas Confederate surgeons discovered that "too few primary amputations were performed on the lower portions of the thigh," which resulted in a high mortality rate among wounded soldiers.[28]

Surgeons usually headed a team that included three assistants. The first assistant administered the chloroform, the second applied pressure to the main artery (a tactic preferred to the tourniquet), and the third held down the limb and prepared to support the flap that would forge the stump after the operation. Though often rushed or fatigued, the team operated as a hedge against mistakes, and each member was expected to give his opinions on whether and how an amputation should take place. One Confederate soldier recalled, "If two of them said amputate it was done at once." Complicated amputations meant that each surgical team member played a pivotal role. One doctor cut the flesh down to the bone and retracted it, allowing the second doctor to saw the bone as the final doctor clasped the blood vessels and created the flap.[29]

Where practical, the most experienced surgeon, or the individual with the most extensive knowledge of the surgical manual, performed the operation. An inexperienced surgeon was expected to ask his superior before deciding on amputation. Then, and only then, could the green surgeon get out the saw. A successful amputation was more complicated than is usually

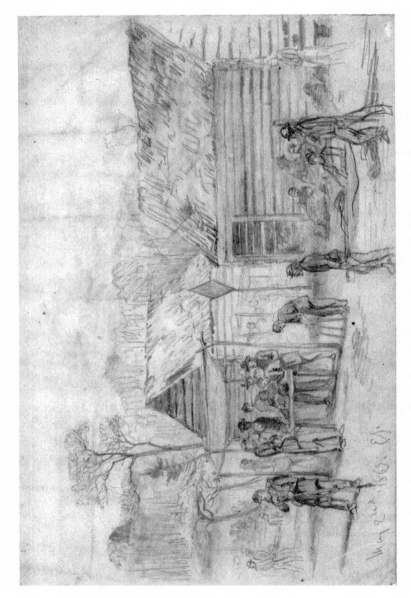

Figure 4. A Civil War field hospital in Chancellorsville, Virginia. Courtesy of the Library of Congress.

allowed. As one medical manual explained, "The surgeon removes the limb, ligates the vessels, and when all the oozing has ceased, secures the stump by points of suture placed at intervals of an inch or a little less along the entire line of the wound." As the surgeon cut, he had to ensure that just enough skin remained to create the flap. As the surgical manual reiterated, "This is the first and most important rule in amputation. You cannot well leave too much skin, and can very easily commit the opposite error. The surplus of skin will be absorbed; a deficiency can in no way be supplied."[30]

There were a number of accepted procedures. The most common, the circular method, called for a circular cut around the limb before utilizing a saw to cut through the bone. If the surgeon preferred, he could administer an oval cut in a similar fashion; this was known as the oval method. Some doctors favored the circular cut because it "required less time and care in dressing, was easily handled, seldom sloughed, that its discharges were less and that it was less frequently followed by hemorrhage." Many found the circular mode also promoted faster healing, better secured arteries, and permitted a patient to travel more quickly after the operation. In addition to oval and circular cuts, surgeons also used the single and double flap method, which consisted of making one or two flaps of skin in order to cover the stump. The flap methods constructed a physically attractive stump but could be time-consuming, and thus surgeons recommended utilizing this technique at hospitals away from the battlefield.[31]

Inexperienced surgeons, those in haste, and especially those recently thrown into a battlefield hospital running at top speed usually made one universal mistake: the protrusion of a bone from the stump, which forced an additional operation. Once the stump healed from a treatment of nitric acid, the surgeon could saw off the protruding bone, rather than perform another amputation. If the surgeon failed to ensure a proper stump had been constructed before dressing the wound, the stump could tear, become infected, cause more pain, or simply appear ghastly. The other common mistake was a failure to take the time to tie off every blood vessel that either was bleeding or might bleed. This process could be time-consuming, as surgeons typically tied off several vessels and could neglect no small arteries. Failure to do so involved a return visit or even death.[32]

Even where the surgeon's work was perfect, medical complications, rampant infections, and disease outbreaks wreaked havoc on recovering patients. Physicians tried to leaven the medical nightmare by vaccinating patients against smallpox. Even so, some vaccine doses produced bouts of blood poisoning. Phoebe Pember, working in a Confederate hospital, described seeing numerous "deep and thick" sores on legs and arms that necessitated amputation to ensure the survival of the patient. Tainted vaccinations also ushered in a flurry of amputations at Andersonville Prison, where Confederate doctors faced accusations of purposefully injecting Union prisoners with a serum that prompted the removal of limbs. A federal official accused Henry Wirz, the commandant of Andersonville, of participating in "implacable cruelty" with the problematic vaccination program.[33]

Some historians have argued that Civil War–era medical personnel had absolutely no understanding of the spread of diseases and pathogens around their hospitals. It is true that, with a limited knowledge of germ theory, doctors did not quite understand the importance of sanitation and cleanliness for avoiding the spread of disease. Some historians have used this fact to highlight the medical quagmire of the Civil War. However, as the war evolved, some Confederate medical personnel did conclude that an unclean environment prompted the spread of disease. Joseph Jones noted that Confederate surgeons conveyed a clear understanding of how dirty instruments, bowls, sponges, and dressings spread some diseases. "When wounds were cleansed with sponges or rags," he noted, "which had been used on erysipelas [gangrene] patients, it was frequently observed that the disease appeared, and such propagation appeared to be clearly referable to the transference of contagious matter."[34]

Gangrene was the greatest infectious threat faced by Civil War soldiers and demanded that a physician work quickly to eradicate or prevent what could be a crippling and deadly infection. Gangrene, a horrendous condition that emerged when a large portion of body tissue dies, resulted from a lack of blood flow or a bacterial infection that slowly invaded adjacent healthy tissue. Doctor Joseph Jones thought that gangrene worked like a contagious disease and offered a serious warning. "As a general rule, no amputation, no matter what be the condition of the wounds, whether gangrenous or healthy, should be performed in the wards of a hospital in which gangrene is prevailing." He labeled the operations "reprehensible," though he conceded that amputation might be required if the joint, muscles, nerves, bones, or blood vessels were exposed, if the wound was large in size, or if the patient faced "a danger of death from hemorrhage."

If the patient had to undergo amputation in a hospital rife with gangrene, Jones directed the operation to take place "isolated as far as possible, and every attention paid to proper ventilation, cleanliness, and diet."[35]

Outbreaks of gangrene forced a surgeon to expedite the removal of a limb. One Confederate doctor, working at Andersonville Prison, noted that "for a while amputations were practiced in the hospital almost daily, arising from a gangrenous and scorbutic condition, which, in many cases, threatened a saturation of the whole system with the gangrenous or offensive matter, unless the limb was amputated." He quickly discovered that in many cases, he had to perform a second amputation, as gangrene regenerated on the new stump.[36]

Once the surgeon had completed the amputation procedure, hospitals found themselves responsible for ensuring the full recovery of the damaged and dependent patient. Confederate surgeon general S. P. Moore issued a strict set of cleanliness standards and rules to regulate how hospitals looked and functioned, with an eye toward establishing a healthy environment. Hospital walls needed whitewashed two or three times per year. Each hospital bed required ample sets of sheets, so the bedding could be changed, cleaned, and hung outside to be aired. A hospital staff member dry-scrubbed the floors with sand on a regular basis. Furthermore, a hospital official inspected the hospital each day to ascertain the cleanliness of the kitchen, the food preparation and distribution, and all matters related "to drainage, removal of offal, water closets, latrines, supply of water, lights, fuel, dry scrubbing of floors, sweeping of premises, ventilation and general cleanliness of the patients, bedding and of the hospital in general."[37]

The Third Georgia Hospital, located in Augusta, specified eleven strict measures, including that a patient had to be in bed when the surgeon visited the hospital ward. Soldiers could not leave or sleep outside the hospital without permission or they would be "immediately returned to duty." Patients could not throw any liquids or bodily fluids out the windows, spit on the floor, chew tobacco, deface or damage the furniture, or mark on the walls and were expected to maintain an orderly and clean living space. Patients, forced to remain in their own beds, could not switch beds or remove the bedding without permission, nor could they "sit, or lie on the bed of any other patient." The attending surgeon had the complete responsibility to set the diet and deal with patient complaints. At the same time, the patients and the staff needed to work diligently in order to maintain a clean hospital in order to increase the likelihood that every wounded Confederate made a full recovery.[38]

Hospitals had the leverage to enforce and even expand on specific directives ordered by the Confederate Surgeon General to keep a tidy hospital. At Fairground Hospital No. 2 in Atlanta, strict inspections took place daily. In addition, patients and staff members could not smoke, gamble, drink, use profane language, or use a sink for other than "appropriate purposes." Furthermore, hospital attendees, forbidden to trespass on adjacent premises, were ordered to avoid all "uncleanly or disorderly conduct." Even with such strict regulations, the hospital promised to provide each soldier with the "kindness and attention due him as a sick man." Visitors to the Fairground Hospital could not eat or sleep at the hospital, nor were they allowed to give the patients any food or drink "without the permission of the medical officers in charge of the ward."[39]

Hospitals, though, did not always live up to the regulations and standards for care and cleanliness. If hospital conditions failed to create an environment appropriate for recovery, the patient could experience enormous suffering. One hospital worker observed men "wounded in every shape and form" dealing with an "abominable diet" that made the recovering patients "look as though they feel like no one in the world cares for them." Sam Watkins, who spent some time in a Montgomery, Alabama, hospital recovering from a gunshot wound to his ankle, remarked, "Everything seemed clean and nice enough, but the smell! Ye gods!" At Chimborazo Hospital in Richmond, a group of 215 Georgia patients petitioned their governor, Joseph E. Brown, about the horrific meals served on a daily basis. The petition catalogued the meals, which included "half-cooked beef or mutton or old fat bacon (such as would make a well hungry soldier blush and wonder if the Confederacy had come to that) with a cup of tea made of something we know not what, but something very sorry." The soldiers complained of having the "abominable tea" at dinnertime with bread that was "worse than you ever saw a Georgia nigger eat." The bread, they claimed, was "the roughest and most impalatable kind" made of "old corn meal, damaged and without sifting."[40]

One of the most stubborn misperceptions of Civil War surgery is that medical practices did not change over time. It is true that the perfect storm of projectiles and pathogens created a medical crisis that the Confederate

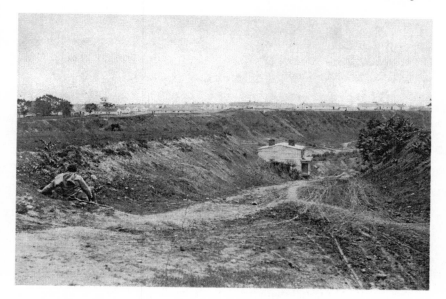

Figure 5. Chimborazo Hospital in Richmond, Virginia, April 1865. Courtesy of the Library of Congress.

Army initially seemed ill prepared to handle, especially given the unexpectedly vast number of patients. The limited number of medical personnel combined with a voluminous number of wounded and ill men left an unending sea of miserables in need of immediate attention. On July 21, 1861, the engagement at the Manassas Railroad junction produced over 1,100 wounded Union soldiers and roughly 1,500 wounded Confederate soldiers. In the aftermath of the First Battle of Bull Run, a resounding Confederate victory, General P. G. T. Beauregard instructed Confederate surgeons to avoid performing amputations on the hundreds of Union wounded left behind. Instead, surgical assistants, with little experience or proper medical training, hacked away at the damaged limbs. One man reported that the operations occurred "in a most horrible manner," while others were "absolutely frightful." Another Union survivor explained that the bone from his severed limb jettisoned through the hasty sutures.[41]

Nine months later, surgeons continued to be overwhelmed, especially after one of the largest battles ever fought on American soil. At Shiloh in April 1862, thousands of wounded patients waited days for medical treatment. Over the course of two days, roughly eight thousand men on each side fell wounded. The nation had never seen so much carnage and bloodshed, and the limited number of medical personnel could not handle the volume of mangled bodies. The damaged limbs of the waiting wounded contracted gangrene, which demanded immediate action. Overwhelmed and exhausted, many surgeons turned to amputation out of necessity. Novice medical personnel endured a horrific trial by fire at Shiloh, many performing operations normally reserved for the skilled surgeons. Unfortunately, they did so, according to one witness, "with little regard for human life or limb." One eyewitness believed that Confederate physicians treated nearly five thousand wounded soldiers.[42]

Although surgical literature recommended a well-planned but speedy operation, some surgeons who worked quickly may have had an ulterior motive. Southern men, who defined their manhood through an honorable reputation, cared about how others perceived them as men and professionals. Abundant evidence reveals the impatience and bravado of young and eager Confederate doctors early in the war who wanted to cut their teeth in the medical profession and felt they had something to prove. Some surgeons boasted that they could remove a leg in mere seconds to "gain the applause of spectators at the expense of the patient's safety," according to one physician. At the start of the war, young doctors assumed that productivity, measured in the number of limbs operated per day, bolstered, rather than hindered, their reputation. Only as the war progressed did a surgeon make his reputation solely "by his successful cases, and not by the number of seconds he takes."[43]

Medical practitioners warned against overeager surgeons who wanted to slice off a limb in order to solidify a reputation for a manly decisiveness. J. J. Chisolm called out many Confederate surgeons, recent graduates from medical colleges, who, early in the war, had brandished the knife and saw a little too quickly "when limbs could have been saved." To correct for this, the medical department changed course and appointed a senior medical official to serve as an examiner to check any overeager surgeons. Another leading Confederate physician demanded that surgeons focus in every case on saving lives and promoting the recovery of patients. He called reports of surgeons removing limbs for their own personal satisfaction as a "sad and humiliating spectacle."[44]

The early instances of surgeons basing their reputation on speed over prudence earned swift condemnation from other medical professionals. One head of a Confederate hospital lashed out at a fellow surgeon for not saving the hand of a patient. The gunshot damaged few fingers, but the surgeon condemned the entire hand to the scrap pile without the consent of other surgeons in the hospital. Likewise, green physicians amputated arms and legs with a compound fracture "with as little hesitancy as if men's limbs, like those of the salamander, were reproduced with great certainty," according to one medical practitioner. In some instances, the young surgeon had no choice, as they felt overwhelmed with a plethora of patients eagerly awaiting medical attention. Surgeons in a field hospital rarely had the luxury of time because they saw amputation as "an everyday occurrence" and it often proved easier to jettison a damaged limb rather than work to save it. Over the course of the war, however, most surgeons evolved and learned to the point "whereby limbs that formerly would have been condemned are now preserved."[45]

Establishing the precise trajectory of the Confederacy's medical evolution is difficult. We have no idea how many amputations took place among Confederate soldiers. By looking at Union records, however, we can get a ballpark sense of numbers. On the Union side, a better medical paper trail reveals 29,980 amputation operations, with 21,753 men surviving (27 percent mortality rate). The 29,980 figure includes 249 additional procedures when more of a limb already amputated underwent further removal. Higher mortality rates – 80 percent – emerged among the 66 patients who underwent amputation at the hip joint and – 30 percent – among the 866 cases of men who faced an amputation of the shoulder joint. Union data sets reveal that a vast majority of amputees survived their amputations, which certainly suggests careful skill on the part of the surgeons, rather than butchery.[46]

There is no reason to think Confederate surgeons were dramatically less successful. Certainly the available medical records force a reconsideration of our impressions of surgeons as saw-happy. The raw medical data that the Confederacy maintained indicate that surgeons followed the guidance of the medical manuals and exercised caution as the war evolved and did not purposefully amputate every damaged or wounded limb that came across their table. In addition, the prudence used by surgeons resulted in a steady decline of the mortality rate among the men who did lose a limb at the operating table. As the war progressed, Confederate hospitals standardized their records, and their previous experiences dealing with dozens of patients prompted more detailed record keeping.

The raw data provided by some hospitals confirmed that surgeons exercised better medical care, as mortality rates continually declined throughout the war. Howard's Grove Hospital, in Richmond, reported the details on twenty-five various amputation cases on Confederate soldiers in 1862. All of the patients fully recovered, although a few faced chronic bouts of diarrhea. At the First Mississippi Hospital at Jackson, Mississippi, from 1863 to 1865 only six men underwent amputation out of a few hundred patients. In the Richmond area from June 1 to August 1, 1862, during the horrific Peninsula Campaign and Seven Days Battles, Confederate surgeons performed only 580 amputations, with 245 soldiers perishing. At Winder Hospital in Richmond, Virginia, between August 1862 and November 1864, the hospital treated 228 patients for gunshot wounds and amputated only about 38 percent of the examined damaged limbs. While 38 percent may seem high in terms of a percentage of men who underwent amputation, most of the patients survived. The Surgeon General's office in Richmond received data declaring that between June 1862 and February 1864, 1,688 amputations took place, resulting in 599 deaths and 1,089 recoveries (35 percent mortality rate). Another set of data, shown in table 1, reveals a 35 percent mortality rate overall among over 1,500 patients who lost a limb in Confederate hospitals. The decline in amputation, coupled with an improved mortality rate, conveyed a vast improvement over both the first year of the war and the 1850s Crimean War (where a large number of amputations took place) in Europe, as displayed in table 2.[47]

In addition to a declining mortality rate, Confederate surgeons performed fewer amputations in the latter half of the war. Major military campaigns from 1863 to 1865 produced thousands of wounded soldiers, many of whom suffered from gunshot wounds. Following Cold Harbor, as Confederate doctors treated 380 gunshot wounds from May 31 to June 7, 1864, they performed twenty-six amputations (6.8 percent). For a portion of the Petersburg campaign, covering June 16 to August 31, 1864, Confederate doctors treated 954 gunshot wounds and performed amputations on only roughly 8 percent of the patients, of whom an equal number lost an arm, a leg, or a finger. Following the Battle of Plymouth, North Carolina, on April 18–20, 1864, Confederate doctors treated 429 gunshot wounds

Table 1. Confederate surgeon general statistics, amputations, 1861–February 1864

Operation	Number of patients	Survivors	Died	Mortality rate (%)
Thigh	507	256	251	49.5
Leg	464	295	169	36.4
Arm	434	339	95	21.9
Forearm	114	96	18	15.8
Foot	34	28	6	17.6

Note: This table reflects only available data from the Surgeon General's Office to the *Confederate States Medical and Surgical Journal.* The journal admits that a wealth of data is missing. *Confederate States Medical and Surgical Journal* 1, no. 5 (May 1864): 77. More data can also be seen in "Paul Eve, Contribution to Hip-Joint Operations, 1867," Joseph Jones Papers, TU and MED, pt. 3, vol. 2, 134–35 and 137.

and performed only thirty-eight amputations. The same level of caution also holds true at Drewry's Bluff in May 1864, when Confederate doctors treated over five hundred gunshot wounds and removed only eight limbs. Throughout the month of March 1865, doctors treated nearly five hundred gunshot wounds after the Battles of Kingston and Bentonville, which required only fourteen amputations. Despite hundreds of cases of gunshot wound victims, Confederate surgeons avoided performing amputations and, in turn, saved hundreds of limbs.[48]

As the war progressed, and as Confederate hospitals became more methodical about record keeping, their reports on casualties and amputation mirror the same level of prudence exercised in field hospitals. Surgeons, away from the chaos of battle, kept detailed records on the number of amputations performed each month. In June 1863, the Blewett Hospital in Monroe, Louisiana, received 685 patients, of whom only six underwent amputation. The surgeons at the Heery and Fairground Hospitals in Atlanta performed only a few dozen amputations amid 4,003 patients treated for a gunshot wound.[49] A survey of eighty-five hospitals in Georgia and Alabama during the months of July through September in 1864 reveals that the various hospitals across the span of three months treated 7,779 gunshot wounds. Many of the Confederate patients in the dozens of hospitals had been casualties of the battles around the city of Atlanta. Despite the high number of wounds, surgeons performed amputations on only 6 percent of the gunshot wound patients. In Columbus, Mississippi, during the fall and winter of 1864–65, surgeons performed only

Table 2. Fatality rates following amputation (selected data)

Location of Injury	British Army in Crimea, 1854–56 (%)	Confederate Army of N. Va., 1861–63 (%)	Entire U.S. Army, 1861–65 (%)
Forearm/hand	5	12	14
Upper arm	26	14	24
Shoulder	33	31	not available
Hip	100	66	88
Thigh	56	38	54
Lower leg	30	30	38
Foot	23	3	6

Note: Bollet, "Amputations in the Civil War," in Schmidt and Hasegawa, *Years of Change and Suffering,* 64–65. Additional statistics are available in Amputation Statistics, box 22, Joseph Jones Papers, TU. Joseph Jones, a surgeon who collected data reports for Confederate surgeon general Samuel P. Moore, revealed a much lower death rate for other amputations in the Confederacy: 27.5 percent for shoulder amputations, 25.9 percent for lower arm amputations, and 50 to 55 percent for thigh amputations, depending on the specific location. In terms of injuries to the humerus, Jones tabulated 7,888 gunshot wound cases, requiring 4,928 amputations, with a mortality rate of 24.1 percent. *CSA Medical and Surgical Journal* 1, no. 6 (June 1864): 89 shows about a 50 percent mortality rate for those who underwent the amputation of a femur and 52 percent for those who did not undergo the operation. Other statistics are in "Primary Surgery of General Sherman's Campaigns," *Chicago Medical Examiner,* June 1866, 340–42, TU. Much of the data presented in that report come from hospital or personal surgeon records. Each month, the hospital counted the number of patients and the physicians listed the number of amputations performed in any given month. In some cases, a patient underwent a second amputation or a few limbs may have been removed from the same patient. Thus, the surgeon would have separately counted each amputation (which may have actually decreased the overall number of amputees). The personal records of a surgeon are a bit more precise, as the surgeon usually listed each patient by name and the course of treatment. Medical furlough records are also useful, as the soldier's name and unit are listed with the specific injury or operation that required a leave of absence. Data shows, for the Confederacy, a 31 percent mortality rate for shoulder, 21 percent for arm, 19 percent for forearm, 38 percent for a primary thigh, and 73 percent for a secondary thigh amputation.

eleven amputations among hundreds of patients.[50] At Ocmulgee Hospital in Macon, Georgia, the hospital surgeon kept detailed counts of operations completed between October 1864 and March 1865. According to hospital records, the surgeons performed amputations on 15 percent of their gunshot wound patients. Some of the data confirm that surgeons exercised caution and maybe did not operate enough, considering the large number of gunshot wounds. Medical practitioners caught their collective breath after the initial shock of so much carnage and suffering and addressed the concerns presented in the medical literature about overeager surgeons and inappropriate operations. Doctors learned, evolved, and persevered, much like their front-line military compatriots.[51]

The desire of Confederate surgeons to earn their own manly reputations by the war evolved from proving their mettle by heroic feats of endurance to a more practical professionalization of the entire Confederate medical corps. Confederate surgeons were conflicted about whether to amputate, and they understood well that a wounded patient's life and livelihood hung in the balance. In addition, physicians related to their patients as fellow men and knew that a medical decision made on the operating table directly impacted a man's ability to function as an honorable man once the war ended. Dr. Thomas Fanning Wood, a surgeon from North Carolina, vividly recalled the very first amputation he performed during the Civil War. He removed an arm right below the shoulder joint and believed the surgery "necessary to save the man's life." While the operation had been a success, Wood worried constantly about the life of his patient and his future after their time together on the operating table. The surgeon wondered if he had made the correct medical decision to remove the arm. Years later, the physician encountered a man named Everett who stopped by regularly to sell oysters. After a few visits, Wood asked the man about his missing arm and inquired as to who performed the operation. Everett responded, "I think you ought to know, you done it yourself." Wood expressed great pride in knowing that his first foray into amputation "recovered and survived the war over twenty years."[52]

In several cases where amputation seemed like an appropriate and routine option, the surgeon reversed course. Captain Charles Knowlton, a member of the Tenth Louisiana, received a gunshot wound that almost cost him a leg but his surgeon jettisoned amputation in favor of saving the limb. One nurse remarked, "Out of many cases of the kind, this was the only one recorded where amputation was avoided and the patient's life was saved." In the midst of the Battle of Bentonville, North Carolina, in 1865, one Confederate officer ended up severely wounded. A projectile hit his leg and cut out "a big chunk of flesh" right at the knee joint. Despite a broken bone and severed tendons and ligaments, the surgeon decided not to amputate and saved the leg. At Fredericksburg in December 1862, Captain Thomas Henry Pitts found himself shot in the leg and hobbled his way behind the lines to catch an ambulance to a local field hospital. Pitts patiently waited for a surgeon, who arrived to inquire about the status of the damaged leg. Despite a horrific looking wound, the surgeon decided to remove the projectile, applied a dressing, and saved the leg. A surgeon decided not to amputate the leg of a private from North Carolina and expected the patient to make a full recovery. However, the hospital at Petersburg ran out of food during the critical recovery time and the patient perished.[53]

Dr. Hunter McGuire, who had treated Stonewall Jackson, recommended that Isaac Trimble not undergo amputation following a moment at Second Manassas when an exploding shell damaged his left leg. Trimble slowly recovered and returned to battle. Another Confederate soldier had his elbow severely damaged during the Battle of Spotsylvania Court House. A surgeon decided not to amputate and the soldier fully recovered with his arm intact.[54]

In some cases, surgeons refused to amputate, even against the wishes of the patient. Silas Ewell, a member of a South Carolina regiment, received a gunshot wound to his arm at the Battle of Jackson, Mississippi, in 1863. Ewell repeatedly demanded an immediate amputation, but his surgeon refused because he believed the patient would simply not survive. The surgeon finally relented and removed the arm. The patient survived. A Union private held at Andersonville Prison begged a Confederate surgeon to cut off his damaged feet. When the surgeon refused, the prisoner grabbed a pocket knife and started to cut through the rotten flesh and damaged tendons all the way down to the bone.[55]

Occasionally patients faced such dire medical circumstances that amputation would not be enough to save their lives. One private from North Carolina received a gunshot wound to his left knee. The soldier languished in a field hospital and survived nearly two weeks before a surgeon examined the leg. Due to the nature of the injury, as well as the extensive amount of time that had passed, the surgeon recommended against amputation. The soldier died after suffering from a high fever, nervousness, sleeplessness, and constant vomiting. The same thing happened to Private J. P. Goforth after he received a horrific gunshot wound to his left knee. Although the soldier avoided amputation and kept his leg, the gunshot wound swelled, and he died shortly thereafter. Another Confederate patient avoided amputation because he suffered from a high fever. Although surgeons hoped that an amputation could be considered once the fever subsided, it never did and the patient died. A private from North

Carolina simply could not physically survive an amputation and he died shortly after his injuries at the Battle of Antietam in 1862.[56]

Surgeons engaged in these internal debates about whether to amputate never expected to become patients themselves, but it happened. Operations took place amid the chaos of battle. One surgeon rushed out of a temporary hospital and shouted to his comrade, "Doctor, Doctor, this is no place for Doctors; a horse got shot in the yard just now." He implored his comrade to move to safety before returning to the patients. During the bombardment of Vicksburg, Mississippi, in 1863, a Union shell tore through the Confederate city hospital, destroying the entire stockpile of drugs and the foot of Surgeon Breets, who underwent amputation. One nurse described Dr. Middleton Michel and an amputation he performed in June 1862. During the operation, the surgeon became "inadvertently inoculated" in the arm and the severe reaction forced the surgeon to spend six weeks "in danger of life and limb." He did not return to active duty for several months.[57]

The experiences of individual surgeons paint a compelling portrait of men who adhered to the medical standards set forth for physicians during the Civil War. Confederate doctor William M. McPheeters served as a surgeon in the Western Theater of the Civil War. Following the military engagement at Helena, Arkansas, in July 1863, McPheeters removed the leg of a patient whose knee had been shattered beyond repair. Two days later, the patient died, which saddened the physician. However, the abundant casualties facing such medical personnel did not give the surgeon much time to mourn the loss of any one patient. Instead, he returned to work and amputated limbs, adjusted fractures, and performed other medical procedures. A year later, after the Battle of Jenkins' Ferry, the surgeon again performed several amputations. The exhaustive work, the unending wounded, and the piles of limbs led the surgeon to reflect, "Let those who prate about the glories of war witness such a scene and then talk of glory— this is the sad part of the picture." The next day, McPheeters remained at the hospital where he spent the entire day and into the late night hours "operating, taking off arms and legs and whatever else was needed to be done." Although he failed to keep count of the number of amputations, he assessed, "I never took off so many in one day before. [I'm] sorry that it was necessary to remove so many."[58]

Surgeons who exercised prudence or performed their duties with a kind and gentle hand received laudatory comments from patients. One experienced physician in the Confederate Army received especially high marks, described by several of his fellow physicians as "courteous, liberal and a high minded gentleman–brave, magnanimous and just and singularly free from the ordinary vices that stain and deform the otherwise exalted characters of so many of our prominent men." Patients made it a point to comment on how the surgeon acted as a "gentleman" and affirmed that the physician displayed the prime characteristics of manhood: a reputable demeanor, a clear and judicious mind when making medical decisions, and a caring countenance when performing difficult operations. He received commendation for his skill as a surgeon as well as for how he conducted surgical operations, especially in the presence of other medical professionals.[59]

Although the image of the surgeon as butcher has appeared in numerous primary accounts and has dominated our historical and popular understanding of Civil War medicine, the record paints a completely different portrait. Patients commonly portrayed field doctors as a devoted group of men who exhibited patience, kindness, and unrelenting skill in the face of trying situations. One man praised his Confederate surgeon as "full of the milk of human kindness." Another rebel private found that surgeons worked "with as much sympathy as familiarity with suffering is likely to leave." Dr. Hunter Holmes McGuire boldly declared that "some of the best military surgeons in the world could be found in the Confederate army." After the first Battle of Manassas, Dr. Darby, from South Carolina was described by another physician as someone who was very kind and "did his very best" to alleviate a difficult situation. Sally Tompkins, a nurse working at a hospital in Richmond during the war, admitted that her head surgeon despaired of "needless amputations" and worked throughout the war to reduce unnecessary operations.[60]

Such praise, though anecdotal, is evidence that not all army physicians became inured to the rigors of battlefield surgery and hospital care. Brigadier General Samuel W. Ferguson recalled having observed an act of kindness by a surgeon as he prepared to remove the leg of a Tennessee soldier. Dr. Chopin, Ferguson recalled, gently kissed the soldier as he was preparing to administer medical care. "It was a touching and unexpected scene, for the surgeons had been operating steadily for hours, and would

I thought, had become callous. Not so however with this great surgeon."
Dr. Walter J. Byrne, described as "social and genial," served with the Kentucky Orphan Brigade during the Civil War. Following the war, a historian observed, "As a surgeon, he was skillful, but conservative; and he saved, through his judgment and kindness, many a limb which, under other circumstances, would have been sacrificed."[61]

In one especially poignant homage to their regimental physicians, members of the Fifty-Ninth Georgia drafted a laudatory poem. The soldiers sought to honor their physicians, Watson and Long, and at the same time assure their comrades that they could fight without any hesitation because a capable physician stood ready to heal them.

> Go, soldier, go, thy country bleeds
> And write thy name in worthy deeds
> And if the ball should make a wound
> Don't tremble at the hurtling sound.
> But onward press—we'll gain the day
> And drive the Vandal hordes away
> While ever onwards in the throng
> We'll shout for Watson and for Long.
> And now the battle rages round
> And freely bleeds the painful wound
> The mournful groan, the painful sigh
> Come startling every passerby.
> Its thunders roar, its lightning's peal
> Then who shall all your sufferings heal?
> We'll fly to Watson and to Long
> And then continue with our song.[62]

Though their impressions have been lost to history, observers recognized the extraordinary work performed by skilled physicians under trying circumstances. Several days after the first engagement at Manassas, Peter Wellington Alexander, a Confederate newspaper correspondent, witnessed a group of surgeons establish a temporary field hospital and then get to work. "I saw legs and feet taken off," he wrote, "arms and ghastly gashes sewed up rapidly and yet skillfully." The patients themselves rarely groaned or complained, leading Alexander to conclude that aside from "a

skillful field officer, the most important man on the day of battle is the Surgeon." Throughout the war, he routinely reported from battlefield hospitals, like Sharpsburg, where he saw more "amputated arms and legs, feet,
fingers, and hands cut off."[63]

The greatest compliments paid to doctors, however, sometimes came
after the war when they encountered their former patients. E. A. Craighill,
a Confederate surgeon, wandered the streets of Lynchburg, Virginia, after
the war. He recalled having no food and no money with only "disap-
pointment and black despair" in his heart. But one day a group of men
approached him in a "cordial" manner and expressed great joy in seeing him. The former patients, members of the Thirty-Fourth Massachusetts, simply wanted to thank their surgeon, whom they recognized, for
his "kindness and attention." They also shared the good news of a fellow
comrade, who had lost his leg at the hands of the surgeon. He claimed to
now have the "best stump in New England."[64]

In the end, many Confederate surgeons were professionalized by the
war itself, which would elevate their stature as men within their communities and among their peers, and they welcomed the extensive knowledge
they garnered in the battlefield hospitals. "I return home a better surgeon, a better doctor," one noted. Multiplying such men a thousandfold,
the South received, when the guns fell silent, "a medical corps which the
war has thoroughly educated and reliably trained," according to another
physician. Thus, wounded veterans would rely for the most part on honorable and reputable men making sound medical decisions for them for
years to come.[65]

The war's medical history, then, presents a mixed record. Most surgeons
were competent, skilled, and compassionate doctors, operating under
sometimes horrific conditions, and saving thousands of lives and hundreds
of limbs. Even so their reputations as a whole could not survive factors
that had little to do with their skill: negative impressions made early in the
war, when medical corps were overwhelmed and shorthanded; the few
examples of doctors who truly were grossly unqualified or who thought
speed and daring were the measure of a medical man; the simple fact that
surgery performed out in the open and in a rush does look like butchery
to the unpracticed eye, especially when performed without chloroform;
and the apparently irresistible urge among Hollywood directors to throw
the added horror of the hospital into their Civil War movies. Weighing all

available evidence certainly suggests that the image of the butcher must be put to rest forever. Instead Civil War surgeons should be understood for who they were: professionals who identified sympathetically with their male patients while plying the best practices of their trade (as they were understood at the time), and men who at least learned significantly from their significant mistakes. The grim irony is they learned so much because the war gave them so much practice.

TWO

The Patients

Enduring the "Fearfulest Test" of Manhood

> To amputate, or not to amputate? That is the question.
> Whether 'tis nobler in the mind to suffer
> Th' unsymmetry of one-armed men, and draw
> A pension, thereby shuffling off a part
> Of Mortal coil; or, trusting unhinged nature,
> Take arms against a cruel surgeon's knife,
> And, by opposing rusty theories,
> Risk a return to dust in the full shape of man.
> —Washington Davis, "To Amputate, or Not to Amputate?"

At the Battle of Gaines Mill, Virginia, in June 1862, Lieutenant H. B. Myatt, a member of the Fourteenth Louisiana, received a gunshot wound to the groin. As an ambulance team removed him from the front lines to a local field hospital, a random artillery shell shattered his left elbow. Surgeons suggested amputation of his left arm, but Myatt refused as he could still move his fingers. Instead, the physicians performed an excision on the elbow joint and removed some of the shattered bone. Myatt experienced some initial pain and swelling in his hand but recovered quickly after adhering to a solid diet and two-daily brandy regimen. Although the operation shortened the arm by about two inches, Myatt retained full functionality, as he could, according to his physician, "hold a fork, a knife or any other small object in that hand; he lifts up a bucket full of water; sensibility and mobility of the fingers are perfect." The patient gloated gleefully, "It seems to me my arm is gaining every day, I can now bend it almost at [a] right angle without the use of the other hand; I can carve my food, tie my cravat, and write a few words with my left hand." While most soldiers succumbed to the inevitable and accepted amputation as a reasonable course of medical treatment, a few soldiers, like Myatt, rejected amputation and not only lived but thrived.[1]

This chapter explores the roles played by Confederate officers and enlisted men in their own medical treatment and recovery. In accepting or refusing amputations, patients laid bare their own practical as well as aesthetic and cultural concerns about how the loss of a limb was perceived by their communities. The operating table and the hospital bed provided an arena where wounded patients assessed their medical, personal, and spiritual condition. Wounded soldiers lay on their backs and meditated deeply about a whole range of issues, including their beliefs about religion, disability, and the male life worth living. Some soldiers decided whether to resist or accept the scalpel and saw based on their own personal notions of honor. For some, a stump was a red badge of courage. For others, it represented a crippling, an emasculation, and a threat to their ability to provide. After all, in the honor culture that held sway in the South, reputation was everything, and the currency of honor rested on others' opinions. Thus, there was much to lose (possibly everything) if a man ended up sized up by a stranger on the basis of his newly compromised physical appearance.

Historian Kathryn Meier has lately reminded us that Civil War soldiers practiced a great deal of "self-care." Doctors were not yet the sole authority over the body, and, from a medical perspective, families and individuals often fended for themselves. As Meier noted, even some of the soldiers who fell out, shirked, malingered, and went AWOL purposely or intuitively *improved* their fighting readiness by avoiding camp diseases, exhaustion, fouled water supplies, and poor diet. Wounded men too often felt that they had a place in the medical decision making, and they often had to tend themselves for hours while waiting for medical attention, especially in the early stages of the war when surgeons found themselves overwhelmed with large numbers of patients. As they waited, some men decided to refuse amputation in order to remain in control of their physique. A potential patient could threaten or use violence against a surgeon in order to avoid the removal of a limb. Wounded men could also run away from a field hospital and potentially desert the army if they feared or distrusted the sawbones. Other patients could beg and plead with the attending surgeon to circumvent amputation. Whatever the reasons for a soldier's decision to deny permission for amputation, resistance assumed major risks, including infection, permanent paralysis, pain, and even the prospect of death.[2]

Officers, more often than regular infantrymen, shunned amputation. Senior officers had the luxury of a personal surgeon with whom they developed a deep, personal trust, and they understood each other as honorable men. Though officers usually accepted the medical advice of that surgeon, the consultation was generally longer, more mutual, and more focused. Commanders were more likely to be concerned that amputation would prevent them from returning to command. A surgeon usually respected the opinion of a senior officer who wanted to avoid amputation, provided the patient understood the potential ramifications and seemed willing to accept the consequences. Lower-ranking officers and common soldiers had to work harder to reverse the traditional power dynamic that existed between surgeon and patient.

The removal of a limb unleashed a plethora of emotions and reactions, including depression, anxiety, self-pity or resignation, and peacefulness that they had survived such a traumatic ordeal. As damaged men recovered in a hospital setting, surrounded by other amputated and mutilated men, a new shared experience among a community of fellow sufferers emerged, as the patients provided support to one another to adjust to the newly forged empty sleeve. Fellow amputees normalized the postsurgical experience and aided soldiers in dealing with the lengthy road of rehabilitation, learning to use a prosthetic limb, and readjusting to society.

Typically, gunshot wounds in battle brought patients to the table, but freak accidents attended any military endeavor. Gervis Hammond Stone, a member of the Eighth Kentucky cavalry, lost his left leg due to a cattle stampede. Before the accident, Stone had been wounded at the Battle of Hartsville and recovered in a nearby hospital. An unidentified man fell from a train carrying Confederate soldiers to Mississippi in 1863. Six different wheels had passed over his thigh, completely pulverizing the bone and prompting a surgeon riding on the train to order an amputation. The train paused thirty minutes and a group of men rushed the patient to a nearby home, collected some saws and chloroform, and quickly removed the leg. The patient remained on the couch in the makeshift hospital to recover as the train sped away into the night. Another soldier in the Sixty-Second Georgia cavalry shot off two of his fingers on his right hand after the accidental discharge of his gun. He nearly bled to death until the fingers could be properly amputated.[3]

Dangerous accidents, piercing bayonets, and unforgiving projectiles sent thousands of Confederate soldiers and officers to the hospital tent. Upon their arrival, the patient had a lot to take in, as the sights, sounds, and smells of a field hospital unnerved even the steadiest countenance. As the patients waited, their thoughts usually drifted among their survival, their family, and their comrades in arms. They assessed their own masculine self-worth, as they posited their past and potential future. The waiting particularly plagued them as they were forced to think about the possibility of amputation for hours or even days. One medical professional noted that men who experienced a significant delay before undergoing amputation felt "a variety of emotions, including depression; suicidal urges, even in those who have never considered suicide before; anger both at themselves and others; fear; worry; and in certain cases, guilt." Jacob Clark, shot in the arm at Shiloh, finally decided that death was the best way out. Although he seemed rather cheerful and in good spirits, he ended his life via a pistol to his temple while recovering in a hospital in Missouri. His wife noted that he ended his life out of fear of losing his arm via amputation.[4]

Of course Confederate patients reacted to the possibility of amputation in myriad ways. Emily V. Mason, who worked in Richmond, watched potential amputees pass by on a stretcher singing "a Baptist or Methodist hymn." Many framed the loss around religious ideals, realizing that their own suffering paled in comparison to that of Jesus Christ and that if they lost a limb, it was simply God's will and should be seen as a blessing, not a curse. Others actively wondered if amputation served as God's punishment for the sins they committed. Historian George Rable argued that "men could almost stand outside of themselves, viewing their suffering and pain as but a temporary phase during which they might glimpse the glories of heaven." An amputee from North Carolina, who lost a leg, now saw himself as more of a religious individual because of his injury. George Allen, a member of the Fourth Texas, lost his right arm at Gettysburg. He relished the removal of his arm, as he truly believed that it strengthened his faith "in God and Christ and Southern rights."[5]

To be sure, religiosity did not remain paramount in the minds of all Confederate patients. At the Battle of Franklin, Tennessee, in November 1864, Capt. John M. Hickey had both of his legs amputated on the battlefield. As he recovered, Rev. E. M. Bounds asked him if "he would like to read from the Bible and pray with him." Hickey refused, asked for "some beer or whiskey," and wished for the reverend to simply tell some anecdotes. One individual recalled about the captain, "The poor fellow was so low that he could not move his head."[6]

In extreme instances, the anxiety of waiting combined with the threat of losing a limb resulted in violent confrontations. At Gettysburg, Dr. Henry Miner dealt with a Captain McMay, who tried not once but twice to shoot the doctor who determined he would need to lose a finger. As the operation commenced, McMay suddenly plunged his hand under his coat and pulled out a pistol, thrust the muzzle against the surgeon's back, and pulled the trigger. Fortunately, a fast-acting fellow surgeon intervened and saved the doctor's life. McMay tried to shoot the surgeon again when the candle that illuminated the hospital scene blew out. Miner wrote, "There we were in the dark, with the angry man trying to shoot again, the doctor struggling to hold him and to hold the pistol." Captain McMay, well aware of the dangers of amputation and the risk that he might never return to the field of battle, resorted to violence to save his finger. After all, the hospital recovery bed sapped away a man's ability to prove his masculine worth in battle before his peers. The size of the amputation ultimately did not matter.[7]

Another Confederate officer threatened violence if doctors followed through on the amputation of his damaged leg. A musket ball at the Battle of Shiloh broke both bones in the left leg of William Brimage Bate, a colonel in the Second Tennessee. While the surgeons insisted on amputation, Bate spurned the advice and ordered his servant to give him his pistols so he could let the surgeons know "he intended to protect that leg." Bate refused to surrender mastery of his own body to a surgeon and kept his pistols at his bedside for the remainder of his hospital stay. Bate survived, kept the bad leg, and returned to the war, though with some difficulty. A veteran remembered, "In the various incidents of horses being killed at Chickamauga, he had to be lifted each time upon another horse, unable to mount alone."[8]

After he received a bullet wound to the foot at the Battle of Chickamauga, Private William Fletcher also resorted to violence at a battlefield hospital. Fletcher witnessed a wide array of injuries among his comrades, including one soldier named Frank, who had been permanently disfigured after being shot in the face. Fletcher chided the unfortunate soul, remarking that he "would make better success courting when he got back, with his back to the girls." The soldier shot back, "That will be better than you; as you can't turn any way to hide your wooden leg." Both men then watched as the surgeon cut off the foot of another unfortunate soldier and tossed it into a "scrap heap." Evidently what had been intended as a humorous exchange had gotten under Fletcher's skin, and as the surgeon approached to investigate his wound, Fletcher kicked the surgeon in the shoulder, prompting the doctor to promise, "I will leave you alone, without treatment." Fletcher replied, "Doc, that is what I want, and the fellow that I considered most to blame would make the mistake of his life if treated without my sanction, as that man . . . has been treated, put under influence of something and when he comes to, his foot gone."[9]

Fletcher escaped the field hospital with his wounded leg still attached, but there were medical consequences to his decision. He traveled by rail to Augusta, Georgia, and recuperated at a local church where the Sisters of Charity assisted him in his recovery. He unsuccessfully tried to obtain a set of crutches on numerous occasions, only to find his name at the bottom of the list each time. When the crutches finally arrived, Fletcher was unable to use them, as gangrene had set in on his wounded foot. He received an acid burning treatment for seven straight days. "If I had been a drunkard I would probably have thought I at least was threatened with delirium tremens," Fletcher said of the treatments, "as the worm or snaky feeling would start at the mouth of [the] wound and make a hurried zigzag run up near the knee, then would return as through backing out, and running out of the wound." The treatment worked, although his foot turned downward, which forced him to now walk on his toes. The doctors suggested either breaking the foot or amputation, since they estimated only a 10 percent chance of saving the foot. Fletcher wrote, "I said I would prefer life with a crooked leg and walking on toes, to an artificial foot; so they said they would consider it no more." When Fletcher made the final decision to resist amputation, the words from the initial hospital visit with a fellow injured soldier rang clearly through his mind. With Fletcher not knowing if women would embrace or resist Confederate amputees in the postwar era, he chose to remain a physically complete man, despite the horrific pain and deformity, and live through the postwar era without having to fear romantic rejection based on an amputation.[10]

Violent reactions to the threat of amputation were both rare and extreme, but they reflect the significant fears soldiers harbored about both amputation and altered manhood, especially with regard to how women and their fellow southerners would look at their damaged bodies. Some men refused medical treatment because they worried about how their family back home would perceive their empty sleeves. One Confederate soldier, wounded at Chickamauga, confided to a chaplain he had been advised that his leg must be amputated and he feared that his mother would never accept him if he were disabled. The chaplain endeavored to help him, and oversaw his transfer to a different hospital where medical attendants determined that his leg need not be amputated. Years later the soldier ran into the chaplain, by now a bishop, and thanked him profusely but still had ill-words for the "saw-bones" physician who first examined him and ordered the amputation.[11]

Confederate amputees often felt a tinge of regret or a burst of panic in the hospital bed as they wondered if women would accept their physical deformities. Kate Cumming, when nursing amputated patients, commented, "I constantly hear the unmarried ones wondering if the girls will marry them now." Despite such overwhelming concerns, the men seemed in solid spirits. Cumming recalled, "We have a room with seven men it, who have lost a limb each. It is a perfect treat to go into it, as the men seem to do little else but laugh." The men routinely told Cumming to call on the women to come see these particular men, since they would make "excellent husbands, as they will be sure to never run away." She hoped that the women of the South would reset their attitudes toward the disabled male and work to end the suffering of the many men who had only performed their duty.[12]

Amputated men sought advice from nurses about how women back home would perceive their injuries. One limbless Confederate asked his nurse, "When do you think my wound will be well enough for me to go to the country?" The soldier requested a speedy return home because he worried that his woman back home might reject him or move on. The nurse confidently predicted, "Ah, but you must show her your scars, and if she is a girl worth having she will love you all the better for having bled for your country and you must tell her that 'it is always the heart that is bravest in war that is fondest and truest in love.'" The soldier seemed content with the response and went back to regaining his full strength to once again return home.[13]

Walter Waightstill Lenoir, a Confederate soldier who lost his right leg at the Second Battle of Manassas in August 1862, also worried about how amputation would now alter his life and romantic prospects. He noted in his diary that his head filled with thoughts of what he would have to give up now that he had lost a limb. "First I thought of my favorite sport of trout fishing, which I would have to give up," he wrote. "Then I thought of skating, swimming and partridge hunting, my other favorite sports which it also occurred to me that I could never enjoy again." Yet, sports did not appear first and foremost on his list of sacrifices. Lenoir confessed that "before all these things I thought sadly of women; for I was not old enough to have given up the thought of women. . . . It may not seem very creditable to me that I thought first of the mere enjoyments which I was to lose with my leg. But such were my poor unworthy thoughts."[14]

The loss of a leg transported Lenoir from a world of independence to one where he had to reassess dependency and accept assistance from those who could facilitate his survival. During his recovery, Lenoir remained particularly dependent on Mrs. Samuel A. Chancellor, who spoke to him "in that sweet, kind woman's voice that thrills the heart of the sufferer as nothing else can, inquiring after my situation and wants." Once he returned home, his greatest fears materialized, as Lenoir did not marry and lacked any true romantic prospects. In order to survive financially, Lenoir spent his first postwar months dependent on some slaves who assisted him in farming. He wrote to his sister, "You know that I had made up my mind before the war that I would not be again a slave owner. . . . Circumstances have made me a slave owner." Prior to his military service, Lenoir wrestled with the morality of slavery and declared he would live an independent life without any connection to the institution. Amputation shifted Lenoir's internal perceptions about slavery and forced him to now remain dependent on his slaves for his health and welfare. While a dependency on slaves compromised Lenoir's principles, he had no choice. His survival necessitated an enhanced dependency on slavery until emancipation forced Lenoir to look elsewhere in order to deal with the difficulties of disability.[15]

This concern for a postwar livelihood also framed wounded Confederates decisions regarding amputation. The removal of a limb could prevent a man from continuing an occupation that had been pivotal in providing for his wife and children. Col. M. D. L. Stephens, a member of the Thirty-First Mississippi Infantry, received a wound in his upper leg at the Battle of Franklin. After an assemblage of surgeons deemed amputation a necessity, Stephens called for Dr. Wall, the chief surgeon of the makeshift hospital. Stephens beseeched, "I am a physician and have a wife and two children at home. Everything is swept away in our country and the Negroes free. I will be compelled to practice my profession if I live to get back there. You know that I cannot practice medicine in my hill country when I am quartered up." Stephens, who decided to serve in the rank and file rather than the medical corps, emphatically declared, "I will go with my leg and my leg will go with me." Dr. Wall offered his own assessment, stating, "I think it best for you to let your leg go." As tears swelled within his eyes, Stephens begged Wall to prevent the amputation and the surgeon finally relented. The decision prompted a sharp rebuke from another physician who vociferously disagreed with Wall, and the two nearly fought over the proper course. Wall, a complete stranger, was willing to shoot a surgeon threatening amputation. He well understood Stephens's plight. While an amputation would remove a limb, it would also diminish Stephens's stature as a man and professional and compromise his ability to support a family. As a man and doctor, Wall understood this.[16]

Without slavery to buttress his household income, Stephens would depend on a profitable medical profession in order for the family to survive. He worried about the practicalities of physically being able to practice medicine without a leg. He also did not think that a doctor missing a leg could construe a reputation that guaranteed a bounty of potential clients. A potential patient would not find credence in the diagnosis and treatment of a physician who looked like a patient. Stephens needed both legs to maintain his honor, protect his reputation, and provide for his family. Wall, in turn, acted honorably through the maintenance of a promise to save the leg of a patient, a pledge he was willing to support with violent means.[17]

As some men worried about their future, others saw death, and their willingness to confront it, as a testament to their honor and thus preferable to living with a damaged body. Brigadier General Matthew Whitaker Ransom refused amputation on his left arm and accepted the declaration from his surgeon that he would not survive. He accepted the fact that if he could not continue fighting, at least he died from injuries sustained in battle. Confederate Lieutenant Colonel Henry Watkins Allen proclaimed similar sentiments. "A man ought always to expect to be killed in battle, and should be willing and prepared for death always before he goes into it." While he survived a gunshot wound at Shiloh in April 1862, Allen refused amputation after he received another gunshot wound to his leg at Baton Rouge on August 2, 1862. Prepared to die, Allen awaited his fate. Although other surgeons strongly advised him to undergo amputation, he continued to remain steadfast in his preparation for death. Allen's decision to await death came with profound ramifications, as men who jettisoned the medical recommendation of surgeons could expect to live severely disabled with constant pain, for a short or long period. He spent months lying in bed and told a friend that he feared the leg "*will never get well!*" Allen recovered and had to use a pair of crutches in order to visit his old comrades, who picked him up and carried him through the camp. He died a physically complete man a few years later from complications arising from his refused amputation.[18]

In addition to contemplating death, many wounded men also feared that amputation might prevent their return to the battlefield. If officers refused amputation, they could immediately return to command. However, if officers accepted amputation and spent time in a hospital recovering from a missing limb, they would be removed from their men, their duty, and their chances for promotion. Some officers expressed this concern before the amputation commenced. Dr. Henry Miner treated a Confederate officer who needed his finger amputated. Initially the officer refused and argued that if he breathed in any chloroform, he would not be able to command his men. The officer confidently predicted another battle the next day and felt he needed to be there. Eventually, he relented, declaring, "Cut this damned finger off." The officer recovered immediately, since he lost only the tip of his finger, and returned to the field of battle. The next day, he was injured again when his horse tossed him and the commander became "lame in both legs, with a ragged finger." Dr. Miner examined the snarled finger once again and insisted on complete amputation, but the officer refused because he thought it would take him out of action for longer. "What do you think of that for courage?" Miner wondered.[19]

Of course men often gambled with their lives when they prioritized a speedy return to the field. Brigadier General John Adams refused to leave the ranks after he was shot in the right arm at Franklin, Tennessee, on November 30, 1864. Rather than seek medical attention, Adams continued in the battle, riding his horse into the federal position, where he endured another wound that took his life. Major Joseph McGraw had his left arm torn away at Spotsylvania Court House in May 1864 by a solid shot that left "only a stump in the shoulder socket." Some of his men rushed to assist him, but McGraw held them at bay, shouting, "Don't mind me, men. I'm alright. Give 'em hell!" McGraw passed out in his saddle immediately after giving the command but later regained consciousness and underwent surgery. McGraw further proved his mettle by refusing all anesthetics, regarding chloroform as unmanly. Instead, he endured the operation without "eliciting a groan," as he puffed away on his pipe. He glibly quipped to his physician, "I reckon I'll be off duty thirty days."[20]

In a similar display of bravado in the face of grave injury, Major General Bryan Grimes refused to follow the advice of his surgeon. Grimes had been severely kicked by a horse, and the surgeon recommended removal of the damaged leg. Grimes declined and continued his military service with great success. In 1863 D. H. Hill described Grimes: "He has been in many pitched battles and has behaved most gallantly in them all. His gallantry, ripe experience, admirable training, intelligence and moral worth constitute strong claims for promotion." Brigadier General Michael J. Bulger of the Forty-Seventh Alabama sustained several gunshot wounds, including one in his arm, which he tied off in order to remain in command. He showed a similarly cavalier attitude when he was shot in the leg, putting a corncob on each side of the wound and tying them off with his suspenders. He fought to exhaustion before a surgeon recommended the removal of his leg. Wishing to continue his military service without interruption, Bulger refused and later commanded at Gettysburg, only to be shot in the chest and left for dead on the field.[21]

Officers understood the risks of declining amputation. Brigadier General Brickett Davenport Fry sustained a hand wound at Seven Pines and then returned to the ranks to receive an even more devastating wound at Sharpsburg, where doctors advised him he would require an amputation. Fry demanded to know his chances of surviving without surgery, and the doctor estimated them at no better than one in three hundred. Fry beat the odds and returned to lead his men at Chancellorsville and Gettysburg.[22]

While more officers resisted amputation in order to get back on the field, some of their lower-ranking fellows followed suit. Common soldiers often saw battle as an opportunity to prove their manhood and resisted amputation in hopes of a quick return to the conflict. One soldier shot in the leg at Spotsylvania Court House in May 1864 vehemently protested his surgeon's recommendation to undergo amputation. Looking on, Chaplain Charles Dobbs tried to convince the patient to accede, but the recommendation fell on deaf ears. The patient knew of others who had resisted amputation, survived, and returned to battle. A month later, Dobbs encountered the patient in a Richmond hospital. "He was a living skeleton, the flesh seemed all gone; he was full of bed sores. His wounded limb was swung up in a cloth; it was four times its natural size and full of worms." Yet the patient continued to resist amputation in order to preserve his manhood and in the end died "in great anguish," according to Chaplain Dobbs, who claimed the man "deeply regretted his folly when it was too late." According to one surgical manual, men were naturally "enthused by the combat" and "willing to submit to anything which gives a promise of future revenge."[23]

Major R. E. Wilson thrived amid the rush of battle and hated to be away from it. He enlisted at the age of twenty-one in the Twenty-First North Carolina at the start of the war. Wilson later became a sharpshooter, refusing to let three gunshot wounds terminate his military service. On April 2, 1865, he lost his left leg at Petersburg and underwent medical treatment in a Baptist church in Richmond, Virginia. The next day, Union forces flooded the city and Wilson found himself a prisoner. Despite having just lost his leg, he allegedly killed three Union soldiers while in prison.[24]

The impulse to return to service after amputation consumed some men to the point that it jeopardized their health and overall livelihood. Brigadier General Adley Hogan Gladden received a gunshot wound on the first day of Shiloh. The surgeon removed Gladden's left arm, but instead of going to a quiet location to recuperate, Gladden returned to his horse and headed back to the field in order to give commands and consult with his staff. After the battle ended, he rode to Corinth, Mississippi, where he underwent a second amputation of his arm. Gladden believed that he would quit his command only when he found himself in a coffin. He was killed by lockjaw shortly after the second operation.[25]

Probably the Confederacy's most famous amputation case was that of General Thomas "Stonewall" Jackson. Jackson had first been wounded on the middle finger of his left hand at the Battle of Manassas on July 21,

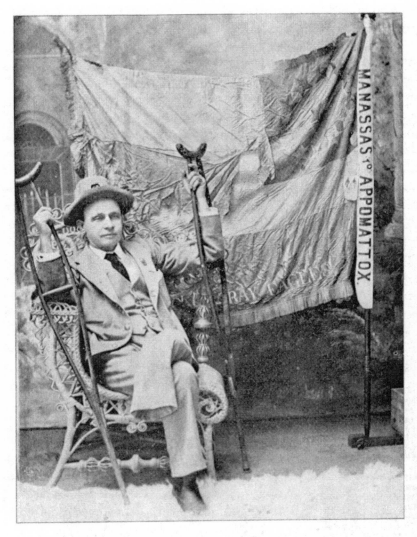

MAJOR R. E. WILSON, FIRST NORTH CAROLINA BATTALION SHARPSHOOTERS.

Figure 6. Major R. E. Wilson. Courtesy of the Kentucky Historical Society.

1861. He waited until the conclusion of battle to receive any medical attention. With a ragged finger, Jackson rallied his men and drove the Federals from the field, sealing a Confederate victory. Although the regimental doctor recommended the amputation of the damaged finger, Jackson refused and galloped off on his horse to find Hunter Holmes McGuire, his medical director, who splinted the finger with two sticks. Jackson and his finger made a full recovery because he preferred the advice of his own doctor.[26]

Jackson faced a second amputation decision on the evening of May 2, 1863, during the Battle of Chancellorsville. A volley of friendly fire raked Jackson and his staff on an evening reconnaissance mission. Jackson, removed to a field infirmary two miles behind the lines, received immediate medical care from his friend and physician, Dr. Hunter McGuire. McGuire asked Jackson if he had permission to amputate the arm if necessary. Jackson replied, "Yes, certainly; Dr. McGuire, do for me whatever you think is best." McGuire noted that a ball had entered Jackson's palm at the middle of his hand and fractured two bones. He said, "The left arm was then amputated, about two inches below the shoulder joint, the ball dividing the main artery, and fracturing the bone." Another physician deemed the operation a great success and thought Jackson would return to command within a few months. The arm ended up buried in the Lacy family burial plot, and visitors today can visit the site simply marked with a granite monument that says, "Arm of Stonewall Jackson, May 3, 1863."[27]

Word quickly spread through the Confederate ranks of Jackson's amputation. Robert E. Lee wrote to Jackson to express his deepest regret and wished that he had been "disabled in your stead," congratulating Jackson for a victory accomplished by great "skill and energy." Jackson appreciated the kind words but remained focused on a speedy recovery so he could once again be in the saddle. To facilitate a speedy recovery, Lee ordered Jackson moved to Guinea Station. As Jackson rested in a comfortable bed in the Chandler House, he viewed his amputation as a positive force. "Many would regard [these wounds] as a great misfortune. I regard them as one of the blessings of my life." Southern civilians and soldiers believed Jackson encapsulated the highest ideals of manhood and honor, proudly displayed in victory and in injury. As Jackson called his own missing limb a blessing, he set the tone for a society coming to see an empty sleeve as a symbol of worthy sacrifice for the Confederacy and not a marker of shattered masculinity.[28]

A man of Jackson's stature certainly had the power to shape southern perceptions of amputated men. He fully intended to return to the field until a bout of pneumonia killed him on May 10, 1863. When Robert E. Lee learned that Jackson's medical condition had taken a turn for the worse, he asked a chaplain to deliver the following message to the ailing officer: "He has lost his left arm, but I my right arm." In using the metaphor, Lee at once affirmed the primacy of working limbs to the performance of masculinity and the honor to be paid the man who sacrificed such a prize on the altar of the Confederacy. (He also set the stage for Jackson's postwar position in Confederate lore.) Although Robert E. Lee underwent a metaphorical amputation after Chancellorsville, he lived to fight another day, as would the Confederacy, as would so many of its most famous officers. Amputation damaged the body, but if the operation was properly "performed," the amputee might underline rather than undermine his reputation. The loss of an arm had secured Jackson's reputation for victory even in the ultimate defeat—death itself.[29]

Jackson's state funeral sent nearly twenty thousand citizens in the city of Richmond to file past the coffin as Jackson lay in state. After a lengthy viewing, city officials asked the crowd to disperse. Suddenly, a man pushed through the departing crowd, demanding a chance to take a final look at his commander. A marshal attempted to intercept the man but before the marshal could seize him, the veteran held up the stump of his right arm, and as his eyes swelled with tears, he declared, "By this arm, which I lost for my county, I demand the privilege of seeing my old general once." City officials acquiesced and allowed the soldier to view the body of his amputated officer, as some of the crowd hung back in appreciation, implicitly recognizing the leveling of two limbless men who had sacrificed so much for them. Jackson's transformation, physical and metaphysical, shifted the perception even of those amputated men who survived the war.[30]

The passing of Stonewall Jackson prompted an outpouring of sorrow from all across the Confederacy. An anonymous writer announced the death of Jackson and commented, "None of us knew how deeply we loved him until the cruel intelligence of his wound taught us all what we felt. To attempt now, while perhaps his maimed body is borne through the streets, to narrate his glorious career, even in brief, is an office from which any one may well shrink." The author wanted his readers to understand that even in losing an arm, Jackson's "body of work" became more complete. No amputation in the Confederacy did more to commend amputees to the public. Southern writers feverishly worked to ensure that Jackson became the very embodiment of how to sacrifice a piece of oneself (and then all of oneself) for the nation. And the "right arm" metaphor would carry Jackson into immortality. He would forever be understood as the Confederacy's most important appendage, its sword arm, its gun arm – the embodiment of its military might, its "right" to bear arms, and the "rights" for which it had borne arms, bled, and died.[31]

Jackson was certainly the most prominent Confederate officer to undergo amputation during the Civil War, but he was hardly the only one. The Confederacy's side of a "Civil War chess set" looks like an army of the walking wounded. Richard Ewell suffered a crushing injury from a minié ball that struck his kneecap during the Battle of Groveton, Virginia, in August 1862. Although some Alabama soldiers offered to assist him, Ewell only growled, "Put me down and give them hell. I'm no better than any other wounded soldier." Initially, Ewell insisted on an amputation, thinking it would actually be the fastest way back to the ranks. The examining physicians refused, however, and sent Ewell to a home near Sudley Ford. A few hours later, Dr. Hunter McGuire examined the leg and agreed with Ewell – the damage was so severe that amputation was the best option. "When the leg was opened we found the knee-cap split half in two," a witness noted, "the head of the tibia knocked into several pieces and that the ball had followed the marrow of the bone for six inches breaking the bone itself into small splinters and finally had split into two pieces on a sharp edge of the bone." Ewell barely survived the operation and clung to life as two other men buried the bloody appendage in a nearby garden.[32]

After an arduous seven-month recovery, including a setback when he took a spill on some ice that split open his leg stump, Ewell was grateful that the leg had finally healed but aggravated that he would need more time to grow accustomed to the prosthetic device before he could return to battle. The recovery time had given Ewell some distance from the war, which he clearly felt ambivalent about. As he told Jubal Early, "I do not want to see the carnage and shocking sights of another field of battle, though I prefer being in the field to anywhere else so long as the war is going on." Following the death of Jackson, Lee recommended that Ewell assume command of Jackson's old corps as soon as he could ride in the saddle. Ewell would ultimately prove a model of stamina, riding several miles a day in front of his men. Sandie Pendleton wrote, "He manages his leg very well and walks only with a stick, and mounts his horse quite easily from the ground." Ewell's return to command was not only necessary because he could not be spared as an officer but also important to send the signal to the entire command that disability did not prevent an officer from returning to ranks.[33]

Yet only a handful of Confederate officers returned to prominent leadership positions after losing a limb. John Bell Hood actually managed to do it twice, suffering major amputations in back-to-back battles in 1863. At Gettysburg, a gunshot wound to the left arm left the limb intact but with limited function. Two and a half months later, at Chickamauga, a minié ball shattered Hood's right femur and prompted the officer to undergo amputation. Dr. T. G. Richardson removed Hood's leg four inches from the hip. By the spring of 1864, Hood returned to command, this time as a corps commander with the Army of Tennessee. As he rode among the men, who now affectionately called him "Old Peg-Leg," Hood displayed a prosthetic leg, dangling from his saddle. He explained how he had tried out several different types of prosthetic devices and confessed that the Yankee leg reigned superior. Even with his prosthetic Yankee leg dangling from the saddle, Hood returned to his military routine and inspired some confidence that a missing limb did not mean a wounded soldier had to forsake his military duty.[34]

As rare as these things were, they were even rarer among the lower ranks. Officers usually had the luxury of a personal physician who could provide the highest level of medical care. They were surrounded by staff members or generous civilians who assisted them during their recovery period. Long hours in a hospital bed provided numerous occasions for the men to openly talk about their injuries and their desires to return to battle. In addition, other officers tended to share their own thoughts about fellow commanders when they underwent an operation and used the opportunity to reflect on the patients' character and bravery.[35]

Rank-and-file Confederate amputees did not leave behind the same level of correspondence discussing the meaning of their empty sleeves, and historians are left with only minimal information about the common soldier and his amputation. While some soldiers revealed their motivations for resisting amputation, others did not, and we are left to wonder what prompted such often rash and potentially dangerous decisions. James William Howard, a member of the Ninth Arkansas, worked as a farmer prior to his enlistment. During the Atlanta campaign on May 13, 1864, a ball struck his left arm about an inch below his shoulder joint. Three different doctors probed his wound with their fingers and confirmed that the ball had cracked his arm and lodged just under the shoulder blade. Howard refused amputation, the recommended protocol, and he also refused to let the doctors remove the ball when they asked him again on May 28. Although complaining of constant pain and sleepless nights, he never reconsidered and managed to survive the war with his arm intact and a bullet lodge under his shoulder as a souvenir of the war. We do not know why he was so intractable, nor do we know why Lieutenant Colonel Jonathan Catlett Gibson, shot in the right shin in 1864 while serving with the Forty-Ninth Virginia, declined amputation. After being sent to Chimborazo Hospital, Gibson resisted form of amputation on his leg, but the Richmond newspapers reported that it "is now thought that he will recover."[36]

Common soldiers, who usually adhered to the advice of senior medical professionals, did not routinely resist amputation and tens of thousands lost legs, arms, and other appendages throughout the war. One soldier lost both of his legs and sustained a gunshot wound to his eyes. Several dozen members of the First Kentucky Brigade underwent an amputation of a leg. Thomas Wingo, a member of the cavalry, lost both a leg and sustained a gunshot wound to his eyes. Private Williamson, of the Thirteenth Mississippi, received a gunshot wound to his right thigh at Seven Pines in June 1862. A surgeon quickly removed the leg within two hours and the patient made a full recovery in six weeks. Another soldier spent months recovering from a gunshot wound that shattered several bones in his leg. When the leg swelled and the wound discharged an enormous amount of pus with a foul smell, surgeons removed the leg and the patient quickly recovered.[37]

In some instances, the Confederate soldier who lost a leg had barely reached adulthood. At the Battle of Pea Ridge in March 1862, fourteen-year-old Billy Wilson had his leg blown off in battle and another soldier carried his wounded body to a local residence. Private John Mather Sloan emerged as the youngest Confederate soldier to lose a limb during the Civil War. At the age of thirteen, he lost his leg at Farmington, Mississippi, as a member of the Ninth Texas. First Corporal John Day Perkins, a member of the Second Florida, laid on the field at Gettysburg for two days before Union crews found his body and transported him to Fort McHenry in Maryland. There, Perkins underwent two operations that resulted in the amputation of a thumb and his left leg. One woman working at the hospital noted, "Oh, he is nothing but a boy. Poor boy, so far from home."[38]

The Confederate men who lost a leg could face bouts of chronic pain that forced them to receive additional medical attention. One soldier, who lost part of his leg, endured a second amputation twenty-two years after the war because of the chronic pain. Private R. A. Vick, a member of the Forty-Third North Carolina, lost the lower third of his right thigh after undergoing amputation as a result of a gunshot wound at Cedar Creek on October 19, 1864. Despite the removal of the limb, Vick faced chronic pain as the stump discharged pus at the rate of four to five ounces a day. Surgeons decided to split the stump open and remove diseased bone fragments. They removed several inches of diseased bone and repaired the stump. Vick consumed a daily ration of whiskey and hospital workers applied a cold compress to the stump in order to prevent a continual secretion of pus. Doctors prescribed a whole host of recovery techniques, including sesquichloride of iron, opium, cod liver oil, and eggs as his main staple of food. The stump completely healed, without any signs of damage, and Vick returned home on July 18, 1865, nine months after his amputation.[39]

While soldiers feared the loss of a leg that created mobility issues, others found their dexterity compromised with the loss of an arm. After a shell shattered his left arm at Frayser's Farm, Virginia, on June 30, 1862, Jesse B. Shivers, a member of the Eighth Alabama, collapsed on the field. As he waited for the battle to subside, he endured an additional six gunshot wounds while lying on the ground. He slowly crawled to the rear, where he underwent two amputations. Another soldier waited on the field for medical attention for nearly twenty-four hours. A surgeon performed an amputation on the right arm of the patient, and he fully recovered.[40]

Although surgeons traditionally removed damaged arms that could not heal on their own, other medical procedures emerged to tackle complicated injuries. Resections, the removal of large amounts of bone in or around a joint, presented some unique challenges for the surviving patients. On May 18, 1862, an unidentified surgeon explained the case of a

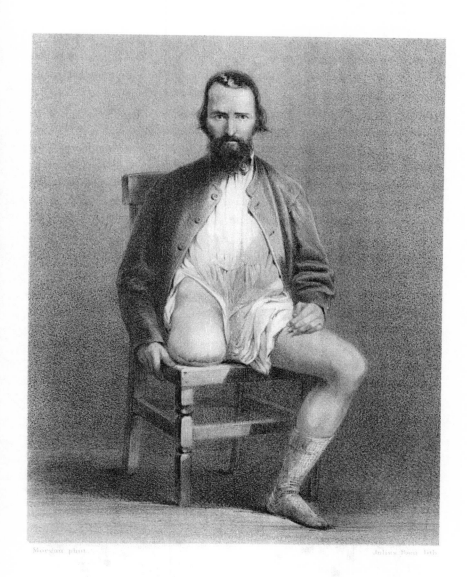

Figure 7. Private R. A. Vick. Courtesy of the Reynolds Historical Library, University of Alabama at Birmingham.

Confederate soldier who fought at the Battle of Williamsburg, Virginia, where a shell "busted and blew to pieces the bone" of his left arm. The surgeon found it remarkable that he could "bend his elbow up and place it upon his shoulder." The surgeon spent the next several days removing bone fragments from the arm and "cutting away the terrible sloughs from mortification." A. P. Carver, who had three inches of bone removed from his left arm after the Battle at Drewry's Bluff, described his arm hanging uselessly by his side, connected now only by muscle and skin. "It hangs perfectly limber and can be twitched round like a piece of rope," he said.[41]

In some cases, soldiers who lost an arm faced additional medical complications, though often of their own doing. Thomas Cavanaugh, a private in the Fifteenth Louisiana, arrived at a hospital about five weeks after breaking his arm at the Battle of Second Manassas in August 1862. His original surgeon avoided amputation, but the limb had failed to heal, as Cavanaugh reinjured the arm after a drunken fall from his bed. Surgeons discovered a series of lesions and an extensive amount of pus around the injury. Persistent alcoholism had rapidly deteriorated his health and the surgeon noted his "great intolerance to pain." Cavanaugh survived the amputation, after a hearty diet and consumption of eggnog to ease his pain, and he recovered fully a few weeks after the operation.[42]

Although arms and legs tend to dominate our impressions of Civil War amputation, the most numerous cases involved fingers, hands, and feet. A private in the Twentieth Georgia suffered greatly from the gunshot wound that resulted in the loss of his index finger and prompted "considerable loss of motion in [the] remaining fingers," according to his surgeon. William A. Russell lost a finger at Cold Harbor and was forced to spend the remainder of the war guarding horses, rather than participating in combat. Foot amputations were usually a result of enemy fire, but exposure and/or inadequate or poorly fitting shoes created horrific conditions that sometimes required surgery. After a cavalry battle in January 1864, Major General Fitz Lee reported that one soldier remained behind "with feet frozen to such an extent that the surgeon thinks they will have to be amputated." Some men accidentally damaged their own feet. Private L. J. Goodwin shot himself in the foot, which resulted in its subsequent amputation three hours after the injury occurred. Goodwin reacted negatively to the operation and exhibited chills and a speedy pulse. Medical records fail to indicate if he survived, although his surgeon, B. W. Allen, reported that he was "barely alive" two weeks later.[43]

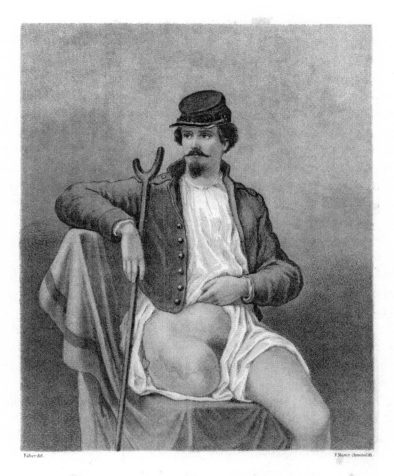

BLACKMAN'S SUCCESSFUL   AMPUTATION AT THE HIP-JOINT.
SECONDARY AMPUTATION.

Figure 8. Private Woodford Longmore ended up shot in the right thigh during a skirmish at Cynthiana, Kentucky, on June 11, 1864. Doctors removed some bone fragments, and Longmore spent months in a hospital bed with his right leg stabilized in hopes that it would heal. In March 1865, he was moved to a hospital in Florence, Kentucky, where Dr. George C. Blackman examined the leg and found a steady discharge of pus oozing from the original wound. A month later, the surgeon removed more bone fragments, and Longmore remained confined to a hospital bed. As the patient's condition steadily worsened and another removal of bone fragments failed, Blackman decided to remove the injured leg on January 18, 1866, eighteen months after Longmore sustained the initial injury. Longmore completely recovered and eventually returned home and married. Courtesy of the Reynolds Historical Library, University of Alabama at Birmingham.

The loss of digits, while seemingly minor in comparison to the loss of an arm or leg, could equally result in serious complications and even death. One Confederate patient underwent the amputation of a toe on his left foot. The newly forged stump discharged pus for several days. Another Confederate who ended up shot in the wrist at Gettysburg spent weeks in the hospital, dealing with a great amount of pain and a regular discharge of pus and water. A surgeon eventually removed the hand at the infected wrist joint. J. W. Hyatt lost three fingers at Gettysburg. His physician recorded that "large quantities of pus had formed in the hand but it was freely discharged" when the physician applied pressure to the "stump of the finger." Hyatt underwent continual water dressings and doses of morphine until he recovered.[44]

Nor was amputation limited to appendages: some surgeons amputated internal organs. One rebel surgeon recalled seeing a patient who had been shot on the left side below the ribs. As the projectile had passed entirely through the body, the gaping wound exhibited a small chunk of flesh protruding from the wound. The physician discovered the chunk of flesh to be the spleen and he tied a piece of silk string around the exposed spleen, sliced it off, and pushed the "stump" of the organ back into the patient. The surgeon named himself the very first to "amputate the spleen or a part of the spleen from [a] gunshot wound."[45]

The time spent in a hospital bed afforded a Confederate soldier, regardless of how he got there, an opportunity to engage in a great deal of reflection. Soldiers and officers who survived the ordeal of amputation now had to struggle to make sense of what it meant to live as a physically altered man. Some refused to allow amputation to alter their internal definitions of manhood and followed a particular rule for discharged soldiers: "What you have lost in body, try and make up in energy, decision and mental vigor." Antebellum southern society had demanded that an honorable man master his emotions. Outbursts of sorrow, anger, or even joy should remain buried in the heart. Yet, the hospital bed was what Whitman described as the "fearfulest test" of the inner man, and the reminiscences and writings of Confederate amputees convey the deep, emotional experience of losing a limb. Men often alternated in single weeks from bouts of joy and sorrow to fear and anger and from cowardice to resoluteness to profound patriotism. Their varied reactions depended both on the circumstances surrounding the amputation as well as how their personality usually dealt with drastic change and trauma.[46]

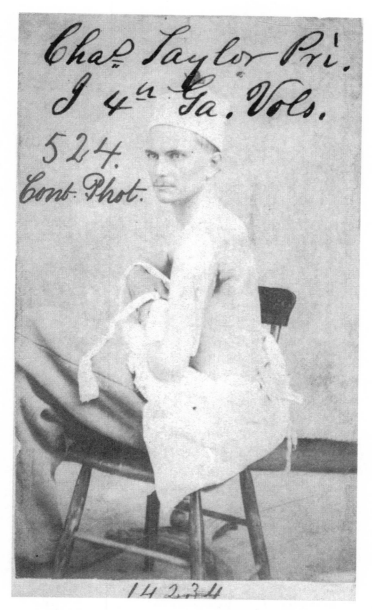

Figure 9. Private Charles A. Taylor from the Fourth Georgia endured a secondary excision of a portion of his left humerus bone on May 10, 1864. Courtesy of Contributed Photographs Collection, Otis Historical Archives, National Museum of Health and Medicine.

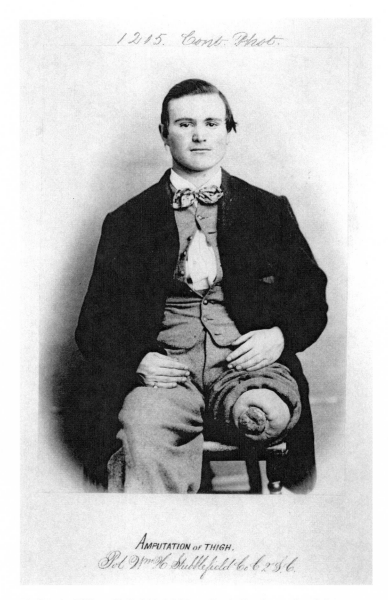

Figure 10. Private William H. Stubblefield from South Carolina endured the amputation of his thigh after he was shot at Cold Harbor, Virginia, on June 1, 1864. He developed gangrene on the stump, which is why the femur bone of his left leg is exposed in this photograph. Courtesy of Contributed Photographs Collection, Otis Historical Archives, National Museum of Health and Medicine.

Some southern amputees tried to laugh off their misfortune and looked for joy and humor in the midst of their hardship. A private from Louisiana lost his leg in 1863. During the operation, a surgeon recalled that the patient acted "cheerful and even jocular." Others saw the loss of a limb as an opportunity to share a joke directly connected to their adversity. At the Battle of Shiloh in 1862, a Confederate soldier had his middle three fingers shot off. In his spare time, both off the battlefield and before the war, the soldier enjoyed playing cards. Now, as he raised up his mangled hand, he stared at it "with a look of ineffable sorrow." He exclaimed, as a tear rolled down his cheek, "I shall never be able to hold a full hand again!"[47]

Some of the humor exhibited by Confederate amputees included a direct reference to Union soldiers. William Jackson, who lost an arm at Seven Pines, stated, "Thank God I have another arm with which to shoot the Yankees." At Corinth, Mississippi, in 1862, a young Confederate soldier, only fifteen or sixteen years old, had been shot in the leg, which prompted an amputation from a Confederate surgeon. Once the chloroform wore off, someone asked the young amputee how he felt. He responded, "First rate! That old leg has bothered me ever since I was born." The patient explained how he had broken the leg twice and spent six months in bed with a sprained knee from the same leg. He jested, "It's been a damned unlucky leg, anyhow; but now I'll have a wooden one, and the Yankees may shoot at that all day." Another Confederate soldier from Alabama lost his foot in the fall of 1864. The missing appendage did not deter him from completing military service, as he spent the remainder of the war on guard duty. He joked that he "did more guard duty than any man in the war."[48]

In contrast, many amputees exhibited signs of depression. S. D. Cannon, a private in the Second Alabama Cavalry, arrived at a hospital with a gunshot wound that required the removal of his leg. His physician described him as "depressed," with a rampant fever and a condition that continually worsened until his death a month later. At the Battle of Chickamauga on September 19, 1863, First Lieutenant John E. Wilson, a member of the Sixth Florida, charged up a hill and took a cannonball in the leg, but it seemed barely to slow him down. As one witness remembered, "With the blood flowing from the wound, he shouted to us to come on, and he led that charge to victory, crawling on his hands and one knee." With victory in hand, Wilson told his men, "We have gained the needed

time. I am willing to die." Physicians removed his leg, and he recovered
in an Atlanta hospital. His brother arrived a month later to transport him
home. Unfortunately, Wilson died on the train ride from Atlanta to Columbus, Georgia, on October 16, 1863.[49]

As recovery periods lengthened, some men succumbed to dependency
or began to despair that they might never recover at all. One chaplain
assisted a Confederate soldier who lost one arm "three inches below the
socket" and another arm had three inches of bone removed from the upper limb that created an "offensive" scene. The chaplain remarked, "He
became very nervous and was completely unmanned, and became as fret-
ful as a little child." The strong emotional reaction of the patient to his
amputation diminished his masculine status in the eyes of the chaplain.
Things did not improve during recovery. The chaplain fed the patient,
who seemed to relish his infantile status. "Of course we had to feed him;
the bits of meat or bread were too small or too large, the soup was too
hot or too cold; the spoon was put too far in his mouth or not far enough;
now he wanted his nose scratched, or his head, or his eye itched, or his
toe." The patient survived his anxious ordeal and eventually made a full
recovery.[50]

A lengthy recovery period usually bred disillusionment and created
jaded hospital patients. Following the Battle of Gettysburg, a twenty-one-
year-old Confederate Lieutenant from Louisiana spent days in a hospital bed recovering from the amputation of both of his legs and the loss of
his eyesight. The Confederate asked a nurse to write a letter home to his
parents and his new wife. The nurse reluctantly agreed, as she routinely
agonized over writing the farewell letters for the soldiers who may never
again return home. The patient freely admitted that his strength evaporated daily and that he was in the midst of his final hours. He asked, "How
does my dying make us free?" He lashed out at the world, declaring, "If
you should ask how I died, and are told 'at peace' it would be a monstrous
lie." Unmitigated pain bred disillusionment, as the soldier angrily questioned why he enlisted in the first place and struggled to deal with "such
maddening pain." He no longer saw any value in his military service and
certainly did not think of his empty sleeves as markers of honor. Rather,
he saw the unmitigated level of death and suffering brought on by the
war as worthless, and he concluded his letter by bluntly asking, "Christ,
what's all the killing for?" Before mailing the letter, the nurse added a

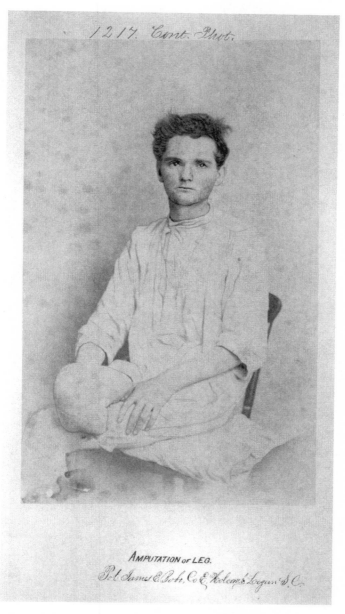

1217. Cont. Phot.

AMPUTATION of LEG.

Pvt James E. Bobo, Co E, Holcombs Legion S C.

Figure 11. Private James E. Bobo lost his leg after he sustained a gunshot wound at Hatcher's Run, Virginia, on March 29, 1865. Although he suffered from a severe infection of his stump, he recovered within a month. Courtesy of Contributed Photographs Collection, Otis Historical Archives, National Museum of Health and Medicine.

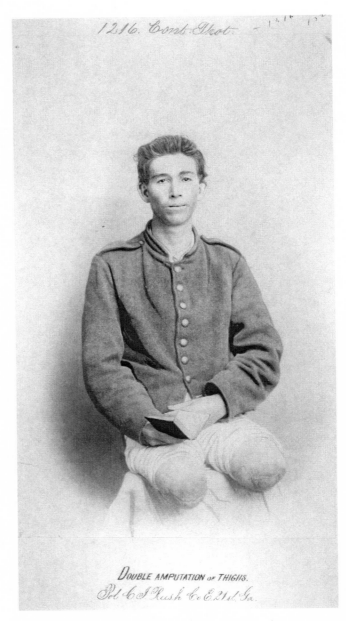

Figure 12. Columbus J. Rush, a member of the Twenty-First Georgia, sustained wounds at the Battle of Fort Stedman on March 25, 1865. He survived a double amputation the same day he was shot in battle. Courtesy of Contributed Photographs Collection, Otis Historical Archives, National Museum of Health and Medicine.

brief rejoinder to inform the family that their son died "protesting violently, not peacefully," as he uttered his final words, "Papa, Missy, weep, weep for me."[51]

Some Confederates viewed amputation as the ultimate symbol of cowardice and submission, as it sapped them of the ability to prove their worth. Such men went so far as to risk death or severe punishment by deserting from the army in order to avoid amputation. Carroll Henderson Clark, a soldier from the Sixteenth Tennessee, endured a gunshot wound at Atlanta that oozed with pus and produced swelling in his fingers and hand. Initially, surgeons applied a simple dressing in order to save the hand, which failed. After moving to another hospital in Macon, Georgia, the wound failed to heal. When his surgeon there recommended amputation, Clark refused and deserted from the army merely to save his hand. He ended up in Dawson, Georgia, where he survived without losing his limb. Clark participated in the dishonorable and unmanly act of desertion in order to save his hand. He viewed fleeing home as a physically complete man more desirable than remaining at war as a disabled individual.[52]

Still, most soldiers who suffered from combat injuries were buoyed by paeans to their sacrifice. Major H. H. Boone, at an engagement at Fordoche, Louisiana, faced an unexpected volley of bullets that tore his right arm to pieces and obliterated four fingers on his left hand. After the officer underwent amputation, a soldier remarked, "A more gallant officer or noble-hearted man never wore gray." Another Confederate officer who lost his leg at the hip joint following the Battle of Cynthiana, Kentucky, in 1864 received universal praise for his sacrifice. His fellow soldiers described him as having the highest qualities of "manliness, gentleness, integrity, modesty and courage, with a personal magnetism that drew all men toward him."[53]

Not all of the remarks about bravery were reserved for Confederate officers, as privates also received accolades for their bravery as the empty sleeve gradually became one of the more accepted markers of patriotism. In an address to the Southern Historical Society after the Civil War that highlighted the sacrifices of amputated men and elevated the empty sleeve to an honorable position, Major H. B. McClellan of Kentucky recalled seeing a young soldier at Chancellorsville "whose right arm was dangling from the elbow by some shreds of flesh." The soldier, in an attempt to convey humor, said, "Mister! Can't you cut this thing off? It keeps knocking against the trees, and it's mightily in my way." Although the officer had no medical experience, he tied a tourniquet above the arm of the wounded private and used a pocket knife to remove the shattered limb. McClellan recalled, "Brave boy! I directed him to the rear, where he no doubt soon met with skillful attention from our surgeons. I saw him no more, but I trust that his sturdy spirit sustained him and ensured his recovery. Such boys grow into men who are an honor to any country." Private James Adams, originally born in Ireland, fought with the First Louisiana. At Malvern Hill in 1862, he lost both of his legs. Once he returned home, he declared, "No epaulets graced my shoulders, on my collar I wore no stars, only a private in the ranks I fought for the 'Stars and Bars.'" A soldier from Mississippi lost his leg and remarked, "I was content to be classed as a private in the noble cause for which we fought, knowing and believing till yet that we were right, and expect to die in the same belief." In 1908, a former Confederate private from Mississippi reflected on the meaning of his empty sleeve after suffering for years with chronic pain. He proudly stated, "Though I am now nearly sixty-seven years old, and have suffered these forty-four years with wounds and am now maimed for life, I have never regretted having been a Confederate soldier, because I still believe, as I did then, that we were right." The rhetoric of remembrance in the midst of the Lost Cause yielded a more nostalgic and heroic view of an amputated veteran.[54]

In their postwar recollections Confederate soldiers evoked signs of their personal notions of bravery and courage in the hospital bed and on the battlefield. In the aftermath of the bloodiest day in American history, a young Confederate captain surveyed the battlefield at Antietam, Maryland, seeking out the dead and wounded. The captain discovered a young Confederate soldier named Watkins, with his head nestled in the hands of an attending surgeon. The captain inquired, "Was he badly hurt?" And before the surgeon could respond, Watkins chimed in, "Not much, Captain, but I've got the flag!" Watkins explained that as he fell from his horse wounded, he tore the flag from its staff in order to prevent the Union soldiers from capturing it. Despite profuse bleeding from a shell embedded in his leg and a wound deemed mortal from the surgeon, Watkins remained in high spirits and "has been so intent upon the safe delivery of that apron into your hands as to seem utterly unconscious of his wound," according to the surgeon. Watkins ignored his own injury and pending

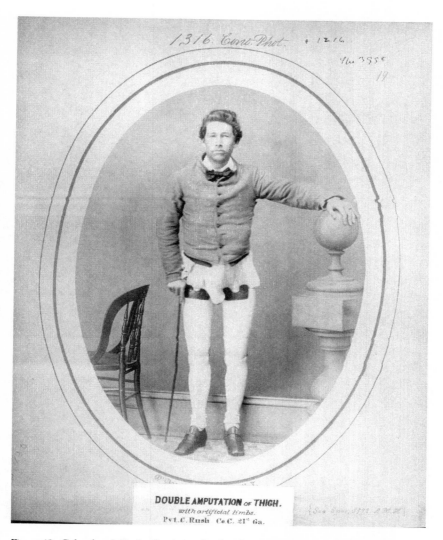

Figure 13. Columbus J. Rush, after being fitted with two prosthetic leg devices, following his double thigh amputation that took place after he was injured at the Battle of Fort Stedman on March 25, 1865. Courtesy of Contributed Photographs Collection, Otis Historical Archives, National Museum of Health and Medicine.

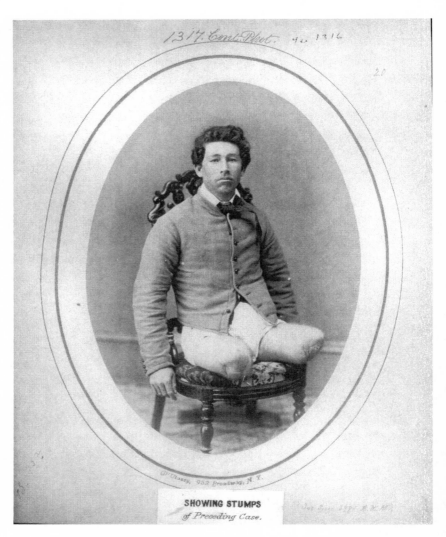

Figure 14. Another photograph of Columbus J. Rush showing off his double amputation that took place on March 25, 1865. Courtesy of Contributed Photographs Collection, Otis Historical Archives, National Museum of Health and Medicine.

amputation in favor of making sure the captain received the small flag. As the captain departed, Watkins's condition rapidly deteriorated and his comrades quickly delivered him to a hospital in Hagerstown, where he underwent an amputation of his leg. Three days later, the young soldier perished in a hospital bed and ended up in an unmarked grave.[55]

If a patient experienced a routine operation without ensuing complications, they expected to survive, but this was not always the case. Private J. H. Wolf, shot through the leg at the First Battle of Manassas, received immediate medical attention on the field by an assistant surgeon. However, the surgeon hurried to catch up to the rest of the Fourth Virginia after he wrapped Wolf's leg. Wolf slowly traveled by train to Richmond, where he experienced a great deal of pain from the movement of the swaying boxcars. After receiving a new dressing, the medical staff informed Wolf that due to a potential surge in patients after the Battle of Manassas, he would have to be moved again. Wolf ended up back on the train, this time headed for Charlottesville, Virginia, fetching up in a former classroom building at the University of Virginia, where another physician examined the wound and determined the leg would need to be removed so close to the hip that it might prove fatal. "I am not afraid to die," Wolf told the doctor, "but amputate for my mother's sake, for she would like to see her boy again." Wolf had his leg amputated a month after his initial injury and died the following day.[56]

In short, amputation was no guarantee of survival. Many seriously wounded soldiers underwent routine procedures and seemed to be recovering but died anyway. Joseph Step underwent amputation of his left arm after receiving a gunshot wound during the Atlanta campaign in 1864. A few weeks later the blood loss caught up to him and he perished. Amputation-related deaths were often blamed on medical ineptitude or malpractice. Take the case of Corporal M. S. Hawkins, who had his right thigh bone shattered by a musket ball. Surgeons decided not to immediately amputate and left the limb intact. Five days later, after Hawkins traveled to Lake City, Florida, a surgeon removed the right leg and Hawkins died. Charles Hentz, a fellow soldier, declared, "It was an outrageous case of malpractice." He believed that had the limb been removed immediately after the battle, Hawkins would have "probably recovered."[57]

While many soldiers survived the arduous procedure, postoperative infections claimed the lives of many recuperating patients. One Alabama private suffered from an outbreak of gangrene after his left leg underwent amputation above the knee. He experienced a painful and extensive round of opium, alcohol, iodine, nitric acid, and morphine doses before he recovered. Colonel Charles Blacknall, from North Carolina, lost a foot at Winchester in September 1864. Gangrene continued to fester around the stump, and Blacknall, described as a man with "ardent patriotism, high conviction of right and principle and an engaging manhood," perished the following spring. H. C. Moore faced a heavy bout of gangrene around a gunshot wound. Although an amputation took place on Moore's shoulder joint, the aggressive case of gangrene consumed his stump, and he died the day of his amputation. J. E. McMillan, who lost a leg at the Battle of the Wilderness in 1864, suffered from a horrific bout of gangrene that killed him a month later. Another soldier perished from blood poisoning after he underwent the amputation of his leg following the battle at Gaines Mill in 1862. Death served as the final notice for several patients who endured and initially survived the horrific process of amputation.[58]

In addition to dealing with the severe consequences of death, some soldiers feared that they would dishonor their family name if they ended up severely wounded or even captured by their Union compatriots. While time spent in a prison camp or federal hospital certainly denied Confederate men an opportunity to prove their masculine worth in battle, it also damaged their own self-worth, as they now had to face medical care at the hands of Union surgeons. A group of Union soldiers discovered a private from Mississippi lying on a battlefield in Kentucky with a shattered thigh. Rather than risk amputation or capture, both symbols of cowardice, the Confederate soldier asked for one request: that his potential captors kill him. The Union men refused and took the injured private to a field hospital.[59]

Some wounded Confederate men selected violence as a course of action to preserve their limbs while receiving treatment from the enemy. A captured Confederate soldier found himself wounded in the leg, and in a Union hospital. A Union surgeon determined the soldier's leg could not be saved. The patient, T. J. McGahee, responded, "I do not want my leg cut off, I would rather die." Unfazed, the surgeon sternly replied, "I don't care what you want, I am going to cut it off," and prepared for surgery. McGahee refused the offer of chloroform, and as the operation commenced, he used his left arm to punch the surgeon in the face. The strike

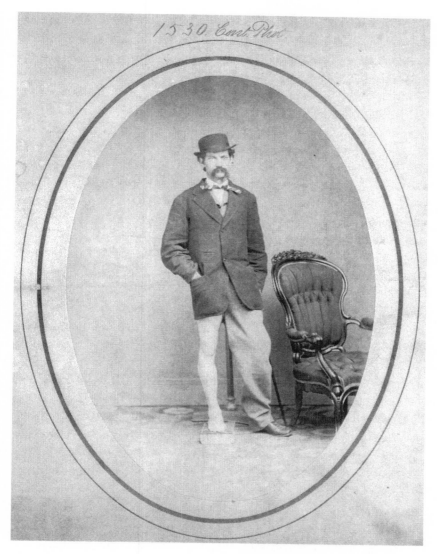

Figure 15. Captain Charles Knowlton underwent an excision of his right knee joint after he sustained injuries at the Battle of Mine Run on November 27, 1863. Although the operation spared his leg, it was now a few inches shorter than his left one. Courtesy of Contributed Photographs Collection, Otis Historical Archives, National Museum of Health and Medicine.

sent the surgeon flying backward, as his nose gushed blood. After the surgeon regained his bearings, McGahee rushed at him with one of the surgical knives and sliced him. The surgeon aborted the operation and the patient left the hospital, leg intact.[60]

Amputated Confederate prisoners filled the wards of several federal hospitals throughout the course of the war. John Cuyler, the medical director for the Department of Virginia out of Fortress Monroe, wrote Secretary of War Stanton and stated, "We have in our hospitals several rebel prisoners with amputated limbs. If not incompatible with the views of the Government, would it not be as well to let these men go home?" Men like T. A. Kelly, a member of an Alabama regiment wounded during the Atlanta campaign on July 22, 1864, spent significant time in federal hospitals. Federal surgeons removed his leg, and he spent the rest of the war in Union hospitals in Chattanooga and Nashville, until August 21, 1865. J. P. O'Rear, a member of the First Texas, engaged Union soldiers about ten miles from Richmond in October 1864. A bullet struck his leg, and he ended up captured. Union surgeons removed his leg and sent him to a U.S. hospital at Fortress Monroe. He remained thankful for receiving excellent care from "good, kind nurses." Although the nurses ensured his successful recovery, O'Rear felt plagued by the constant groans and crying of the wounded men who surrounded him in the hospital. It stayed with him, day or night.[61]

Sometimes care provided by federal physicians on captured Confederate patients had disastrous results. William Moxley, captured in Georgia, underwent the amputation of his leg by a federal surgeon, who quickly performed the operation and fled the region, leaving the patient alone to eventually die. While incarcerated at Camp Chase, Henry Hupman, a member of the Twentieth Virginia Cavalry, refused to extinguish his light after a guard at the prison gave the order. The guard opened fire, hitting the arm of Hupman, who underwent an immediate amputation that killed him. Another Confederate survived the war largely unscathed until February 1865, when a bullet entered his leg. Confederate medical personnel moved the patient to a hospital in Richmond, which ended up besieged by Union forces when the city fell on April 3. Federal surgeons removed his leg on June 5, resulting in death.[62]

Confederate patients tended not to trust the medical advice provided to them by Union surgeons, especially with the horrific ramifications of what imprisonment could mean. When a shell tore through his left arm, S. P. H. Ewell, a member of the Twenty-Third South Carolina, found himself undergoing an amputation at the hands of a federal surgeon. Rather than accept the loss of a limb at the hands of a Union official, Ewell tried to escape into the swamps. However, he did not get far, arriving at a house that served as the headquarters of the federal surgeon. The surgeon provided the Confederate soldier with appropriate medical care and did not banish him to a prison camp.[63]

The very threat of imprisonment at the hands of Union soldiers forced some Confederate men to take drastic actions. Albert Mellen, from Natchez, Mississippi, found himself captured and held by Union forces at Vicksburg, Mississippi, in 1864. The federal officials ordered Mellen to work on roads and fortifications around the city, under the watchful eye of black Union troops. He refused, and when the black troops arrived, pointing their bayonets at Mellen to prompt his obedience, he "suddenly seized a hatchet that happened to be in reach, and, throwing himself upon his knees, quickly extended his left arm along the floor, and with two bold strokes of the hatchet completely severed the hand from the arm." Mellen, a bloody mess, held the mangled stump up to his face and asked the white federal officer commanding the black soldiers, "Now sir, will you make me work for your rotten government under a Negro guard?" He admitted that he did not regret his decision. He did not define his manhood through the complete male physique. Instead, he saw working for the United States under the watchful eyes of black soldiers more degrading to his manhood than a missing arm.[64]

Confederate men who doubled as both amputees and prisoners had few options to avoid care by federal officials. A Confederate soldier at Gettysburg spent three days lying on the field, hoping that someone would arrive to care for his damaged body. He ended up in a federal hospital where he lost a leg and thumb and spent several months in a prison camp. Will Coffee, a soldier from Florida, sat in a Union prison in Ohio with his right leg still unmended and shorter than his left leg. A fellow soldier, who called him a "cripple for life," remarked, "Will is yet compelled to use crutches, though he thinks he can walk without them for a while." Another Confederate amputee who lost a leg found himself a prisoner in Baltimore. The Confederate pretended to be a prison official and convinced a German guard, who could not speak any English, that he should be immediately released. The guard fell for the charade and released the prisoner.[65]

For the Confederate soldiers who underwent amputation and had the ability to survive away from the hands of Union captors, the recovery period served as a critical time for them to begin contemplating the next step in their own lives. Damaged Confederate men could continue their military service as honorable members of the Invalid Corps. Army officers used the Confederate Invalid Corps, created in February 1864, to replace able-bodied men who filled provost and desk positions, which also included naval personnel, musicians, noncommissioned officers, and privates of the Marine Corps. Confederate president Jefferson Davis had recommended the creation of the group in his annual message to Congress because he thought the men "could be made useful in various employments for which efficient officers and troops are now detached." Members of the group, who received clothing and food rations, had to undergo a physical examination every six months in order to determine whether they should remain in the Invalid Corps or be sent back to the front lines. If they failed to show up, they ended up dropped from the discharge/retirement list and could be conscripted. However, if soldiers' disability prevented them from traveling to see the medical board, they could get certification from a local or army surgeon to prevent possible conscription. The Confederate Invalid Corps did not resemble their Union counterparts, as they lacked any clear organization and were void of companies or regiments. The Army of Tennessee and Leonidas Polk's Department of Alabama, Mississippi, and east Louisiana used physically damaged men to fill various positions behind the lines. William Mooney, a member of the First North Carolina, lost his arm at Malvern Hill in the summer of 1862. He ended up in the Invalid Corps after its creation in 1864.[66]

Other amputees filled other vitally important positions. Brigadier General John Decatur Barry, who lost two fingers at Deep Bottom, Virginia, on July 27, 1864, worked desk duty for the remainder of the war due to the inability of his right hand to heal properly. Zebulon York, who lost his left arm at Winchester on September 19, 1864, served out the rest of the war in a recruiting office. At the same time, amputation meant avoiding military service altogether. J. D. Bohannon lost an arm at Gettysburg and left the war. In Alexandria, Louisiana, on February 14, 1863, military officials declared, "A person incapable of bearing arms, as one having lost an arm or a leg, or being paralyzed or bedridden, is exempt by law," in terms of enlisting for military service. In most instances throughout the war, amputation allowed a Confederate soldier to live a long and healthy life beyond the battlefield and well into the twentieth century.[67]

Many surviving amputees, as they prepared to adjust to a world away from the battlefield, never forgot the final resting place of their dismembered body part. John C. Portis, a member of the Eighteenth Mississippi, lost his right arm during the Atlanta Campaign on May 14, 1864. In 1896, he remembered, "My good right arm lies about a mile south of Resaca, Georgia, just north of a church at the root of a large oak or chestnut tree. It was put in a board box and buried by a comrade." Brigadier General Albert Gallatin Jenkins underwent the amputation of his arm in 1864. A young black boy buried the arm in a family orchard, which allowed Jenkins to know the precise location of his missing appendage. Some believed that the entire body needed to be buried together in order for the spirit to be physically whole on judgment day. Others believed they would experience pain in the location of their missing limb if the dismembered appendage did not receive a proper burial.[68]

Some men had to make a decision as to whether or not they wanted to keep their dismembered appendage. After John Bell Hood lost his leg at Chickamauga in 1863, he traveled to his recovery location with his leg. The way he figured it, if he perished from the amputation, which had an 80 percent mortality rate, his body could be buried physically complete. Hood survived and his leg ended up at the family cemetery near the home in north Georgia. Confederate medical officer Joseph Jones remarked, after a visit to the Medical Museum, "The Yankees have preserved an immense number of fractured bones and even entire limbs. Generals have sent their amputated legs with their compliments." Confederate officer Matthew Galbraith Butler saved his embalmed foot in the family attic. As a Catholic, he believed he needed to go to the grave as a physically whole man in order to pass into the afterlife as a complete entity. On many occasions, the neighborhood children, who routinely frolicked in the attic, used the foot as part of their childhood games.[69]

As an army of amputees made their various recoveries and turned toward home, they felt deeply conflicting emotions. No one could deny that they had done their duty as men. But the war had literally taken its pound of flesh. They had been blown up, shot to pieces. They were not the same men who left their farms and families. They had been dependent on their surgeons to perform skillful amputations and forge clean stumps where prosthetic limbs could be attached. They had been dependent on female nurses to provide medical and emotional support as their bodies recovered from the physical and emotional shock of a major operation. Back home, they would now be dependent again and in new ways on the women in their lives, on their communities, and on state governments to provide the love, support, and economic means to help them navigate what it would mean to live a disabled life. The war was supposed to complete them as men; instead it had left them partial, and they could hope only that their empty sleeves would serve as red badges of courage and visible reminders of all they had sacrificed for honor.

THREE

The Women

Reconstructing Confederate Manhood

You must bind up the wounds of a Nation
Nor falter, nor shrink from your part
Up and down through the wards where the fever
Stalks noisome and gaunt and impure
You must go with your steadfast endeavor
To comfort, to counsel, to cure
I grant that the task's superhuman
But strength will be given to you
To do for the dear ones what woman
Alone, in her pity can do.
–John B. Lightfoot, Jr., 1910

With her husband Will away fighting the American Civil War, Emma Shannon Crutcher had a dream. She dreamed of receiving word from an army surgeon that her husband had been shot in the leg, but his life spared. Crutcher reacted to the news with "maximized joy," remarking, "Now, thought I, he will never leave me again, for he will be of no use, in the army, and–if I die, he will never marry again, for no one but me would love a lame man–he is mine now." While she worried about the welfare of her husband, Crutcher realized that her newly amputated husband would be dependent on her for the rest of his life, and this was a reversal of gender roles she rather relished. Confessing the dream to her husband, she defended her reaction by writing, "But you came home and the meeting was all my imagination pictured, and I awoke, sighing that it was not reality, lameness and all. If I only regarded my own feeling without thinking of duty, I had rather take you now, lamed for life, than wait for months and maybe years longer, with the chance of [not] having you back with me." Crutcher's dream captures the mental transition that many white southern women were making during the war to accept a physically disabled man as somehow more whole, and more worthy. Women would

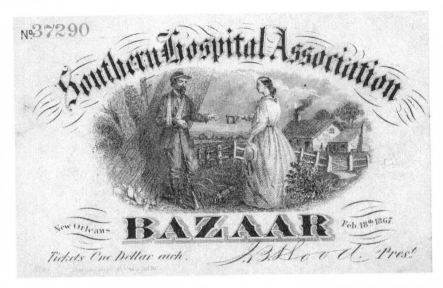

Figure 16. An invitation to the Southern Hospital Association Bazaar held in New Orleans on February 18, 1867. The Southern Hospital Association raised funds to care for wounded Confederate veterans. Courtesy of Louisiana Historical Association Collection, Louisiana Research Collection, Tulane University.

serve on the front lines of the process by which the amputated reconstructed their image of themselves and their postwar lives.[1]

As George Fitzhugh, a prominent proslavery writer noted before the war, if a woman wanted to gain the love of a man, she needed to be "weak, helpless and dependent." Historians have echoed Fitzhugh's notion, arguing that young women understood both their dependent position in a marriage and their need to submit to the will of their husband. Historian Victoria Ott has pointed out how white women's dependency on their husband, before the Civil War, "helped to buttress the patriarchal or paternalistic power of white men both in and outside the home." At the same time, southern men needed to secure a desirable wife in order to cement their status as male providers and protectors. Thus, southern elite white women remained by definition and in practice dependent on their husbands. Yet, the Civil War altered traditional notions of dependency, and in many cases turned this old arrangement on its head; returned home, amputated men reverted to the role as helpless and dependent on a willing woman to care for their altered bodies and maintain both their health and welfare.[2]

This chapter focuses on the female response to the damaged white male body and the vital role women played in dealing with war-related disabilities. Although most women accepted the challenge to care for and rejuvenate amputated men, others remained ambivalent about their men who returned home missing a limb. Some women recoiled in disgust and rejected their husbands and fiancés and shunned handicapped men as potential spouses. Other women feared that being with a disabled man damaged the potential livelihood of their family, as men missing limbs made poor choices as providers. Still others, consumed with sympathy, brushed their personal concerns aside due to their patriotic duty by staying with and caring for a veteran amputee. As historian Libra Hilde noted, "Women saw a direct connection between healing soldiers, healing the nation, and healing memory." And women were integral to the rehabilitative process: propping up amputated men in both the domestic and public realms of society as nurses, benevolent workers, wives, and potential spouses. Southern women emerged as the crucial first step in reconstructing the damaged manhood of amputated veterans as they returned home to face the newfound challenges of dependency and disability.[3]

Confederate women had, from the outset of the war, well understood their role in the war effort. Caring for wounded soldiers, whether as nurses or doting family members, was broadly accepted as a woman's province. Some southerners did wonder, especially as body counts began to rise, if white women would be able to handle the rigors of nursing, not to mention the presence of pus, excrement, and bloody and naked bodies. Others believed the exact opposite, feeling that southern women were suited by temperament to serve as caregivers. As one Confederate mother noted in 1861, "The young ladies are exceedingly anxious to imitate Florence Nightingale, and distinguish themselves in the Army." Soon enough, however, the realities of the hospital emerged, and it was widely understood that there was little romance in the wards. J. L. Underwood, in an essay that chronicled the sacrifices of southern women, reminisced about women who tirelessly worked to care for southern soldiers as "very much battered and worn by long service." They were, said Underwood, like a tired old hoopskirt that "had been wounded and broken and mended and spliced until it was hardly its former self." In Underwood's opinion, such women had sacrificed just as much as the soldiers who had marched off to war.[4]

To be sure, not every southern woman was a would-be Nightingale.

Morbid curiosity sent many off to see battered and damaged men for themselves. Such a spectacle occurred in Charleston following the Battle of Fort Wagner in July 1863 when scores of wounded, both Confederate and Union, flooded the city. The newspapers reported on numerous amputations, estimating on July 20 "probably not less than 70 or 80 legs or arms were taken off." Trying to patch all these men up, a volunteer nurse remembered that "troublesome and obtrusive persons in female garb" crowded around out of "morbid curiosity for seeing wounded men and naked bodies."[5]

Soon enough, such women could not escape the sights of amputation. Cordelia Scales, residing in Holly Springs, Mississippi, noted five hospitals in the area with every home occupied by wounded or ill soldiers. She said, "You can't cross a street or turn a corner, but what see wounded or sick soldiers. Some . . . their leg shot off and walking on crutches and some with their arms shot off. . . . [I have] seen so much suffering lately that I feel like I could stand almost anything." Janie Smith, who lived in North Carolina, noted the horrific sights she saw, including that "under every shed and tree the tables were carried for amputating the limbs." Her heart broke as she watched men return from battle in a mangled state, the puddles of blood around the grove and the usage of her Aunt Mary's piano as an operating table. Smith wrote that the agonizing sounds and horrific screams of the "poor suffering soldiers" left a painful impression on her. She called her sacrifices her "trial" as she used her time and energy to roll bandages and send food to the mangled soldiers.[6]

The vivid recollections of Confederate nurses' experiences with observing amputations and treating amputated patients suggested a deep level of trauma experienced by women on a daily basis. Sally Louisa Tompkins recalled "the trail of blood that oozed drop by drop from the human veins" as a wagonload of men passed by, scurrying to the hastily arranged hospitals in the region. Later during her service, Tompkins evoked a sight that she would never forget: "Wooden legs tapping the corridors, so many amputations, stumps of arms and legs, some still oozing, spreading the deadly pyemia and effluvia." Cornelia McDonald, a southern woman who worked in a hospital, explained how a surgeon ordered her to wash the damaged face of a patient. McDonald wanted to reach deep down and find the courage to wash the wound. Instead, she staggered toward the door and experienced another horror as her dress "brushed up against a pile of amputated limbs heaped up near the door."[7]

Circumstances forced many women into the medical arena in order to ensure the safety, health, and survival of thousands of men. Many southern women, despite a call to assist with wounded and sick soldiers, found they were not up to the task and simply could not handle the grim reality of a hospital ward. A volunteer nurse found herself in an old warehouse in Mechanicsville, Virginia, in 1862. She remembered, "As I passed by the rows of occupied cots, I saw a nurse kneeling beside one of them, holding a pan for a surgeon. The red stump of an amputated arm was held over it. The next thing I knew I was myself lying on a cot, and a spray of cold water was falling over my face. I had fainted." The hospital matron declared her unfit for medical service and she returned home, distraught and embarrassed.[8]

Obviously many such women overcame their fears and became old hands at the difficult work of Civil War medicine. Betty Johnson, a nurse from Kentucky, relished the chance to assist a surgeon. After she assisted with a rather bloody amputation, Johnson lifted up the skirt of her dark calico dress to show off to her friends and fellow hospital workers where the blood of an artery had bespattered her garments. However enthusiastic, nurses still faced daunting challenges. The process of amputation and the piles of limbs emerged as one of the toughest challenges for women volunteers. Confederate nurses regularly reflected on the impact amputations had on them in their letters and diaries. Nurse Fannie Beers called amputation her "greatest dread." She hated how surgeons gravitated toward the saw so quickly without giving the patients "the benefit of the doubt." She remarked, "It was easier to amputate than to attend a tedious, troublesome recovery. So, off went legs and arms by the wholesale."[9]

Nurses were usually the first and most constant faces injured men saw after they experienced the removal of a limb. The newly forged dependent relationship between the disabled patient and his nurse prepared a Confederate man for the alteration in gender roles that would usually continue when they returned home. Hospitalized men, who relied on their nurses for food, beverage, and fresh bandages, began the process of coming to terms with their newfound level of dependency and what it meant to be handicapped. In turn, nursing prepared southern women for their postwar duties, which would include an immense amount of physical and emotional care giving to help rehabilitate men physically as well as psychologically. As the nurse made her hospital rounds, she viewed mangled and deformed physiques, bloody bandages, and gangrenous stumps, and could often claim to have seen more gore than the soldiers themselves. Daily contact with such horrors forced many southern women, as Drew Faust has argued, to abandon their support for continuing the conflict. They knew full well that the mammoth task that awaited them of caring and rehabilitating some thousands of men, and they were rather keen to keep that number as low as possible.[10]

The Confederate women who worked as nurses forged close bonds with patients who underwent the removal of limbs and demonstrated deep sympathy for their condition. Ada Bacot, a nurse working in Charlottesville, Virginia, recalled seeing a patient named Forester. "'Tis a sad sight to see his pale haggard face, so young too," she remembered. "If he lives he will have to go through life with one leg, he can never walk again without a crutch." He died only a few days later, "with but little or no pain," according to Bacot. She marveled at a young man who arrived with him, working as his personal nurse, who acted in a manner that was "most attentive to him, so kind and gentle with him." As she continued her nursing duties, Bacot casually stared out the window and saw two men passing each other on the street. One of the men had lost his right leg, while the other lost his left leg. Both men hobbled past one another with their crutches gliding down the street in a better manner "than could be expected," according to Bacot. She reflected, "It is sad to think of the hundreds of disabled men this war is producing, many will be of no possible use to themselves or anyone else." Bacot knew how difficult it would be for amputated men to survive without any help, much less play a meaningful role in society on their own.[11]

Nurses like Mary Jane Lucas, who had firsthand experiences with amputees, emerged from the hospital ward more sensitive to the personal sacrifices and unprecedented level of physical suffering produced by the war. "No one will know," she said, "what the people of Virginia have suffered and what they are still suffering but they bear it with remarkable fortitude." Lucas told the story of a soldier named Barrow who lost his leg and survived because of the women who watched over his bedside day and night. As Lucas witnessed other women care for amputees, she found her own family coping with the same situation as James Martin Ashley, a family member, lost his arm at the Battle of the Wilderness in May 1864. Josephine Crump, working in a Little Rock, Arkansas, hospital, wrote, "And that evening as I made my daily round from cot to cot in the hospital, finding a man here with a leg already in the grave, another mere boy with both arms gone trying to prop himself up to drink the nourishment his nurse had brought him, I felt the conditions of the soldiers was far more pathetic than mine." She found herself overwhelmed by so many patients. Gertrude Thomas, in Georgia, described seeing men lying on the floor on beds constructed out of straw "with their arms and legs cut off." The horrific conditions did not deter her from fulfilling her medical duties.[12]

Women cared for patients before and after the operations severing their limbs, and so well understood the amount of care they needed and the extent of their suffering. Phoebe Yates Pember, who worked as a nurse in Richmond, Virginia, during the war, recalled the case of a young "stalwart" soldier from Alabama who would require amputation. The attending physician gave her the task of feeding him in order to "give him strength to undergo amputation." Pember knew that the young man would have a difficult time eating anything, especially since "irritability of stomach as well as indifference to food" arrived hand and hand with gunshot wounds. She chopped up a pound of beef and mixed it with "a half pint of water" and stirred it until the "blood was extracted" and then she added salt for taste. Pember did this for ten days and the soldier gained his strength and underwent surgery. She wrote, "After the amputation, which he bore bravely, he looked as bright and well as before, and so on for five days – then the usual results followed. The system proved not strong enough to throw out the pus or inflammation." The soldier died shortly thereafter, and the nurse noted that her "heart beat twice as rapidly as ordinarily whenever there were any arrangements progressing for amputation, after any length of time had elapsed since the wound, or any effort made to save the limb."[13]

Nurses' direct contact with surgeons and the wounded gave them a platform, informed by their own experiences, to advocate for patients and even criticize surgeons for their decisions. Pember actively questioned the practices of amputation throughout the war to herself, rather than the attending surgeon, noting that "often when a hearty, fine-looking man in the prime of life would be brought in minus an arm or leg, I would feel as if it might have been saved." Unfortunately, the conditions the men faced on the battlefield did little to help. "Poor food and great exposure," she noted, "had thinned the blood and broken down the system so entirely that secondary amputations performed at the hospital almost invariably resulted in death, after the second year of war." Another soldier "had his leg cut off in pieces," as he underwent three separate amputations. Pember again questioned if the surgeon had taken the appropriate course of care since it had resulted in so much continual suffering.[14]

Experiences with amputees profoundly affected the life of Kate Cumming, a nurse who began work in a hospital after the Battle of Shiloh. Cumming recounted stories of two soldiers who had died following amputation. Each had lost a leg and longed for the day he could return home to his family; both died a few days after their operation. Cumming also remembered Isaac Fuquet, a soldier who had lost his arm and predicted his death because "all who have had limbs amputated in this hospital have died." He perished a few hours after the operation. Another soldier arrived, and the doctors diagnosed that an amputation of the arm had to commence at once. Cumming usually stayed as far away as possible from the operating table, but on this occasion she walked by and saw the horrific scene. "A stream of blood ran from the table into a tub in which was the arm," she remembered. "It had been taken off at the socket, and the hand, which but a short time before grasped the musket and battled for the right, was hanging over the edge of the tub, a lifeless thing." Cumming longed for an end to amputations, but they gradually became a routine part of her day. "Our sins must have been great," she prophetically wondered, "to have deserved such punishment."[15]

Cumming tended to a steady stream of young men who had faced the bone saw. She remembered entering an area about one hundred feet long in a hospital in which every single patient was missing a limb. One man had lost a leg at Chickamauga and was suffering from gangrene, but he had a "smile on his countenance." A thirteen-year-old boy named Sloan lost his leg and remained in a rather cheerful disposition, as his father arrived to stay by his bedside. While Sloan survived, several other amputees perished after their operations, including a Mr. Jones, who lost a leg and had been tended to by a woman named Miss Henderson. Before his death, Jones listed several names that Henderson had to contact should he die after his amputation. Only eighteen years old, he "died the death of a Christian," according to Cumming.[16]

As difficult as the experience was for Confederate women, the mere presence of women fortified the spirits of most wounded men. William Beavens, a member of the First North Carolina, recalled going to Winchester, Virginia, to recover from the removal of his leg at Snicker's Gap in 1864. In his diary, Beavens noted that the "ladies were very kind." He died less than two weeks later. James Beaty expressed his gratitude toward local women after the Battle of Fredericksburg in December 1862. "The ladies here have been exceedingly kind and attentive to the wounded. They go into their tents and nurse them and that well." In some cases, young children visited the wounded soldiers in the hospital. Lily Rosalie Pilkington, who resided in Manchester, Virginia, came to the local military hospital daily, where she sang and passed out flowers to the soldiers. Berry Benson, recovering in Manchester, recalled, "She was four or five years old, and could sing sweetly, having a fine voice. She was petted by all, and there was no eye that did not brighten at her coming." Although Berry survived the war, young Lily Pilkington did not; her father wrote Benson shortly after the war to inform him of her death.[17]

Women intuitively understood their importance in both the physical and emotional recovery process of amputees. Emma Mordecai, who volunteered in Virginia in 1864, recalled one "splendid-looking" Confederate soldier who had his arm blown to pieces by an artillery shell. The soldier underwent amputation, and as he recovered, Mordecai plied him with humor. "This is a bad way of getting a furlough," she joked. The soldier simply sighed and forlornly remarked, "Ah! The worst of it is, to think of our families."[18]

In addition to caretaking, nurses also provided important services to recuperating amputees, especially helping with letter writing. Part of their job, they knew, was to assist family members back home and prepare them to welcome a disabled veteran. They also framed how the soldier's sacrifice should be interpreted, whether he lived or died, emphasizing the masculine characteristics of how a soldier had faced his operation and his recuperation afterward. Mrs. Joseph S. McGruder, a nurse in a hospital in Richmond, Virginia, cared for Asa T. Martin, a Confederate soldier who lost an arm at the Battle of Fair Oaks in 1862, who revealed that he feared returning home with only one arm. Shortly afterward, McGruder found herself writing a series of letters, emotionally preparing the wife back home to deal with the reality that her husband was now an amputated man. The nurse knew Martin to be a kind, affectionate husband and father, and she genuinely felt that his missing arm did nothing to diminish his stature as a worthy man. Unfortunately, Martin died a few weeks later, which forced her to write another letter, announcing the death of a husband. He had been, she assured his wife, as "good, humble, patient, grateful, [and] kind hearted [a] soldier as ever died in Richmond." McGruder added that she hoped someday to find "another good man like him." In another instance, a nurse assured the family of Junius C. Battle, a Confederate soldier who died after an amputation, that he had every attention "except the matchless love of a mother or sister to watch over him with their soothing words and gentle attentions of whom he often spoke to me and particularly his mother."[19]

Apart from nursing, women actively participated in benevolent groups during the war that sought to help take care of their amputated men. Participation in such ladies' aid societies grew naturally out of prewar work with benevolent reform organizations. The work was by no means simply symbolic, as the gathering and movement of medical supplies ensured that the Confederate military could effectively orchestrate the war on the front lines. Thus, as one historian noted, "Confederate women understood that their unremunerated labor produced supplies most quickly, cheaply, and effectively."[20]

In Greenville, North Carolina, dozens of women joined the Ladies Association, whose mission was "to provide hospital stores and clothing for the soldiers of the Confederacy." The group of women, who wanted to provide "the aid and comfort of the sick and wounded," started on July 19, 1861, requiring their members to pay $5.20 to join. When women could not afford the high dues, they were simply encouraged to give as much as they could. The funds raised and items collected, including clothing, bedding, food, and bandages, ended up in hospitals in the region to help wounded Confederate soldiers, suffering from disease, gunshot wounds, or amputation. Simultaneously, women in Warrenton, North Carolina, joined the Sick Soldiers Relief Society in August 1861, holding their meetings six times a week. Within five weeks, the women had gathered and donated "140 shirts, 54 pillow cases. 60 pairs of socks, 2 comforters, 44 sheets, 33 pillow licks and 83 towels."[21]

In many instances, women gathered to support the men on the lines as soon as the war commenced. The city of Richmond, Virginia, witnessed the emergence of the Soldiers' Aid Society, which called on all their "sisters" to form benevolent groups "in every county and every community." In Charleston, South Carolina, Margaret Ann Meta Morris Grimball wrote in her diary on July 26, 1861, "The ladies are all as busy as possible forming themselves into relief societies for the wounded soldiers, and also to prepare clothing for them in the winter, which will soon now approach." The Soldiers Relief Association in Charleston worked, according to their Constitution, "to provide garments for our soldiers in the field and hospital stores and other comforts for the sick and wounded." Local newspapers carried the local rallying cry: "Let us not forget our sick and wounded soldiers." The organization requested donations of materials, money, and time, and an individual only had to donate in order to become a member. Men and women united behind the organization, and many women processed dozens of donated items, including socks, quilts, bandages, soap, candles, and a wide variety of food items, including pickles, brandy, tea, coffee, spices, fruit, wine, and rice. As stores of items diminished, the women of South Carolina requested additional goods from their friends in England and the Bahamas because the massive amount of wounded soldiers had exhausted much-needed supplies.[22]

Even though women rallied behind the cause of providing medical care and relief to amputated men, they sometimes struggled in considering a wounded veteran as an appropriate mate. Women certainly gravitated toward soldiers as potential husbands. Yet as the war dragged on and eliminated many eligible single men from society, some women eschewed a long courtship in favor of quickly attaching themselves to any man that had at least some desirable qualities. The escalating pace to select a spouse alarmed some members of southern society. Emma Holmes in South Carolina commented on "the strange marriages and matches made by the war." She stood aghast at how many young women showed a profound willingness "to take any offer, without regard to suitability." Historian Amy Murrell Taylor has argued that marriage served as a mechanism to demonstrate that Confederate men and women were united together as they prepared to deal with the political and economic difficulties of Reconstruction. But the process of marriage would not be easy, as at least 20 percent of the white male population in the South died during the war. Statistically speaking, scholars have argued that white women married at roughly the same rate as they did before the war. Thus, in order to reach the same statistical level, southern white women had to lower their criteria for a marriage partner out of necessity, which fundamentally changed the nature of a potential relationship.[23]

Some women gravitated to veterans as potential mates, as their military service represented the prime characteristics of manhood. One southern song assured women that a soldier who went off to war would never forget "the girl he left behind." As for the young men who marched off to war, they were expected to "go to the field where honor calls and win your lady there." The returning soldiers who tried to prove their manhood in battle excited several southern women. Loula Kendall, from Georgia, described soldiers she encountered as "handsome and commanding," "an ideal picture of a soldier," "a noble, commanding soldier," and "a gallant soldier." She noted, "We did not condescend to receive particular attentions from any but those who wore uniforms." Amanda Worthington declared, "I love all Confederate soldiers," while Alice Ready loved and prayed for all the soldiers because the decision to enlist "entitled them to our warmest sympathy, and gratitude."[24]

Although some women showed a great amount of enthusiasm toward veterans as potential spouses, many of the veterans returned home physically or emotionally altered by a war they had lost. Thus, some women avoided veterans and married much older men, who did not bear the physical and emotional scars of war. Such aging noncombatants, though, might not survive long enough to adequately care for their bride. Women also looked at men of a lower socioeconomic status as potential mates but impoverished or working-class southern men might have financial difficulty in supporting a spouse. Finally, southern women also considered disabled men, as thousands returned home with empty sleeves or visible gunshot wounds. Women responded to amputees as a spouse or a potential spouse in a variety of ways. Some embraced their loves and felt grateful they returned home alive. Others found it difficult to hide their contempt and revulsion and rejected the handicapped men. Most women, though, were conflicted, especially since disabled individuals raised questions about the economic sustainability of a family now reliant on an amputated breadwinner. Cultural cues prescribed acceptance of amputees for their sacrifices, and women internalized this patriotic notion, but it contributed to their anxieties and inner conflict about what to do about prospective mates who lost a limb.

During the course of the war, southerners realized the important role that women would play in caring for the handicapped men of war. Confederate president Jefferson Davis ordered a crowd of disillusioned women in Macon, Georgia, on September 23, 1864, to recognize the "limping soldier" as the new aristocracy of the South. He declared, "To the young ladies I would say when choosing between an empty sleeve and the man who had remained at home and grown rich, always take the empty sleeve." Jefferson Davis knew that southern white women must play an active role in rebuilding the shattered white male physique obliterated by the onslaught of war. After all, as historian Mark Wetherington noted, women needed to put "their soldiers and the new nation above all else" in order to assert both their patriotism and womanhood. Davis solidified, in the minds of his audience, that the amputated war veteran would hold an honorable place in society and that women had an important task in ensuring that the wounded returned heroes, rather than dishonored failures.[25]

Southern writers employed metaphors, such as images of the damaged landscape, to describe the role women should play in the postwar period of healing and recovery. Men appeared as the strong, sturdy southern oaks, which can survive for centuries despite the challenges brought on by Mother Nature. At the same time, women appeared as the gentle vines, which wrapped themselves around the damaged oak tree in order to ensure their survival. In the poem "Blighted Hopes," the writer described an oak tree "scathed by lightning's sudden stroke," but it stood tall to face "the coming storm." Then, around the trunk, a vine curled in order to save the damaged tree. One southern writer in the years following the war noted, "Do you see that tender vine binding up the shattered tree and hiding its wounds? That is southern woman clinging closer and more tenderly to father and husband when the storms beat upon him, comforting as only such Christian women can comfort." If women wanted to represent the "tender vine" that would hold together the southern oak of manhood that had been "riven by the lightning" after the war, they needed to accept the call issued by Davis and honor the noble sacrifices of the amputees by ensuring their health, welfare, and ultimate survival.[26]

Other southern writers championed the idea that amputees should be honored for their sacrifices by the women they encountered on a daily basis. Women had to assist damaged men with the simple daily chores of life. In a poem written during the war by Dr. G. W. Bagby, titled "The Empty Sleeve," the author describes Tom, a Confederate soldier who lost an arm during the war, declaring that his wound would serve "as a badge of honor." Yet Tom begins to cry, stating, "She deserves a perfect man" and also noting that he is "not worth her" in his "prime." Although Tom had an internalized fear of women not recognizing his sacrifice, men and women praised his sacrifices on the street and he returned home to "a nation's love in proud remembrance" of the sacrifice that he gave "for freedom's sake." Tom, ordered at once to return to his sweetheart, returned to a loving relationship with a "tender" and "strong" woman who committed the rest of her years to "helping as hard as she can, to put on his coat and pin his sleeve, tie his cravat, and cut his food." Because of their physical sacrifice in the Civil War, Confederate men should not fear but rather embrace their newfound dependency on women, who stood ready to serve.[27]

If official and literary authorities prodded Confederate women to embrace the returning amputees, southern society applied various forms of community pressure that left no doubt how women should receive men with the "empty sleeve." In a newspaper account of an incident that occurred in New Orleans several years after the war, two women traveled by streetcar through the city. A gentleman, described as a "Knight of the Crutch," despite his amputated limb, took the women's tickets to a box at the front of the car, a traditional act of chivalry in New Orleans. As the amputee hobbled toward the front of the streetcar, the women sat silently, ignoring both the man and his actions. One eyewitness vented his frustration in the local newspaper, decrying the insensitive actions of the ungrateful women and argued that at least the man adhered to societal definitions of manhood and womanhood because he had been polite to the women, even though he lost a leg. For women to convey their true femininity, according to the observer, they needed to show courtesy and "delicate thoughtfulness and consideration for the comfort and convenience of others, especially the unfortunate." Granted, the women allowed the man to complete the act of chivalry, but their marked indifference, combined with a failure to recognize the virtue, indeed nobility, in the disabled status of the Confederate amputee, prompted the eyewitness to harshly judge the women in the newspaper. The witness concluded with a sarcastic prediction, asking, "I wonder if you two are 'Women's Rights' women? If so, how will you manage to get your 'tickets' into the ballot box independent of the assistance of a gentleman with or without a crutch?" In refusing to act in a cordial manner to the injured gentlemen, the women left no mistake, in readers' minds, that such behavior undermined a lady's status and reputation. The two women failed to heed Jefferson Davis's call to recognize the empty sleeve as a marker of the new aristocracy, let alone an appropriate sign of manhood.[28]

The women on the streetcar were not alone in expressing a negative reaction toward physically altered men. Although some southern men believed that the Confederate cause glorified any wounds garnered on the battlefield, not everyone could overlook physical deformities. Martha Bird, the wife of Samuel A. Bird, ended up in a South Carolina mental asylum. She expressed the cause of her insanity as her husband losing his right leg during the Civil War. Mary Lucas did not hold out much hope for her sister Emma to find a suitable spouse. She told her sister that she would be very "lonesome" because "you will see nothing but one legged and one arm soldiers." Clearly, Lucas saw the war destroying any suitable able-bodied men for her sister to pursue. Ellen House, a young girl from Tennessee, received an offer to correspond with a Confederate lieutenant, but she rejected the invitation, noting, "[Just] because I felt sorry for him on account of his being a Confederate soldier and having lost a leg, was no reason why he should presume upon it and write me." For House, the empty sleeve solicited not sympathy but rather derision toward the veteran who thought of her as a suitable romantic prospect.[29]

A physically scarred man prompted some women to end a relationship that had been established before the soldier marched off to war. Nurse Fannie Beers wrote a letter on behalf of a Confederate soldier from Mississippi who lost a leg at the Battle of Franklin and suffered from a gunshot wound to the face. The soldier described being engaged to one of "the prettiest" women in the state but worried if his future bride would accept him in his "murdered up" condition. Beers assured the soldier that his fiancée would accept him, as she knew of several women who remained steadfast in their love for their men, despite their deformities. She described a girl who married her "mangled" lover because he still had "enough of his body left to contain his soul." However, Beers found herself having to break the cold news to the soldier that his fiancée rejected him because she would never "marry a cripple." The woman had already found a man who could support her. Although the soldier fell into despondency, he quickly recovered and shared his assessment of the situation with Nurse Beers. "I've been thinking over the matter and I reckon I've had a lucky escape. That trifling girl would never have made me a good, faithful wife." Beers felt enraged at the woman who rejected her fiancé because of his disabled condition and could never forgive the "faithless girl."[30]

Although some women could not handle being romantically involved with a disabled man, others remained ambivalent and internally torn over whether or not they should accept an amputee as a potential mate. Probably no one fits into the category of internal conflict in trying to love an amputee better than Sally Buchannan "Buck" Preston, the love interest of Confederate general John Bell Hood, who lost the use of his left arm and his entire right leg during the war. Although Preston showed minimal interest when the couple met in 1863, she did enjoy being courted by a Confederate officer. However, one afternoon, after Hood departed, she admitted, "I never cared particularly about him, but now that he has chosen to go with those people, I would not marry him if he had a thousand legs, instead of having just lost one." Preston did not show any true sympathy for an amputee early on and remained lukewarm about the relationship, especially since she had a plethora of male prospects who had all their limbs intact.[31]

Regardless of several women who either admired him or pursued him during his recovery in Richmond, Hood remained focused on Preston, despite the fact that she had the ability to cast "a spell upon her lovers" that resulted in them being "killed" or having "died of the effects of her wounds," according to Mary Chesnut. Hood, aware of the flirting tendencies of Preston, remarked to Preston one afternoon, "I think I will go set a mantrap near your door and break some of those young fellows' legs, too." Hood seemed to think that Preston would not show affection to any other physically altered man. Despite the realm of ambivalence conveyed by Preston, Hood enthusiastically pursued her as his love interest for several months. Although Preston and Hood materialized as a staple in Richmond's social circle, she did not reciprocate any affection for him and even declared during a party, with her romantic pursuer within hearing distance, "Engaged to that man! Never! For what do you take me?" Although Hood felt heartbroken and would rather die than endure continued rejection, the couple mysteriously announced their engagement a few weeks later. Mary Chesnut remained convinced that Preston did not love Hood but rather had mustered up nothing more than some "sympathy for the wounded soldier."[32]

However, the engagement ended up on hold, as Hood headed back to the active duty and Preston continued her ambivalence about wanting to be with a disabled man. Preston received abundant criticism from the elite women in Richmond, who sided with Hood. She declared to her detractors, "Don't waste your delicacy! Sally H[ampton] is going to marry a man who has lost an arm, so he is also a maimed soldier, you see; and she is proud of it. The cause glorifies such wounds." Preston thought that mentioning Sally Hampton would prove that she was not rejecting Hood because of his physical disability. In fact, several women in the social circle pursued physically damaged men. Yet, there seems to be a deep level of inner conflict within the women in terms of how they felt about being romantically linked to a wounded man. One member of the Chesnut circle stated, "What a glorious assortment of noble martyrs and wrecks— heroes I mean." The unnamed woman quickly corrected herself when she referred to the damaged men as "wrecks." While other members of her social circle may have been willing to attach themselves to a wounded or amputated man, Preston shifted back and forth, from steadfast opposition to Hood masked by the guise of an engagement to genuine feelings of love and care, exhibited by a continued correspondence with the officer, public prayers for his safety, and the wearing of a diamond ring. Preston eventually moved on and ended her ambivalence about whether or not to marry a Confederate amputee.[33]

Men well realized the new burden their injury would have on suitors and wives and offered some women, who may have been ambivalent about their feelings, a way to end the relationship. John Redding, a Confederate soldier shot in the leg at Chickamauga, received word from a surgeon that he would lose his leg. After the amputation, Redding called for his fiancée, Carrie McNeil, who had traveled to see him. Redding offered to end his engagement due to his amputation but his future wife refused, declaring, "No, no, John, I can't give you up and I love you better than ever." Another amputee returned home from the war and offered to end his engagement with Miss Maggie Pharham because he did not feel he could financially provide for a family in his physical condition. Pharham refused to end the relationship and believed the couple could survive. In both cases, the women embraced their role as caregiver. While it is possible that both women felt guilty about the possibility of rejecting a damaged man who needed help, they ultimately decided not to allow a missing limb to be the reason for diminishing their love for their future husbands.[34]

As some southern women rejected amputated men or felt unsure about the relationship, many embraced their disheveled, wounded, and bedraggled veterans simply because they had served in the war. Eliza Andrews noted that the war had created an unceremonious time when social distinctions vanished and damaged and ragged men seemed entitled to more honor than a king. Yet, in order to grasp the thought of marrying an amputee, women reconceptualized their expectations of the perfect man. They had to, as historian Victoria Ott argued, "accommodate the bodily damage to southern manhood." In some cases, women eagerly accepted the challenge. In Savannah, Georgia, Whitelaw Reid, when visiting the city in 1865, overhead a man immersed in conversation with a captain who returned home missing a hand. The man reassured the captain that not all was lost returning home with a missing limb. "A hand is a bad thing to lose, but it won't hurt you among the ladies of Savannah. There are plenty that you can persuade to give you one." Women throughout the city rushed to meet their returning soldiers from war, even if they had lost a limb. Reid witnessed the reunions filled with "warmth," even though the South failed to achieve success in the Civil War. In addition, Frances Dallam Peter witnessed elite women who before the war "wouldn't have touched [poor white men] with the hem of their garments" now flocking to the returning soldiers.[35]

Southern women who remained committed to the man they fell in love with before he marched off to war set aside their own misgivings in favor of providing care for an amputated soldier. A soldier named Hurley asked a young girl from South Carolina for her hand in marriage before the Civil War. At the end of the war, Hurley returned home missing an arm. However, his fiancée embraced him and his amputation, and the two married because "the woman's soul rode roughshod over everything." Another Confederate captain from North Carolina lost his arm at a federal field hospital after the Battle of Gettysburg. Nervously, the amputee constructed a letter to his wife to share the news of his newfound disability. His wife accepted the news, and their relationship remained strong and stable, especially since a federal surgeon also assured the wife that her husband seemed positioned for a quick recovery. The amputee joked that he could not wait to embrace his children in his arm and "bestow in person the kisses I now give through Mama."[36]

Other women who accepted the challenge of their patriotic duty occasionally found themselves having to defend their decision to marry amputated men. One woman approached a female friend and expressed her sympathy because she was about to enter into matrimony with a one-armed soldier. The potential bride fervently declared, "I want no sympathy. I think it is a great privilege and honor to be the wife of a man who lost his arm fighting for my county." Alice Bailey ignored her detractors and willingly married Simon Boozer, who had his leg amputated at Gettysburg. The missing leg failed to derail a lengthy courtship strengthened through continual correspondence throughout the war. In another instance, a southern woman also stood steadfast in her relationship and married her veteran who lost his leg at the Battle of the Wilderness.[37]

Southern women who accepted amputated veterans defended their relationships to family members who questioned how an amputated man could support and provide for his potential wife. James H. Berry, a Confederate officer who lost his leg in 1862, agreed to marry Lizzie Quaile after the war. However, he had little to offer his potential bride, with no money and no future prospects. Although Berry acted in a chivalrous manner and asked Quaile's father for permission to marry his daughter, the request was summarily rejected because the father did not want his daughter marrying a man who could not financially support her. Quaile's father instantaneously equated amputation with the prospects of an impoverished and worthless life. Berry asked if the marriage would receive approval if he could "provide a way to make a good living." Quaile sternly replied that there "was no use in holding out hope that would probably not be realized" and recommended that Berry "let the whole matter drop."[38]

Berry refused to accept the denial of marriage and promised his potential bride that if she disobeyed her father's wishes, he would buy her diamond earrings and he would someday be governor of Arkansas. Lizzie Quaile agreed, and the day after her father rejected the marriage proposal, she married James Berry at the home of his sister. Mr. Quaile refused to speak to his son-in-law or even acknowledge his presence until 1882, seventeen years later, when Berry received the nomination for governor of Arkansas. Berry won the election, served one term, and then ended up in the Senate for twenty-two years. One man remembered Berry by stating, "He limped back to his state after being maimed on the battlefield for life. He spent his remaining days with the high ideals of southern manhood always before him." Berry did not let his injury deter him from his life pursuits, whether in his quest for political power or his relationship with Lizzie Quaile.[39]

The fears expressed by Lizzie Quaile's father appeared all throughout the former states of the Confederacy. Many Confederate amputees limped home to diminished financial prospects and needed women more than ever because they had transitioned from being "brave men" to "more prostrate and helpless than infants," according to one southern woman. Prior to the Civil War, the notions of marriage within the patriarchal society rooted in paternalistic ideology demanded that women receive protection and financial support. Yet as the war concluded and damaged men returned to their prewar relationships, southern white women faced a mix of emotions, as they worried about their livelihood but also saw their role in caring for amputated men vital to the sustainability of an altered sense of southern manhood.[40]

Some women found the role reversal of dependency as an exciting prospect and welcomed amputated men into their homes, where they could provide medical care and assistance with the daily rigors of life. After Richard Ewell lost his leg in 1862, he traveled to a home known as Dunblane, where he emerged as a minor celebrity among the women whom he depended on in order to recover. One woman recalled Ewell's arrival and said, "I remember well the maimed figure on the litter, covered with a sheet, and the pale haggard face upon the pillow." Once Ewell regained his senses, another woman remarked, "He impressed us all as not only heroic and strong but as having the nicest consideration for others." After he departed the home, the women expressed how much they missed him, especially his "fortitude and patient endurance."[41]

After Ewell departed a congregate of devoted women, his fiancée, Lizinka Campbell Brown, emerged as his primary caregiver. Ewell's status as an amputee had clear ramifications on his relationship with Brown. As Brown wrote to Ewell, "While I sympathize in your terrible suffering and loss, it is only womanly to remember that one of its consequences will be to oblige you to remain at home and make me more necessary to you." Brown worried that Ewell would have had a host of women to choose from after the war, especially since he served as a Confederate officer. The empty sleeve changed everything and provided Brown with an enhanced level of personal security in her relationship because Ewell remained dependent on her in order to survive. Ewell's dependency on his fiancée also guaranteed that the engagement transitioned into a permanent marriage. Brown confessed, "That whereas I thought before you ought to marry and could very well marry a younger woman, now I will suit you better than any one else, if only because I will love you better." Brown admitted that her own sympathy for Ewell's injuries heightened her feelings toward her fiancé and created a unique codependent relationship that only she could replicate. If Ewell returned from the war physically intact, his relationship most likely would have mirrored pre-war relationships rooted in a patriarchal system. Amputation allowed a woman like Lizinka Campbell Brown to feel a heightened sense of security in regard to a romantic relationship with a physically dependent husband. She watched over Ewell, according to some witnesses, "with sleepless vigilance, and cheering him up by hopeful and recreative converse." The two married on May 26, 1863, right before Ewell rejoined the Army of Northern Virginia. The empty sleeve allowed a loving partnership to ensure both a stable marriage and a successful postwar career, as Ewell lived on and made money off his wife's farm in Tennessee. Both Ewell and his wife died within a few days of one another from pneumonia in January 1872.[42]

The shifted notions of dependency forced some Confederate amputees to seek another spouse if they outlived their first wife. In several instances, Confederate amputees quickly remarried, usually within a year or two. John L. Cathey, who lost his right leg during the war, returned home to his wife who now had to assist her handicapped husband on a daily basis. After his first wife died in 1878, Cathey, entirely dependent on the care of someone else, quickly married another woman, who died seven years later. Rather than seek a third wife, Cathey remained dependent on his oldest son.[43]

Many amputated and chronically ill veterans remained entirely dependent on their wives. Men who returned home with damaged bodies faced continual bouts of chronic pain that prevented them from earning enough money to support their wives. Charles Klem, who lost his leg at Dallas, Georgia, on May 28, 1864, had no property or income and relied on his wife, who had an estate worth $350. Sarah Jane Klem earned the only income for the family at a rate of $50 to $60 per year from some sewing work. Her husband remained in a dilapidated condition, as he succumbed to glaucoma that blinded him in both eyes and endured searing pain in his lungs from an additional gunshot wound sustained at the Battle of Stones River. Although Klem secured a pension from Kentucky that financially assisted the relationship, he died a few months after his pension application had been approved. Thus, his wife found herself forced to apply for a widow's pension and worked as a clerk in a local store in order to support herself and their daughter.[44]

The amputated men who returned home to their wives and families struggled financially, largely because of their disabilities. Disabled men faced chronic health issues, usually related to their amputation or other nagging wounds that sent many to an early grave. Southern women, who stood by their amputated men and sacrificed a portion of their own livelihood, faced rampant poverty and limited means for survival. Dr. Joseph Jones, the Surgeon General of the United Confederate Veterans, insisted that the states recognize the "forlorn and struggling widows of those who yielded up their lives to a just and righteous sense of duty to their native States." Thus, the southern state governments had to remain proactive in caring for many impoverished widows who needed a pension in order to survive. Once again, notions of dependency shifted, as widows now remained dependent on the state and a pension in order to survive. In addition to needing the financial capital, widows also welcomed the pensions because it served as a way for the state government to thank the women for their patriotism and service during the war. In 1912, the state of Virginia recognized all southern women who worked in a Confederate hospital for at least a year with an annual pension of forty dollars.[45]

As southern states established pensions to care for Confederate widows, each state established specific criteria that eligible applicants had to meet. Widows needed to provide thorough documentation of their former husband's military service, remain unmarried, meet residency requirements, and not exceed a certain amount of income and property, which varied from state to state. Widows stood before an elected official to verify under oath that all of the pension application information could be verified as factual. Some states, like Louisiana, initially offered widows large land grants of 160 acres in the years preceding the passage of pension legislation. Emilie Verret lost an arm during the Civil War and drowned after the war when his ship sank and he could not properly swim. His widow applied and received a land grant from Louisiana. Texas extended a massive land grant of 1,280 acres in a program that lasted two years. Tennessee transitioned the Hermitage, the home of former president Andrew Jackson, into a home for damaged veterans and their widows.[46]

The land grants, residencies, and pensions proved pivotal, as scores of women applied for the financial assistance they so desperately required. Ada Green lost her husband in 1901 and required a pension to survive because her husband left her with no property. Another widow in Kentucky applied for a pension to care for her two children after being left penniless following the death of her disabled husband. After Nannie Douglas's disabled husband died in 1901, she managed to receive a pension because she had no children to assist her. If the husband died before the state passed a pension program, several widows ended up completely impoverished without any visible means of survival. Susan Lanthrip had to rely on her neighbors to support her and her three children after her amputated husband died in 1884. Mariah E. Dehart faced the same exact situation, as her husband, also an amputee, died before he received any funds. Josephine Robinson's husband died shortly after he had filed an application for an artificial arm. The General Assembly in Virginia attempted to rectify the situation by paying Robinson forty dollars (rather than the standard sixty). The state later revised the policy in order to allow any money not paid to the veteran applicant to go to either a widow or, if she had passed, their respective children, beginning in 1886.[47]

Other widows who lost their amputated husbands faced a few obstacles in securing a pension due to paperwork delays inside a bloated state bureaucracy, violation of the application requirements, or verification issues, as state officials ascertained the validity of the applications. The wife of Andrew J. Dowless had her pension application denied because her amputated husband had deserted from his command and swore an oath to the United States before hostilities ceased. Samuel B. Rawls, who lost a leg in 1864, traveled to Texas after the war from Florida to work for a telegraph operator. He and his wife, Hannah, communicated regularly through letters. Suddenly, Hannah received no further correspondence from her husband, and every letter she sent him ended up returned. Left on her own, Hannah tried to secure a pension but needed proof that her husband had died. She eventually heard from the telegraph company, who informed her that Samuel had vanished. Local authorities located a dead body that may have been her husband. With some proof from the Texas authorities, Hannah received her pension from Florida in 1903.[48]

In some cases, the widow of an amputee had her pension revoked once evidence emerged that she had tried to illegally defraud the system. Henrietta and her husband, James Robarts, faced numerous accusations of trying to unlawfully garner a pension. Robarts lost a thumb and a large portion of his right hand at Seven Pines in 1862. When he applied for a pension, it was denied because records indicated he had been absent without leave. Robarts produced a witness for the Pension Board in the form of a former surgeon who emphatically denied the desertion charge and claimed the man in question had spent the rest of the war working as a nurse during the latter part of 1864. The Pension Board in Florida, convinced by the sworn statement, approved the pension but then ceased payments because Robarts collected a pension from the United States for fighting Native Americans after the Civil War. After his death, his wife applied for and received a widow's pension. Once their daughter received word of this, she notified the state that the couple had been divorced for a number of years and her mother married another man five months after the divorce. Other children stepped forward to offer harsh testimony about how their mother treated them and deserted their handicapped father. Henrietta Robarts had violated her patriotic duty by leaving her husband but then wanted to financially benefit from being married to an amputee for a period. The children despised their mother's actions and motives and told the state of Florida that she did not deserve a dime. The state followed the wishes of the children and rescinded the pension.[49]

In addition to acknowledging the sacrifices of women through pensions, numerous speakers across the South in the postwar period extolled the vital role women played in healing amputated men. In December 1910, John B. Lightfoot Jr. delivered a dedication address for a small tablet at the site of the Robertson Hospital in Richmond, Virginia. Lightfoot used the rhetoric of the Lost Cause in order to highlight the heroic role of southern women. Amid a lengthy discussion on the paramount role of the hospital during the war, he turned his attention to the women whom he described as "fearless and brave, enduring beyond belief, self-sacrificing, patient." The "tender and gentle" women, who also possessed a "fearless and brave" character, allowed for a "victorious defeat, a thing unique to war." In other words, Lightfoot credited the women who stood by the bedsides of the wounded and amputated men as crucial in shaping not only men but also the mythology applied to men that reflected a "victorious defeat."[50]

Lightfoot praised the sacrifices of southern women who "typified the perfect woman." In another dedication speech at Christ Church in Matthews County, Virginia, on June 3, 1925, Lightfoot again relished the opportunity to delve into the Lost Cause rhetoric in order to both highlight the "conviction of the righteousness of the Confederate cause" and argue that all women possessed the "strength and the will" to achieve a paramount task: the revitalization of wounded Confederate soldiers. Lightfoot did not reminisce about the women who failed to assist amputated men. Rather, he saw all women involved in rehabilitating men to the point where they were "ready again to take the field and fight for the Southern Cause." Women not only cared for the wounded, but also ensured that the men "returned to duty freshly imbued with patriotic resolve to serve their flag."[51]

The destructive power of the Civil War changed the very nature of dependency for amputated men and their supportive wives. Debilitating wounds created a new class of men who remained dependent on a spouse to help them navigate through the challenges brought on by their newfound disability. Most southern women embraced a missing limb as a noble badge of sacrifice and either maintained relationships with their injured mates or married amputated men in significant numbers. Men and women recognized some dependency on women as a buttress, rather than a hindrance, in personal definitions of male identity and self-worth. As amputees adjusted to a new form of manhood in the postwar period, so did women. Confederate women sacrificed throughout the war with their service in hospitals and in benevolent societies to assist amputated men. Once the amputees returned home, women, for the most part, continued to provide steadfast support and love that assisted men in reconstructing their shattered lives.

Confederate women understood the vital role they played in healing both broken bodies and the broken expectations of secession and war. They struggled and fought to ensure that amputated men received recognition for their injuries, while benefiting from a newly forged relationship that provided many women with more self-worth and security and a man who now remained dependent on her for survival. The love and sacrifice came at a cost to some women, who were left impecunious and dependent on the state to provide a pension as a means for survival. Yet, could women alone care for wounded men? Southern society at large and individual state governments needed to step in and assist southern women with the enormous challenge of caring and providing for an entire generation of disabled men. In the midst of these economic challenges, women still forged the necessary crutches for amputated men to cope with both their altered physiques and an altered society constructed by victorious Union armies in the Civil War.

FOUR

The Return

Adjusting to Dependency and Disability

> I see the people in the street
> Look at your sleeve with kindling eyes;
> And know you, Tom, there's naught so sweet,
> As homage shown in mute surmise.
> Bravely your arm in battle strove,
> Freely for freedom's sake you gave it;
> It has perished, but a nation's love
> In proud remembrance will save it.
> –G. W. Bagby, "The Empty Sleeve"

> This old coat don't fit me Mary, as it did when I was young
> Don't you remember how neatly to my manly form it clung
> Never mind the sleeve that's empty, let it dangle loose and free
> For I am going out parading with the boys of '63.
> –S. Fontaine, *Parading with the Boys of the Sixties*

Bill Hicks did not get over the amputation of his leg during the Civil War. Described as "a fine young man, an Apollo in form, and a model of strong physical manhood," Hicks returned home to work as a lawyer. Even though his legal practice seemed promising, the absence of a leg preyed on Hicks's mind, prompting him to make a rather rash decision. Rather than live the rest of his life as "a cripple," as a doctor noted, "in a fit of despondency, he blew out his brains." He was not alone. Charles Minnigerode received a gunshot wound in his leg at Appomattox in 1865. Although the doctors allowed him to keep his leg, he limped for the remaining days of his life. With his business endeavors failing and a mountain of debt consuming his ever-growing family, Minnigerode took his own life in 1888. In another case, A. G. Ewing, a Confederate cavalryman living in Nashville after the war, decided that he no longer could live his life as an amputated man. Ewing sacrificed his leg at Fort Pillow, Tennessee, in 1862 and took his own life via an overdose of chloroform in

1872. John Campsen, a Confederate artilleryman, shot himself in the head while standing in front of a looking glass. Campsen, who lost an arm during the Civil War, ended his life after it had been proven that he severely beat a child.[1]

Taking one's own life or the very thought of suicide constituted one response, albeit an extreme one, to living as a disabled man. The very notion that many veterans contemplated suicide and took their own lives reveals the depths of the challenges they faced as they attempted to reintegrate into civilian life. Summarizing the life of the veteran, one member of the Eighth Georgia noted at war's end, "It was all over but the empty sleeves and wooden legs." War unmade men. It damaged them physically, emotionally, and mentally; it battered their bodies, their souls, and their very identities. At the conclusion of the Civil War, Confederate amputees returned home with visible markers of both their sacrifice and their failure. As historian John David Smith noted, amputees disproportionately displayed the symptoms of posttraumatic stress, exhibiting "hostility, superficial self-confidence, rationalization, compulsivity, extreme pessimism, delusion, and the setting of excessively high goals."[2]

This chapter examines the daily physical and emotional challenges of disability and dependency among Confederate amputees after the Civil War. Damaged and defeated men, coping with chronic pain, abundant health issues, and difficult transitions in a depressed postwar economy, found it often difficult to reassert their masculine identities. Amputated men still faced a crisis in manhood, as the notion of masculinity inherent in the Lost Cause limited the use of Civil War memory to help these men. Some southerners still rejected the idea that a real man, even an honorable veteran, should be dependent on society or the state in order to survive. As one disability historian has noted, "Many men, perhaps all men, could not sustain masculine ideals—unfaltering, a heroic warrior, a successful breadwinner and able to stand strong despite all—which undermined their status in society."[3]

As the reality of defeat set in, southern communities found themselves coping with an unprecedented and staggering amount of death, destruction, and dashed hopes, creating a kind of cultural depression that lingered for decades after the war's end. The death toll left numerous empty chairs at dining tables across the South. Many of the men who did survive returned disfigured and dilapidated and remained dependent on fellow southerners to recognize the value of their sacrifices. A damaged body ran counter to prewar notions of masculinity, which forced southern society to eventually recognize disability and dependency as a new part of what it meant to be a man. The sentiments of acceptance were not universal. While white southern women paved the way for others to accept disabled men, not all damaged veterans returned home to a supportive environment. Some returned and resided alone, without a supportive family. Others depended on friends and neighbors to help cope with the empty sleeve. Thus, members of southern society remained absolutely pivotal in helping to rebuild the white male body—and with it white patriarchy.

Prior to the extension of prosthetics and pensions from state governments, amputated men struggled first to find meaningful employment. Ramshackle veterans tied themselves to a plow in order to prepare their farmland; they begged for money and sold items on street corners, hoping that their missing limb would elicit sympathy and sales. One historian, who examined the impact of World War I on amputees, noted that gainful employment was the most significant means of transforming disabled veterans from "unproductive cripples into independent, manly citizens." The same idea applied to Confederate men, who needed a steady income for their families and to reclaim their sense of themselves as providers. Of necessity, some amputees had to look to benevolent organizations to help them survive when they could not find meaningful employment. However, the benevolent organizations had staunchly positioned themselves as disseminators of the Lost Cause, which grated against some amputees less romantic memories of their war experience. Furthermore, while the Lost Cause eventually fostered the image of the heroic veteran and his empty sleeve, it failed to provide meaningful assistance to assure that the very men honored in speeches or through monuments actually survived. Benevolent organizations, particularly those that raised large sums of money to hold reunions and dot the landscape with bronze and marble markers of memory, also quickly found themselves limited in the amount of assistance they could provide to a large population of disabled dependents. Southern amputated men needed a strong medical and governmental infrastructure in order to rebuild their shattered lives. Gradually, as they aged, amputated men emerged as dependent wards of the state and relied on funds from the state legislatures in the waning decades of the nineteenth century.[4]

Amputees faced continuing medical and physical complications in the immediate aftermath of their amputation. Chronic pain handicapped some of them on a daily basis, as they adjusted to a newly acquired prosthetic device or faced the prospect that nagging injuries would never completely heal. Men were encouraged to face such difficulties in stoical silence, leaving historians with few accounts of how such men dealt with chronic pain. Charles McCall, who lost a leg, suffered from a stump that remained so painful an artificial leg was not an option. Richard Ewell, the Confederate officer who lost a leg in 1862, remembered cautiously walking down a street wearing his wooden leg when he encountered another officer who, upon seeing the prosthetic, inquired, "Does it hurt?" Ewell thought the officer to be jesting but then noticed that his compatriot also wore a wooden leg. Amputee to amputee, Ewell felt he could respond honestly for a change: "Yes. Does yours hurt you?" It was one of the few occasions in which Ewell even spoke of his discomfort.[5] Confederate veterans suffering from chronic pain found it especially difficult to work. Some literally could not stand; one veteran, for instance, had crippled both feet by extreme marching during the war. James Dyer of the Tenth Missouri reported suffering ever since he lost his right leg. Other Confederate veterans suffered chronic health problems and infections around their stumps. Charles Frank Pascoe found it difficult to work on crutches, which he required to stand after he lost his right leg as a member of the Sixteenth Mississippi.[6]

As medical research expanded after the Civil War, physicians discovered additional challenges facing amputated men. Silas Weir Mitchell, a neurologist who published *Injuries of Nerves and Their Consequences* in 1872, researched a condition known as *Causalgia*, described as a "burning pain" that made "the most amiable grow irritable" and turned a brave soldier into a "coward." The pain continued long after the wound had healed and appeared usually in feet or hands. He also described a condition referred to as *Sensory hallucination*, known today as *Phantom Limb*, in which amputees feel pain in a part of the body that has been removed. "Nearly every man who loses a limb carries about with him a constant or inconstant phantom of the missing member, a sensory ghost of that much of himself, and sometimes a most inconvenient presence, faintly felt at times, but ready to be called up to his perception by a blow, a touch, or a change of wind." He discovered that amputees rarely felt the presence of the entire missing limb but rather just a hand or foot.[7]

A number of amputees described feeling the ghostly presence of their whole limb. Chaplain Charles Dobbs cared for a young soldier who lost his right leg above the knee. One morning, the patient awoke extensively sobbing. Dobbs asked him what happened and the patient responded, "I thought I was sleeping with my little brother at home, and my foot, the one that was cut off, itched and I tried to rub it against the other, and I moved this stump." The pain caused by the movement of the stump awoke the soldier and he now had to deal anew with the emotional pain associated with living life as "a cripple." After being shot in the leg at the Battle of Chancellorsville in May 1863, Berry Benson traveled to several different hospitals and met a soldier named Hurley, who had lost an arm. Benson wrote, "He lay on a cot not far from mine, and every now and then he would bring his right arm across his body as though to take hold of something." Hurley laughed at this constant motion, as he claimed he still thought his left arm "were hanging down by the side of the cot," and tried to use his right arm to raise the now absent appendage. Hurley also claimed to still "feel all the fingers in his lost hand." The presence of constant bouts of pain and sensations of an absent limb made it difficult for amputees to ever fully adjust to their loss.[8]

In addition to phantom or chronic pain, Confederate amputees had an additional psychological burden during their transition from soldier to civilian: they returned home under a cloud of defeat and lacked the benefits, financial and psychological, that met those of their Union counterparts upon their return home—a Grand Review (where Union amputees received excessive cheers and support from the enthusiastic crowds), an aggressive pension and prosthetic system, and the knowledge that their physical sacrifice had resulted in glorious victory. As one Union amputee recalled, "Suffering is unpleasant; but, if one must suffer it is better to do so in a good cause: therefore I had rather have my leg blown off by a rebel shell, than crushed by a locomotive, or bitten off by a crocodile." Another Union amputated soldier reflected a similar sentiment: "Understand I don't regret its loss, it has been torn from my body that not one State should be torn from this Glorious Union."[9]

While northern amputees had the benefit of associating their missing limbs with victory, limbless southerners became a highly visible reminder of all kinds of loss, as the empty sleeve marked failure for all to see. During the Civil War, many southerners recognized amputated men, like Stonewall Jackson, as patriots sacrificing a part of their body for a glorious cause.

When, after four horrific years of war, the glorious cause failed to produce a victory, the meaning of the empty sleeve shifted from a symbol of sacrifice and patriotism to a visible reminder of defeat and failure. Although southerners carefully reiterated in Lost Cause speeches and writings that their masculinity had not been diminished by defeat, rhetoric failed to grasp the reality among damaged veterans. Southern men failed the ultimate test of manhood by losing the Civil War and returned home as "living symbols of this defeat," according to historian Mark Wetherington.[10]

The presence of thousands of amputated and disfigured men ran counter to notions of manhood established in the antebellum period when, as historian E. Anthony Rotundo has noted, the ideal of the white male body provided the foundation and embodiment of patriarchy and mastery. Although the Civil War destroyed the institution of slavery and dramatically altered notions of mastery within the southern household, the need to control African American men and women and white women did not evaporate, which placed amputated veterans, who remained disabled and dependent, in a position where antebellum notions of honor and mastery no longer applied. Altered and dependent veterans, who had failed in the ultimate male quest to protect home and homeland, could not easily fit the antebellum ideal, forcing a cultural reconception of the white male body.[11]

The tension in reconciling the battered and reliant body with notions of manhood ebbed and flowed throughout the postbellum period. On April 19, 1865, two children, ages nine and eleven, encountered a drunken man on the streets of Macon, Georgia. In an act of depravity, "unparalleled in the annals of civilization," according to a newspaper, the children grasped a rusty saw, cut off the man's leg, and left the leg behind. However, the patient would recover as the children had severed his wooden leg. While the newspaper reporter remarked about these events in horror, the children involved had operated from a different frame of reference. Rather than seeing the man as a veteran, the children had punished a drunk for violating societal perceptions of manhood. The outrage from the newspaper reporter reflected anger over the parents' failure, and maybe even southern society's failure, to sensitize children to the new symbolism of the white male body.[12]

The potential negative reaction toward amputated men, as exhibited by children and others, led some veterans to thank their lucky stars they had returned home in one piece. Charles Rainwater came home from the war with all his limbs, but he only slowly recovered from a gunshot wound that forced him to use crutches and a cane. When finally he could walk unaided he proclaimed, "I am so thankful that although I carry a reminder of the war in my body, in the shape of a leaden bullet, no one can tell it." Amputated men had a harder time hiding their injuries.[13]

Southern civilians who encountered amputated men offered some clues as to how the altered male physique impacted thinking about manhood. In her diary on March 31, 1863, Kim Rowland recalled a visit from Richard Ewell and Brigadier General Charles W. Field. She remembered that the two men "hobbled in on their crutches" and that "it was quite a touching site, these two brave, strong men – crippled the one for life and the other still for some time I suppose." Despite their shattered limbs, she saw them as "agreeable and fine-looking martial physiques." However, Rowland made sure to note that Field's physique impressed her a bit more than Ewell's. Considering Ewell had permanently lost a leg and that Field would recover from his gunshot wound, Rowland's confession is rather telling. Although she recognized the manhood and physique of both men, she could not help but note that one man stood physically complete and the other incomplete.[14]

Again southern women who had worked as nurses or care workers remained crucial in fostering an environment in which southerners accepted amputated men as honorable (and marriageable). Such an environment was not created overnight, however, and it was never perfect. Southern civilians exhibited a variety of responses to amputated veterans, from hilarity to apathy to empathy, as they navigated through fluctuating postwar definitions of manhood. On one side of the emotional spectrum, women used humor to help amputated men adjust to postwar society. One woman jokingly wished her husband had lost two legs rather than one, jesting that a second amputation would have secured a larger pension and allowing them to paint the house, pay off the mortgage, and buy their daughter Mary a piano. The wife told her husband about another amputee who lost both legs, and his wife "holds her head high, dresses fit to kill, and goes in the best society." On the opposite side of the spectrum, as the novelty of returning amputees wore off, one woman from South Carolina remarked that because a plethora of amputees roamed the city streets, "the cork leg and one armed men have ceased to attract special attention."[15]

For the most part southern communities embraced their disheveled and injured veterans. In his postwar visit to Savannah, Whitelaw Reid witnessed ample reunions of Confederate soldiers and their family, friends, and well-wishers. The crowds who gathered around the veterans "seemed in nowise tempered by contempt for their lack of success." In fact, Reid noticed that men dressed in their gray uniforms with missing legs and arms received extra attention. He noted, "The compliments would rain upon him [veteran] till the blushes would show upon his embrowned cheeks and he was fairly convinced that he had taken the most gallant and manly course in the world." Families gathered around the "long vacant" chairs that now contained "a crippled soldier, home from the wars, with only his wounds and his glory for his pay." Robert Somers, a British visitor, observed, after traveling about the region, "Southern gentlemen have a singular habit of wearing their coats without putting their arms in the sleeves. I have caught myself several times in a full flow of tender feeling for the gallant fellows who had lost both arms in the war."[16]

The return of amputated men elicited a wave of sympathy from most southern civilians. Eugenia Babcock's husband returned to South Carolina in 1865 and opened a hospital due to the large number of wounded men still suffering from Sherman's march through the Carolinas. She remembered, "One had been used as a carriage factory; it had a second story, which was soon occupied by the sick, and, more pitiful still, men whose wounds had been so long neglected that many an arm and leg had to be amputated."[17]

Edward Pollard, a newspaper writer and one of the original Lost Cause writers, wrote an impassioned and sympathetic description of Richard Ewell, who emerged as a public face of amputated men in the postwar South, as he spent a hefty amount of time in the public eye. He stated, "The spectacle of a worn and mutilated man looking prematurely old, mounted on a white horse that had often snuffed the battle with defiance, but was now scarcely more than a crippled skeleton." Despite the "sorrowful picture" created by Ewell wandering the streets in a "dilapidated sulky," Pollard recognized the devotion too. The skeleton warrior was "a sorrowful picture," he admitted, "but a nearer view disclosed a man remarkable even in the ruin of health and constitution, whose gray eye was as sharp and fierce as ever, and whose precise conversation showed that the vigor of his mind was as yet untouched." Pollard used the description of a man who suffered and sacrificed to not only frame Richard Ewell but also the former Confederacy writ large. Despite the negative physical ramifications of war on the body, Confederate veterans survived and remained mentally alert and willing to discuss their participation in the war. Pollard called on his fellow southerners to look beyond the empty sleeve and broken body and see the noble and honorable soldier now masked by disability.[18]

Many amputees did feel genuinely appreciated. Major John C. Haskell, who lost his right arm, spent some time with a group of women on a porch in Richmond. Haskell, described as being "very handsomely dressed," had a "short military cloak thrown over his shoulders." As Haskell conversed with the ladies, a group of Confederate soldiers marched by and admired Haskell's impeccable taste in clothing. Suddenly, Haskell "wheeled and faced them and threw back his cape showing his empty sleeve." The soldiers "took off their hats and one continuous cheer greeted him as the whole corps passed, each regiment catching inspiration from the one ahead of it," according to an eyewitness. In 1905 a Memorial Day service in Albany, Georgia, brought "tears to hundreds of eyes." As one eyewitness recalled, "Every head was white or streaked with gray and nearly every form was bent. Here was an empty sleeve, there was a leg of cork." Another Confederate soldier returned home to Alabama and noticed dozens of men who waited for their wounds to heal and looked like they had traveled through "some kind of butchering machine" that trimmed away arms and legs or created holes all over the human body. The veteran felt sorry for his physically altered compatriots, feeling that they were in a class by themselves.[19]

This initial wave of sympathy certainly had the potential to benefit veterans who struggled financially after the war. On one occasion, Richard Ewell spoke with Duff Green, who had also lost a leg in the war. As their conversation commenced on a street corner in Richmond, a factory owner from Georgia saw them looking "homely" and offered them jobs at his factory. It is suggestive that the factory owner, while well-intentioned, assumed that their missing legs meant Ewell and Green were probably lower class. When Ewell and Green turned him down, he responded, "Well gentlemen I beg your pardon but you looked like common folks mightily." Interestingly Ewell and Green did not interpret the remarks of the factory owner as an insult to their honor. In the antebellum era, such remarks might even have precipitated a duel or a cowhiding for failure to recognize an honorable gentleman. But in the postwar period, where the economy was broken and white bodies with it, such mistakes were forgivable.[20]

The interplay between Ewell and Green and the factory owner conveys a small sense of the muddying of white male symbology in the postwar South. With the system of slavery destroyed, the landscape of the South in shambles, houses fallen and fortunes with it, men broken psychologically and physically, the elite southern gentlemen could no longer guarantee that they would be recognized. Jefferson Davis's call on southerners to treat amputees as a new aristocracy only blurred class lines further. For generations, as Elliot Gorn has argued, scars reflected the marks of lower class men who resorted to fist fights and brawls to protect their manhood. Thus, the factory owner was trapped between an older symbology and a new one, between old and new ways of reading class and status in the New South.[21]

There is another reason the factory owner assumed Ewell and Green were poor: most amputees probably were. Southern culture could say what it might about elevating amputees to a new aristocracy, but in reality thousands of impoverished or middling-class men who relied on manual labor struggled financially in the postwar period. During the war, one chaplain had tried to explain to a Confederate amputee how God would give a good Christian man meaningful employment after the war. But it was not that simple. The southern economy was decimated and had never placed tremendous emphasis on manual labor jobs for whites. As veterans returned to farms they could not work, and in their town searching for social, economic, and medical support, they often found they had nothing but charity to rely on.[22]

Such economic struggles were represented in various cultural venues throughout the South. *The Ku Klux Klan; or, The Carpet-Bagger in New Orleans*, a play published in 1877, told the story of Peter Plucky, a Confederate veteran who lost both arms in the Civil War and lived with a lame leg. He bemoaned that his children had to pick up "rags for their livin'" and found their breakfast in "the gutters." Plucky called himself a "poor piece of a man" and wished he had been "shot in the head" instead. As the Confederate veteran contemplated suicide, a Union amputee approached him. In an act of reconciliation, the Union man thanked the tattered Confederate for saving his life at a battlefield near Richmond. Both men shared a distinct commonality, a missing limb that brought them together again in a moment when past scores had receded into history. Captain Tommy Truegrit, the Union officer, told the distraught Confederate, "Don't look at life through such blue glasses. The sun shines yet. You can eat, drink, and sleep, as well as if you had a dozen arms." Truegrit also optimistically predicted the end of Reconstruction and a lousy economy with Democratic victories across Louisiana. He also invited Plucky to join him as partner in a new grocery business.[23]

After all, Truegrit, unlike his southern counterpart, received a lucrative government pension and he wanted to bury the sectional hatchet, permanently, in the ground of mutual endurance. "[Your sons]," Truegrit declared, "shall have two pieces of men for their daddy—[and] two pieces make one pretty good whole." Plucky accepted the offer and soon discovered that the generous Yankee had fallen in love with his daughter, Polly, who despised Yankees. Although Polly appreciated the warm gesture of Truegrit financing the new family store, she knew she could never love "a mean Yankee." While Truegrit wondered if his empty sleeve had ruined his chances with Polly, she reminded him that an empty sleeve was "not the worst defect" but rather his Yankee identity. Truegrit wished that "an ocean of love" could wash away the bitterness of the Civil War. As in any love story, in the very end, Polly changed her mind and married the Yankee amputee who saved her destitute family.[24]

The theatrical tale of Truegrit and Plucky reveals a wealth of issues facing Confederate amputees in the postwar era. The Confederate veteran struggled to find meaningful employment and could not support his children. Many nonelite amputees returned home unable to continue in their professions because of their disability, which threatened their ability to earn a living. The inability to support his dependents turned the Confederate veteran into a psychologically distraught dependent, who contemplated suicide and wished he had just died on the field with all the others. The play reminded southern audiences that while Union veterans received pensions, their own veterans waited decades for any financial assistance. Indeed, Peter Plucky's survival remained dependent on an act of kindness from a Yankee, whose grocery store business emerged as a symbol of reconciliation between North and South. Amputation was the common bond in this popular play, the symbol of the mutuality of sacrifice and the petty pointlessness of holding grudges. Erasing African

Americans from the picture, the fiction depicted a white America that was all broken alike and needed to come together for patriarchy to be again whole ("Two pieces of men for their daddy, and two pieces make one pretty good whole").[25]

To be sure many Confederate amputees did make adjustments and were able to continue as farmers. John Bunyon Samples of Georgia lost his leg but persevered, utilizing his prosthetic device to help him navigate around the fields. Another armless Confederate veteran had no other economic opportunities and found himself forced to farm to support his wife and four daughters. John Read, who lost a leg during the early part of the war, returned home and worked in a tobacco house in a "greatly reduced" condition, laboring at a slow but persistent pace. A Confederate soldier in Georgia, missing both arms, spent his postwar years hitched to a plow that his wife guided; supplying all of the muscle and none of the direction, he must have felt like a mule.[26]

Many men, though, were simply too disabled to farm. Some of these eventually found employment through their pen when memoir writing became potentially lucrative in the 1880s. John Robson, who served in the Fifty-Second Virginia Infantry, wrote a memoir detailing his wartime experiences. Grandly echoing Lost Cause principles, Robson crafted his memoir to serve the greater glory of Thomas "Stonewall" Jackson, a fellow amputee, rather than focusing on his own difficult readjustment to society. As Robson noted in his preface, "My chief object in this work is to get something to support myself with—in fact, it is a scheme founded on food, raiment and shelter, which I find hard to come at by one in my situation." Robson, who lost his right leg at Cedar Creek on October 19, 1864, had little education and job training and refused all charity. His memoir allowed him to strike one last blow for his cause (and allowed those who wanted to offer charity do so through the purchase of his book).[27]

Other disabled veterans sought solace in education, taking classes and even taking up teaching positions at a variety of schools and universities around the South. The University of Virginia in 1864 agreed to offer free courses to any Confederate veterans discharged from the war due to severe injuries. Georgia set up a progressive educational opportunity for all disabled veterans, as members of the legislature argued that education might be necessary for those indigent and maimed soldiers who could no longer perform physical labor. Such handicapped veterans received three hundred dollars to cover their educational expenses at one of five Georgia colleges and universities and agreed to work as a teacher following their education. Outside of Georgia, amputated veterans taught at a variety of public schools and institutions of higher learning. One veteran who lost an arm at the Battle of Winchester taught Latin at the Virginia Military Institute and his colleague, who also lost an arm during the war, taught mathematics. Columbus Washington O'Hara, who lost his left arm while fighting with the Eighteenth Alabama, taught in the public schools for a decade, using his work as a teacher to support his wife and six children.[28]

Teaching was an attractive alternative to many amputees no longer able to work in their prewar professions, but some were not suited to it temperamentally, having unresolved issues related to wartime trauma. James Fraser, who lost his right leg in 1862, returned home after his amputation to a society he no longer recognized. Unable to farm or participate in manual labor, Fraser turned to teaching as a means of economic survival, but he routinely lashed out at people and, as one acquaintance understated, "He has not led a very enviable life since the war." Despite his bitterness, Fraser eventually married a widow, Eliza Crenshaw, who had children. After Eliza's death, the court removed the children when accusations of physical abuse surfaced. Fraser also faced murder charges for allegedly killing the man who had taken the children in, Dr. Joseph Dunwoody.[29]

There were some success stories, however, and in the class fluidity after the war, some men who might otherwise have always been farmers were given new opportunities to rise into the professional ranks. Thomas W. Dodd, who lost an arm during the Atlanta campaign, went to law school after the war and emerged as a prominent attorney in Texas, while another Confederate officer, who lost a leg, emerged as an important lawyer in Arkansas. Alfred Flournoy Zachary, who lost his left arm at Spotsylvania, worked in a dry goods store, while another southern amputee did not let the loss of an arm during the war deter him from working in the railroad industry. John Manly Richardson lost his left leg and spent his postwar years establishing Bowdon Collegiate Institution in Georgia, where he served as the school's president. Another armless veteran somehow continued his medical practice after the war.[30]

William M. McGalliard, who lost a leg at Gettysburg, emerged as another economic success story among Confederate amputees. As a traveling physician, McGalliard used a buggy, but his prosthetic leg made it difficult to get in and out on a daily basis without bumping into the wheels. He wrote to the Wheeler Carriage Company about designing a specific vehicle to accommodate his injury. The company responded that their doctor buggies had been designed with wheels at a higher location that allowed the doctor "to get in or out without coming in contact with the wheels." The new carriage took about six weeks to construct and cost two hundred fifty dollars.[31]

With a better mode of transport in hand, McGalliard traveled around New Orleans but found his prosthetic leg broke on a regular basis. Although he found someone willing to fix the limb, the repairer eventually abandoned the business and returned to working as a carpenter because the dearth of patients hampered his financial prospects in the prosthetic limb industry. With his usual repairer gone, McGalliard sought out A. C. McDermott and urged him to start an artificial limb business on Camp Street in New Orleans. McDermott agreed, and McGalliard became one of his first customers, as the amputee received a new prosthetic device from the state of Louisiana in 1884. The new leg allowed for a greater range of motion and made McGalliard's days of travel from patient to patient a more comfortable and bearable enterprise.[32]

While some amputated men found economic success in medicine, others entered the political arena, partly to earn a living and partly to advocate for other amputated men through the passage of legislation caring for damaged veterans and their widows. Like the "bloody shirt," the "empty sleeve" was a mainstay of southern politics in the postwar period. During the April 1866 elections in Natchitoches, Louisiana, for instance, the local newspaper endorsed three amputees for office. All three men had lost an arm during the Civil War and thus, according to the paper, deserved the victory. However, one reader protested. He stated, "There are other noble Confederates before the people and to make such an issue against them . . . simply because they were fortunate enough to return from the conflict of arms with sound limbs, is in bad taste." For this particular writer, being an amputee did not immediately qualify a man for office, and he expressed outrage that a newspaper would endorse a candidate simply because he lost a limb. It is interesting, however, that his anger stemmed from the fact that the limbless should rank above other men, merely above other *Confederates*.[33]

The politics of the empty sleeve was not peculiar to the South. Northerners also elected large numbers of amputated men and used partial men as a rallying cry for political action. Two months before the presidential election of 1868, for instance, an editorial appeared in the *New York Tribune* titled "Empty Sleeves." The author recalled seeing a wealth of Union amputees, all living reminders of the suffering, torture, and starvation in southern prison camps. The author then turned to the election and demanded that amputated veterans cast ballots for Republican Ulysses S. Grant, who recognized the meaning of sacrifice still embodied in the thousands of empty sleeves all over the North.[34]

Southerners followed suit, using the empty sleeve to rally voters and backing numerous amputated men for electoral office. When white southerners went to the polls and cast ballots for disabled Confederate veterans, they were working, in part, to restore the white patriarchy that had been undermined by defeat and Reconstruction. Southern white men used the electoral process to restore elite men, who served as officers and may have lost a limb during the war, to positions of political power. As time passed and southern society embraced the empty sleeve as a symbol of sacrifice rather than defeat, they reaffirmed the shattered manhood of their wounded veterans and granted them electoral success at all levels of local and state government. Indeed, over time, the empty sleeve, partly because it is visually available but not visually repulsive, trumped other injuries as a decided political asset.[35]

The politics of the empty sleeve ran deeper and broader than electability, however. As historian William Blair notes, "Speakers used the image of the crippled veteran to prevent disgruntled white men from breaking party ranks and to build a new Democratic Party that was once again national." The new Democratic Party, built on the rhetoric of the damaged veteran, included several amputees who won gubernatorial elections all across the South. Francis Redding Tillou Nicholls lost his left arm and left leg during the Civil War, and he asked the voters of Louisiana to elect what was left of him for governor, which they did twice. He joked that he needed to go into politics because he "was too one-sided to be a judge." Wade Hampton, who lost a leg, won the governorship of South Carolina, and James Lawson Kemper, who dealt with an attached but paralyzed leg, secured the governorship in Virginia. James Berry, who predicted his own electoral success as governor of Arkansas when marrying Lizzie Quaile, received numerous accolades for his political leadership.

One eulogy praised Berry for limping back to his native state as a maimed man, declaring that his missing limb was not a symbol of shattered manhood but gave Berry a platform to reinforce the highest ideals of southern manhood through his work on behalf of damaged veterans and in marking the graves of the war dead.[36]

Thus did southerners send limbless men to all levels of the political process. Amputees found success as city treasurers, judges, tax collectors, registrars of deeds, and state legislators. Jesse Malcolm Carmichael, who lost his hand during the war, had failed at farming before he made a successful run as a state legislator in Alabama. Another amputated veteran worked behind the scenes on political campaigns and routinely engaged legislators in Tennessee on behalf of destitute and damaged veterans. Charles L. Sowell, born and raised among the aristocracy on a South Carolina plantation, lost his left arm during the Civil War. Although he had been described after the war as "hopelessly maimed, penniless, tattered, and without promise of a future," he secured a position as tax assessor, which allowed him to rise above his injury and depressed condition.[37]

Some Confederate amputees held multiple elected positions at the state and national level and used their electoral fame to foster an environment of reconciliation. William C. Oates, who lost an arm during the Civil War, held several political positions, including governor of Alabama and U.S. congressman. After he lost a bid for U.S. Senate, President William McKinley asked him to fight in the Spanish-American War. As a staunch Confederate, Oates pondered the invitation. "Times change and we change with them. I believed implicitly in the righteousness of the cause of the Confederacy and served it to the best of my ability until it went down in smoke and blood." However, the acrimonious memories of the war receded and he stated, "The United States is now my government and with my one arm I will serve it as faithfully as I did the Confederacy. I now don the uniform and wave the flag upon which many times from 1861 to 1865 I ordered my command to fire. I am now a Yankee general, formerly a Rebel colonel, right each time." (Oates had long desired a brigadier general position during the Civil War, and now he accepted the rank, though in a U.S. uniform.)[38]

The presence of so many amputated men in political office drew sharp criticism from political opponents. In the state of Virginia in 1879, the Readjusters, a biracial political movement led by William Mahone, stormed into power in the state legislature. The political movement supported public education, shunned government corruption, and worked to secure some civil rights for black voters. A newspaper editorial envisioned a new place for amputated veterans in politics now that the Readjusters had assumed political control. "Make way there, you crippled Confederate soldiers. . . . You fought and bled in defense of Virginia; you served her faithfully in war and peace; you are crippled for life, and performed the duties of your office well and faithfully, but you must now limp out on your remaining limb and give your place to an able-bodied man." The harsh editorial noted that while amputated men may have found some electoral success after the war, the era of the "crippled soldier" had ended in favor of a new vision of political dominance on behalf of African Americans.[39]

Behind of all of these success stories and paeans to the disabled vet, however, lurked a large number of men who never really recovered from their war service, men who languished in the alms houses, the insane asylums, the drunk tanks, the prisons, and the graveyards. After returning home following the loss of his leg at Fort Donelson in 1862, Marion Albertis Misenheimer stated, "But the war coming on—knocked me out of an education such as I wanted as well as disabling me from manual labor therefore. I have had kind of an uphill pull [since]." One Confederate amputee arrived at the poor house and demanded financial assistance because he had sacrificed a limb for the "lost cause." Another veteran wrote the state government in Virginia to point out how many "crippled soldiers" are starving on the streets or residing in the poor house. Exasperated, he declared, "I for one am a one legged man all most on starvation." Another amputee in Virginia feared he would end up sent to a poor house because he lacked a few dollars.[40]

More amputees, however, fell back on their family, perpetually trying and failing to eke out a living. Charles Moore Jr., who lost a leg at Gettysburg while fighting with the Fifth Louisiana, found himself unemployed twelve years after the war. He noted, "Truly it seems to me that the time has come when 'No Maimed Confederate Need Apply.'" Moore, who lost his position as a clerk, felt he had failed as a man because he had not been able to financially support his family, which resulted in their eviction from their house. Other amputated veterans never found work, earned not enough to survive, or ended up fired from their job due to their disability. R. B. Clements, who lost an arm, found himself fired from his job as janitor and mule watcher at the Richmond armory because of his physical condition. Another veteran in Louisiana worked as an impoverished carpenter and expressed his frustration about trying to financially survive with a disability. "A man with one arm cannot be expected to make as much as one with two." Another one-armed veteran tried to work as a police officer but was not hired. Instead, he slowly painted homes in order to survive.[41]

With few employment options, forestalled educations, or disabilities that prevented manual labor, some Confederate amputees turned of necessity to begging. Thomas Drinkard, who lost an arm during the war, worked as a policeman and city tax collector in Richmond, but when he lost his job, he struggled to pay his mortgage. He begged the governor of Virginia, also disabled as a result of the war, "*Please do what you can. I am very much in need.*" The governor agreed and paid Drinkard sixty dollars for his military service. An unnamed Confederate veteran, who lost his leg at Atlanta in 1864, was a fixture at the steps of the capitol in Austin, Texas. A physician who saw him reflected that begging had emerged as a routine practice across the South, as ex-Confederates stumped their "weary way through life on crutches or a wooden leg; so common that it does not challenge a remark, or hardly a notice; we do not give it a thought." Of course, the decrepit, grizzled, and gray veteran on the capitol steps could not afford an artificial limb, which partly explains why he ended up selling pencils on the steps of the capitol. Depending on the manufacturer, artificial legs cost anywhere from seventy to over a hundred dollars, at a time when the average laborer earned about a dollar a day. When the doctor approached the veteran, he felt a tinge of guilt for a man "neglected, despised, alone," and asked for several pencils, as he claimed to have run out at home. As the physician reflected on the meaning of the empty sleeve, he declared, "Poor old Confed. Despised old 'rebel.' They told you a wound would be an honor, and you a hero. Cruel mockery. Bitter deception. Your life blood shed, your youth wasted; all in vain."[42]

Even begging had its barriers, however. In 1879, the city of New Orleans cracked down on street beggars, especially those who had been wounded, injured, or diseased. Men were particularly forbidden from "wandering abroad and endeavoring by the exposure of wounds or deformities to obtain and gather alms." One New Orleans newspaper decried, "The whole community is shocked, disgusted and sickened that these maimed

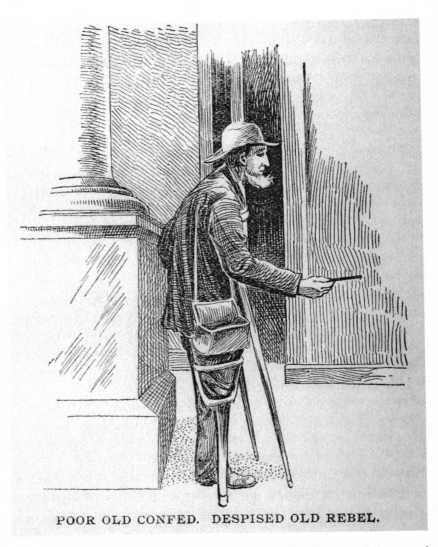

POOR OLD CONFED. DESPISED OLD REBEL.

Figure 17. An unnamed Confederate amputee on the steps of the Texas capitol. Courtesy of the Reynolds Historical Library, University of Alabama at Birmingham.

beggars may secure a few nickels." In 1883, the city organized an event known as "Corralling the Cripples," wherein city officials picked up disabled beggars, including Confederate veterans, and placed them in the Shakespeare Alms House. Realizing that Confederate veterans faced punishment under strict begging laws across the South, many southern cities amended legislation to protect war veterans from excessive fines or imprisonment related to begging. Even with such exceptions made, the lines between wounded veterans and imposters were difficult to draw. The state of Georgia effectively licensed maimed and disabled veterans to allow them to peddle in the towns and cities free and unmolested provided they did not sell spirits and had a certificate issued from the county of residence stating they were a disabled Confederate veteran. (The legislature approved the new licensing law on September 26, 1883.)[43]

Confederate amputees forced to beg for money exhibited a heightened level of dependence not merely on family and community but on strangers. The preferred arrangements for this kind of assistance were the benevolent organizations that sprung up across the South during and after the Civil War. Asking for such help came at a price, as some men decried admitting that they had failed to support themselves and had no one else to fall back on. One former Confederate noted, "The thought of having to go to the Paupers Home is a horror and a dread to many of us old vets, to beg, we are ashamed; to accept the charity of friends in case we have them is humiliating." Some amputated men shuddered at the thought of having to spend their waning days on earth reliant on a charitable organization or group of individuals who financially supported their very means of existence. Yet men had few options, especially when they faced dire economic opportunities and lackadaisical state legislatures that did not quickly reach consensus on how to support their veterans.[44]

Benevolent groups saw their greatest success in the supply of artificial limbs. On January 22, 1864, citizens in Richmond formed the Association for the Relief of Maimed Soldiers (ARMS). The organization wanted to seek out the "benevolent and patriotic Confederate citizens" to unite them in the cause of providing artificial limbs to Confederate veterans, as many had witnessed "the sight of empty sleeves and of men hobbling on wooden pegs, or swinging on the gallant crutch." ARMS stressed that providing limbs was an act not of charity but of "esteem, respect and gratitude" and hoped to provide nearly ten thousand limbs. Their scope of assistance extended far out of Richmond, as they requested "that the mayor of every city, and county judge of every county, in the Confederate States" be named "an assistant treasurer" to help collect membership dues. Through the payment of ten dollars annually or a lifetime membership of three hundred, ARMS purchased and distributed hundreds of artificial legs across the South. Many members and companies donated several hundred dollars beyond the membership-level dues, including E. M. Bruce, who donated five thousand. Early after its inception, the group accounted for nearly twenty thousand dollars in donations.[45]

The members of the benevolent organization believed they had to supply artificial limbs to amputated men because no one else would. The leader of Richmond's relief organization worked quickly to produce prosthetic devices and asked a carpenter in January 1864 to immediately begin construction of one thousand artificial legs. Even if the carpenter was not willing to fill the order, the director asked him to make at least one for display in the Richmond office. Ultimately, he wanted the craftsman to construct "some cheap, simple, strong and durable apparatus, to supply the loss that battle has caused to so many of our brave soldiers." Although the leadership presented the artificial limb construction job to several people, they eventually selected Wells and Company, which produced artificial legs at three different prices: $125 for amputations below the knee, $150 for those at the knee, and $175 for those above the knee. With prosthetic production a relatively novel enterprise, some board members feared that Wells could produce only two hundred prosthetics a month for the nine thousand veterans in need. Furthermore, with battles raging in Virginia in the spring of 1864, more men found themselves in dire need of a prosthetic device.[46]

With thousands of Confederate veterans initially dependent on benevolent groups to furnish an artificial leg, leadership within the groups felt overwhelmed and dependent on the generosity of Confederate citizens to rally behind their patriotic duty to care for the men who bore the scars of war. C. K. Marshall, president of ARMS, believed that citizens needed to donate money rather than participate in "unproductive and idle sentimentalism" and constant crying at the sight of amputated men across the South. Marshall asked that if civilians "cannot offer our limbs in the holocaust demanded by the blood-thirsty spirit of our barbarous invaders, may we not furnish the poor substitutes of human contrivance to those who need them?" The organization raised $113,464 and bought the legs from either overseas or from manufacturers in North and South Carolina, Alabama, Georgia, and Virginia. As long as the Confederate veteran swore an oath and provided documentation on their military service and the nature of their injury, they received the complimentary prosthetic.[47]

In addition to wartime groups that bestowed prosthetic limbs, Confederate veterans found multiple organizations that embraced their sacrifices and worked to maintain their health and welfare in the postwar years. The United Daughters of the Confederacy organized themselves around a principle of benevolent care "for the maimed and indigent soldiers of the Confederacy, their widows and children," as well as maintaining Confederate homes and their subsequent hospitals with delicacies "in order that our soldiers may answer to the last roll-call surrounded by the comforts of life." In 1906, H. A. Sommers delivered an address that later appeared in the written proceeding of the United Daughters of the Confederacy. Sommers used the occasion to draw a sharp contrast between the Union and Confederate postwar experiences in the American Civil War. He stated, "The Northern soldier returned to prosperous homes and full granaries, to a land that had not felt the touch of marching armies, and to pensions from a grateful government." At the same time, Confederate soldiers "returned to a home burnt by the ravages of the enemy to a land desolated by tramping thousands and conquering hordes." Southern men faced a shattered world "without money, without provisions, without pensions, with his slaves freed and unaccustomed to work." On another occasion, B. S. Grannis spoke similar sentiments to the Daughters of the Confederacy. He pointed out how southern men did not return home and sit about and cry. Instead, they worked and taught their children to embrace hard work, while their northern compatriots "loafed away their time and waited for the pension check to arrive."[48]

In addition to the United Daughters of the Confederacy, the United Confederate Veterans emerged to assist the war's wounded. Since the group was composed of veterans, it functioned as a self-help and fraternal organization. By 1893, according to Joseph Jones, the UCV had nearly 25,000 members in 251 camps across the nation. Leaders in 100 of the camps revealed the presence of only 270 disabled members, signifying that damaged men, if still alive, did not share a desire to join a group that would force them to relive the memories of a war that had produced so much personal suffering. A year later, the UCV Constitution provided a specific article declaring that the organization would "relieve the deserving veterans who may be in distress." In addition to caring for the widows of soldiers and sailors "who bore themselves honorably and gave life to the cause," the UCV worked to "educate and assist the orphans of veterans." The UCV did not specifically mention the care of amputees. Rather, the constitution stipulated that a "Committee on Relief and Donations" would be formed consisting of five members who would oversee the collection of "material aid and assistance" for veterans, widows, and orphaned children. The organization held several reunions across the South. In June 1917, the members gathered in Washington, D.C., and one of the invited guests was James E. Hanger, the very first Confederate amputee, who was wounded at Philippi in Barbour County, Virginia, on June 3, 1861. Hanger developed a successful prosthetic leg still in production today.[49]

When a national organization like the UDC or UCV had little direct impact on bettering the life of an amputee, some dependent men had no choice but to look to local organizations for assistance. The Confederate Survivors Association, organized in Augusta, Georgia, gathered yearly, beginning in 1879, with Charles C. Jones Jr. serving as the organization's president. In his presidential address on April 26, 1880, Jones recognized Private William M. Dunbar, who lost his right arm during the war. Jones announced that Dunbar had received unanimous election to the post of color bearer for the organization. The group also passed a resolution that named all members "who lost a leg or an arm in the service" to the Color Guard. Jones worried about the amputees who could not access pensions and residencies in a home for veterans. However, when the organization reconvened a year later, the talk shifted from care for amputated men to the broader Lost Cause. Jones called for monument construction, the remembrance of the dead, and the end of all vestiges of Reconstruction, rather than caring for the living. Although they remained committed to benevolence and camaraderie, the Confederate Survivors Association cast its lot with the political and social dimensions of the Lost Cause.[50]

Confederate amputees participated only marginally in events that smacked of the Lost Cause. This limited participation may have been the result of a number of factors, including difficulty traveling to the celebratory location and the financial burdens of dues and traveling to events. They may also have had a genuine disinterest in organizations that celebrated veterans better in rhetoric than in practice. After all, while the Lost Cause organizations hailed the honorable sacrifices of an entire generation of veterans, they failed to raise a substantial amount of capital to help those very veterans survive, outside of commemorating their sacrifices. Paeans to the dead, apparently, were easier to deliver than alms to the living.[51]

As they aged, many Confederates turned to residence in a Confederate home as their only viable option for medical care, sustenance, and shelter. The Texas Confederate Veterans Home, located in Austin Texas, admitted, according to records, thirty-six amputees between 1887 and 1919. Among the amputees, twenty had lost a leg, thirteen an arm, one a hand, and two their feet during the war. In addition to missing limbs, some of the veterans suffered from arthritis, blindness, and natural old age. Over half of the patients had been farmers prior to their entrance into the home. The rest of the amputees had worked in a variety of vocations, including carpenter, blacksmith, lawyer, physician, rancher, clerk, merchant, mechanic, saddle and harness maker, and auctioneer.[52]

Willis Parsons, who lost his left leg at Peachtree Creek in 1864, moved into the Kentucky Confederate Home at Pewee Valley in December 1904 and lived there for two years until his death. W. H. Arnold, who lost a leg at Chickamauga, and Thomas B. Cheatham, who lost his left leg below the knee, also resided in the Kentucky facility. Cheatham needed a veteran's home because he owned no personal property and constantly suffered from the ramifications of his amputation as well as an enlarged prostate and rheumatoid arthritis. Ultimately, though, even with dozens of benevolent groups and assisted living facilities helping thousands of dependent amputees, the problem, as men aged, became simply too large and ultimately demanded a concerted effort from the state.[53]

The loss of a limb during the American Civil War traumatized the mind and body of thousands of Confederate soldiers and produced numerous challenges, beyond the mere healing of broken limbs and bones. As men hobbled home to shattered communities, these onetime masters of worlds, large and small, became dependent on families, communities, and southern society at large for psychological support and economic opportunities in order to care for themselves and their families. As amputated men struggled to cope with chronic pain and the limitations of the postwar economy, southern society evolved to recognize the empty sleeve as a symbol of sacrifice, rather than defeat, and exceptional amputees were elected to political office, were offered employment, and helped to direct benevolent organizations that sought to maintain the health and welfare of an entire generation of men traumatized by the experience of war. Ultimately, it was not enough; Confederate amputees needed additional help to survive, and state governments became the only entities capable of responding to the needs of an aging, ailing, deeply symbolic population.

FIVE

The State

The Politics of Paying Damages

War unmakes legs and human skill must supply their places as best it may.
—Oliver Wendell Holmes, 1863

In 1876, at the opening of the Centennial Exhibition in Philadelphia, controversy swirled over the inclusion of Peter Rothermel's painting, *Battle of Gettysburg: Pickett's Charge.* In addition to reigniting sectional animosities that many had sought to bury, the dramatic and violent painting drew criticism for historical inaccuracies, including placing the July 2 Battle of Little Round Top in the background and putting Union general George Meade on the scene. The controversy generated its own cartoon: a one-legged Union and one-legged Confederate veteran argue before the painting. Each man supports his body weight with a crutch in order to wildly gesture in front of the painting. The text accompanying the image reads, "Two one-legged relics of the late war, both of whom claim to have taken part in the original, stood before it, wrangling and almost fighting it over again."[1]

By 1876, amputated men had become the symbolic embodiment of the Civil War and its legacy. Veterans' need for financial and material support particularly triggered intense and important debates. In the immediate postwar years they had struggled to secure gainful employment, prosthetics, and health care. In the fall of 1865, a Confederate veteran, identifying himself as "One Arm," lashed out at the politicians in North Carolina for neglecting his fellow veterans from the Civil War. Appalled at the silence coming from political candidates on what would be done to "comfort the poor unfortunate man who has his feeble scarred body suspended on crutches," he wondered what would become of the "poor creature who has hanging by his side an empty coat sleeve." With the former

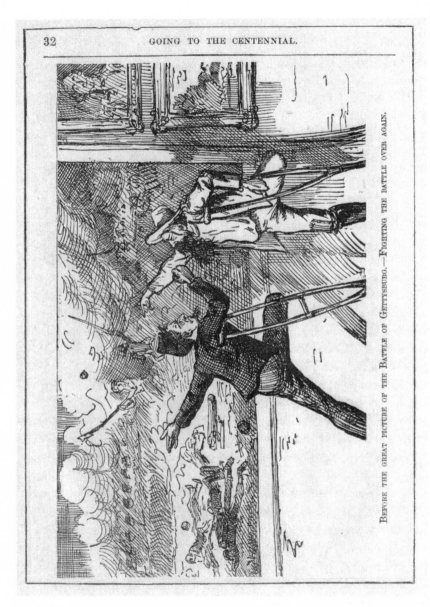

Figure 18. Bricktop Stories, *Before the Great Picture of the Battle of Gettysburg.—Fighting the Battle over Again*, from *Going to the Centennial, and A Guy to the Great Exhibition*, 1876. Courtesy of the Print and Picture Collection, Free Library of Philadelphia.

Confederacy sapped of economic productivity and potential by the collapse of slavery and the hard hand of war, the "maimed of the land" faced "hard times." The veteran pleaded, "Give us a chance and we will not be a burden to the country."[2]

Clement J. Moody followed the lead of his fellow veteran in North Carolina when he pleaded with the Tennessee legislature to care for the veterans, who had been neglected since the end of the war. "When the Southern Confederacy had been wrapped in her bloody winding sheet, and the formally cherished hope of the South had gone down in darkness and in death," he argued, the transition had begun for veterans to return to public life. He noted the men "stacked their guns at Appomattox and began their lonesome journey home" in "sorrowful sadness." Moody observed, "Some came home with empty sleeves, some came hobbling home on one leg, some left both legs on the battlefield, some with sightless eyeballs groped their way home in blindness, in darkness—all came in tatters and rags to look upon the ashes of their ruined homes." He pleaded that veterans needed care as they already had started perish "and will soon be gone."[3]

Ultimately the plight of the dependent veteran could not be met by the support of women or traditional, prewar sources of aid from voluntary contributions and associations. The scale of the problem demanded a larger solution, which could be overseen only by the state. This of course was mimicked in the North, as the U.S. government provided Union amputees with the opportunity to procure artificial limbs from 1862 until after World War I. Each veteran received free transportation to the limb fitting and also got fifty dollars to purchase an artificial foot or arm and seventy-five for a leg. Oliver Wendell Holmes echoed the importance of northern amputees receiving prosthetic limbs. "A plain working man, who has outlived his courting-days and need not sacrifice much to personal appearance, may find an honest, old-fashioned wooden leg, cheap, lasting, requiring no repairs, the best thing for his purpose." In addition to providing prosthetic limbs to Union veterans, the federal government had instituted an elaborate pension system in the 1860s and 1870s that paid up to thirty-one dollars per month to injured and diseased Union veterans. Caring for the wounded victors remained a dominant item in the U.S. budget, as pension programs accounted for nearly 40 percent of the federal budget by the 1890s. Thus, the U.S. government set the precedent for the state supporting those who arguably sacrificed themselves for it.[4]

At the same time, the U.S. government had blocked any financial support, prosthetic limbs, or pensions for Confederate veterans through stipulations built into the Fourteenth Amendment. Section 4 prohibited the U.S. government from paying any financial obligations tied directly to the aid of those who had participated in the rebellion against the United States. During the war, Confederate veterans had turned to the Confederate Congress, which voted in 1863 to permit injured soldiers to continue collecting their salaries as soldiers if the "wounds or injuries received in service" prevented them from finding meaningful employment. Legislators had also agreed to help cover transportation costs to move disabled soldiers from hospital beds to homes.[5]

Obviously the destruction of the Confederacy and the position of the federal government had forced damaged men to look elsewhere for help, with mixed results, as we saw in the last chapter. This chapter focuses on Confederate amputees' "court of last resort"—their state governments. While the nature of the debates varied from state to state, the dire financial condition of virtually all of them made meaningful support of disabled veterans difficult and the federal politics of any such effort remained particularly treacherous. Some legislators questioned the constitutionality of providing benefits to a class of men who were either branded as traitors in the eyes of Unionist politicians and elected officials or seen as undeserving of support because, as some believed, dependency dishonored a man and stripped him of his dignity. Many legislators initially expressed opposition to state support for amputees because they remained rooted in rigid notions of manhood that did not permit outside assistance and had no room for a new class of dependent citizens.

Yet, in a handful of states, legislators agreed to provide prosthetic limbs, land parcels, and educational grants to the men who could prove they had honorably lost a leg (and later an arm) in their military service to the Confederacy. The three early modes of assistance were specifically designed to help amputated men remain self-sufficient. Postwar southern legislators clung to a prewar notion of masculinity and offered prosthetic limbs because they increased the mobility of a man who could now seek employment on his own accord. Land and educational grants provided mechanisms for amputated veterans to have a plot of land for the family to work or a degree that may open up career opportunities. All three areas of assistance, although they cost several thousand dollars, emerged as a relatively small financial commitment from state budgets trying to rebound from the chaos of war and reconstruction.

However, as we saw in the previous chapter, a vast number of veterans begged on the streets after they found limited economic opportunities. Aging veterans, who were no longer self-sufficient and were unable to provide for their families, forced a reconsideration of state policy. While it may have been unseemly or unmanly for men to accept help from the government, it was necessary in the postwar years. Following redemption, when southern state legislatures started to consider wide-scale pension programs, gender standards underwent a reconstitution across the South that would permit a measure of dependency. With so many destitute men unable to provide for their families, which had been a central tenet of traditional masculinity, the state stepped in to help restore men's bodies so they could be self-sufficient, or even, in extreme cases, stand in as the ersatz patriarch. Ultimately all former Confederate states acquiesced to the demands to help reconstruct the shattered male body and provided small-scale financial assistance in the form of prosthetic limbs, land parcels, veteran homes, and/or pensions.[6]

The extension of a massive amount of aid to a dependent group of citizens marked a new chapter in the history of social welfare policies in the South. Like their northern counterparts, antebellum southern states had provided assistance for the poor through local tax funds as well as creating almshouses and mental hospitals, but these programs had always been underfunded and the conditions often relatively poor. The outbreak of the Civil War had prompted southern state governments to issue an unprecedented amount of aid because, as one historian noted, "it was unthinkable that the wives and children of the brave fighting forces should have to accept the indignities of pauper relief." Thousands of residents had looked to their state governments as the only potential mechanism to get them through the difficult war years. Several southern states even created food programs through levying taxes or issuing bonds to ensure that needy residents survived. Once the Confederacy collapsed, the federal government, through efforts of the U.S. Army and the establishment of the Freedman's Bureau, stepped in to prevent mass-scale starvation. Hospitals and soup kitchens sprung up that transformed the lives of both white and black southerners. As one historian noted, the appearance of federal assistance allowed state governments to shift "their attentions exclusively on veterans and their families, leaving problems of freedmen and other poor whites to the state agencies."[7]

Such attention began with state-level artificial limb programs. Confederate amputees faced a cornucopia of choices, as the prosthetic industry exploded following the Civil War. James Hanger, himself a Confederate amputee, opened up artificial leg factories in Atlanta, St. Louis, and Richmond. As one historian noted, "Never had prostheses manufacturing possessed such commercial value as the artificial limb industry of the postwar South, where numbers of needy veterans far exceeded those who had been maimed in prewar farm accidents." Prosthetic devices earned 133 patents between the years of 1861 to 1873, representing a wide variety of styles, comfort, and feasibility. The variety of limbs also created a potential bidding war in some states, as companies lobbied members of the pension and prosthetic boards extensively to have their devices provided exclusively to all the wounded veterans in the state.[8]

One option among amputees was the Anglesea leg, constructed of brass and leather that allowed for a seamless fit, but a problematic ankle joint made the leg rather unsafe. Others purchased a Benjamin Franklin Palmer leg, which received numerous awards and endorsements from surgeons on both sides of the Atlantic. Other limbs, constructed out of willow, easily absorbed the shock and strain placed on the limbs through everyday walking. After a horrific wounding at Fredericksburg, Brigadier General George W. Price used a simple cork leg.[9]

Perhaps the most popular option was the prosthetic leg manufactured by Douglas Bly, which consisted of rubber with ivory balls to serve as sockets all tied together with cords. Bly's prosthetic devices received enormous attention, and he won awards at the state fairs of New York, Ohio, Indiana, Missouri, and Illinois, as well as larger fairs in Chicago and Cincinnati, where his patients stepped forward to both endorse and praise the mechanical legs and arms. Confederate officers emerged too as product spokesmen encouraging veterans to try out a Bly limb. Even John Bell Hood wrote Bly on January 11, 1867, "Sir, it is with pleasure that I state, that of all the artificial legs that I have used, I prefer that of Dr. Bly. I have tried the French, English and American. His has given me more satisfaction." Bly's company took great pride in Hood's endorsement. In

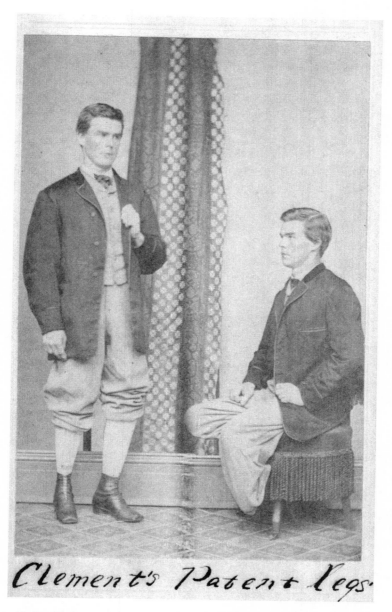

Clement's Patent legs.

Figure 19. In addition to providing testimony and sketches of the prosthetic devices, surgeon Richard Clements also provided this before-and-after photo that shows a veteran with and without his artificial legs. Courtesy of South Carolina Department of Archives and History.

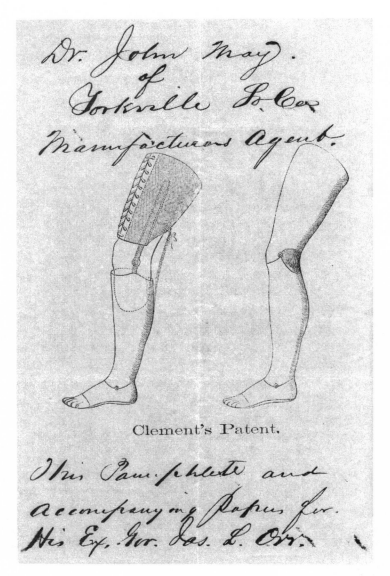

Clement's Patent.

Figure 20. Surgeon Richard Clements wrote the governor of South Carolina on numerous occasions in 1866 to secure a contract as the exclusive prosthetic limb manufacturer for all Confederate amputees in the state. He provided the governor with sketches of the prosthetic limb (shown here). He also offered abundant testimony from other Confederate veterans who acquired the prosthetic device and found it to be comfortable and superior to others. Although Clements made a strong case, Douglas Bly received the exclusive contract. Courtesy of South Carolina Department of Archives and History.

one advertisement, the company noted, "The late Brigadier General John Bell Hood wore one of these legs and praised it highly, after trying others which were not satisfactory." Captain J. S. Penet remarked, "The people around here don't know me anymore; before they used to know me two or three blocks away." Penet admitted he no longer recognized himself due to the high quality of the limb. "I will say that your name will go down to posterity—among the cripples at least—as a public benefactor," he noted. "I wish every soldier and sailor in the United States that needs an artificial limb had one of yours."[10]

Some limb manufactories, like Bly, competed nationally; others strove to work with individual states to become an official and exclusive supplier. Strasser and Callahan in Montgomery, Alabama, for instance, emerged as the official prosthetic limb company of the Yellowhammer State. Strasser and Callahan ostensibly boasted a prosthetic leg that was "equal if not superior to any other artificial limb" and excelled in "utility, durability and price." One exuberant Alabama citizen and prosthetic wearer vouched for the company, writing, "I have been wearing artificial legs and have worn one of Callahan and Strasser's and in my judgment those manufactured by them are, for general use, superior to any I have seen." Another appeal of the Callahan and Strasser prosthetic was that it could be easily repaired by any skillful mechanic. In an advertisement for the legs, the manufacturer declared, "The work that I turn out for simple construction and peculiar and skillful adaptation of the joints as well as superior durability and lightness cannot be surpassed by any yet brought to the notice of the public." The Strasser contract remained the premier distributor of artificial legs in Alabama until 1874.[11]

Another industry leader was the A. A. Marks Company of New York City. Marks forged an artificial leg containing rubber feet that increased the self-sufficiency of the amputee. The company showed off their prosthetic limb in an advertisement showcasing an amputee climbing a ladder. The ad noted, "With his rubber feet he can ascend or descend a ladder, balance himself on the rungs, and have his hands at liberty. He can work at the bench and earn a good day's wages. He can walk and mingle with persons without betraying his loss; in fact he is restored to his former self for all practical purposes." The Marks prosthetic won numerous awards, and the company claimed to have sold over nineteen thousand prosthetics across the globe, completing many an ex-Confederate man.[12]

As limb manufactories multiplied, local benevolent societies, then municipal and state governments, moved in to organize distribution. In New Market, Virginia, men and women gathered together in the Methodist church at six o'clock on the evening of February 1, 1864, to gather money in order to establish "a manufactory, at some suitable point within the limits of the Confederacy to furnish artificial limbs." The audience raised $650 that evening to care for any soldiers "who may have been, or may hereafter be so unfortunate as to be deprived of a limb."[13]

Despite the best of intentions, the New Market model simply would not work on a large scale as wounded vets poured back into the South. At varying times and with varying degrees of intensity, the states of North Carolina, Georgia, Mississippi, South Carolina, Virginia, Alabama, and Louisiana all instituted their own prosthetic limb programs. Prior to their legislatures taking up legislation, state officials requested a census to ascertain the number of disabled men residing within their state to understand the scope of financial commitment. Alabama called for a disabled census in 1865 so that they might provide care for "the illustrious men who, in the hour of peril, counted not their lives dear in the discharge of what they believed and felt to be their duty." Mississippi conducted a similar effort in 1865–66. J. L. Power, the superintendent of army records, predicted that Mississippi had at least three hundred veterans who lost a leg during the Civil War.[14] North Carolina called on each county sheriff to ascertain how many veteran amputees resided in each county and whether they lost an arm or a leg. County tax collectors in South Carolina counted amputees and returned rather uneven lists, as some collectors counted just legs while others counted arms and legs. Some officials tabulated all war injuries, including gunshot wounds, abdomen wounds, broken bones, paralysis, resections, and otherwise useless limbs that remained intact. The initial tally revealed 498 amputees in South Carolina.[15]

As state officials fanned out across the South to tabulate the number of amputated veterans, legislators began work on aggressive prosthetic programs. In early 1866, North Carolina authored the first state initiative to care for amputated men, and the legislature gave each veteran who lost a leg either an artificial limb or a one-time cash payment of seventy dollars. Both measures provided a means of self-sufficiency to the disabled veteran without making the man entirely dependent on the state. The newspapers heartily endorsed the resolution, the *Raleigh Daily Standard* championing the measure as one that could "make the man over again" and allow him to transition from consumer to producer. As the *Raleigh Sentinel* noted, "The State owes them, at least this small token of her appreciation." Because the legislators looked at economic livelihood only through mobility, however, the state ignored men who lost an arm, requiring them to purchase one through the state for fifty dollars. In December 1866, E. G. Cranford, who lost his arm at Spotsylvania Court House, vented his frustration in a letter to the governor. He pointed out, "It would be bad for a man to fight four years for his country and lose an arm and then have to pay for a wooden one." Cranford needed the prosthetic in order to find a job. State legislators had assumed that only legs would be required for men to find work and rectified their error on February 15, 1867, when they amended the program to provide free prosthetic arms or a one-time cash payment of fifty dollars.[16]

The assistance provided to Confederate amputees in North Carolina drew fire from some of the local citizens. John Robinson, a Unionist residing in Goldsboro, North Carolina, vented his frustration that traitors should be rewarded for their misdeeds during the war. "This sort of Compulsory Charity for treason may suit the palate of some," he complained, "but the Union men of this State would rather be the dispensers of their own bounty—What! Get legs and arms for wretches who, when our poor fellows sick and helpless fell into their hands, buried them alive in pits." Despite the objections of some Unionist citizens, North Carolina remained diligent in providing artificial limbs designed to ensure self-sufficiency to Confederate amputees, spending over eighty thousand dollars over the course of five years.[17]

While Georgia, Virginia, Mississippi, and Alabama constructed prosthetic programs similar to that of North Carolina, two other states became so embroiled in Unionist objections that their programs were delayed or suspended.[18] In September 1866, doctors George Trescott and Samuel Logan petitioned the state senate in South Carolina to follow the lead of their sister states across the South and provide prosthetic limbs to disabled veterans. The physicians noted how many destitute veterans simply could not afford a prosthetic device and they concluded, "We earnestly trust that our own state will not deny to those of her sons who have suffered on her behalf the means of obtaining relief at her expense." Three months after the impassioned plea, the legislature started an artificial leg program that later ended in 1869, as funds diminished, applications dried up, and the Republican Party rose to dominate the state legislature. After redemption, South Carolina state legislators once again returned to veterans' issues with new legislation passed at the end of 1879 that allocated more funds for assistance for amputated men.[19] Louisiana, controlled by the Union military through large portions of the Civil War through Reconstruction, faced similar Republican opposition, and thus Louisiana's prosthetic program did not appear until 1880. As one New Orleans paper observed after the state's redemption, "The war veterans who received as holiday presents artificial legs and arms, may be said to have been truly remembered."[20]

The amounts spent on prosthetic limbs in each state depended on the number of amputated men and the state's financial resources. Historians routinely cite the state of Mississippi as an example of large-scale assistance for amputees to note how citizens across the state embraced their wounded veterans and lifted them up with aggressive care. Prominent historians have declared that in the year after the Civil War, Mississippi spent 20 percent of its state budget on prosthetic devices. However, historians have routinely misread the law, which allocated 20 percent of the budget to care for "the relief of disabled veteran and destitute persons, with *preference* being given to widows and children of Confederate soldiers." Hard budget data display a dramatically different situation (see table 3). Beyond the data outlined in table 3, the state spent another $626.00 to purchase limbs from 1870–71, leaving $2,834.75 from the original allocation. In comparison, during budget year 1867–68, the state allocated $20,000.00 to mount a defense for former Confederate president Jefferson Davis. Clearly Mississippi spent an average amount compared to other southern states.[21]

Once a state government allocated the funds for prosthetic assistance programs, artificial limb companies engaged in a ferocious competition to win the lucrative contracts. While North Carolina's governor quickly selected Jewett's Patent Leg Company of Washington, D.C., as the state's official provider, Mississippi received several requests by manufacturers, each making its own case for sole supplier status. B. Frank Palmer, the head of the Palmer Arm and Leg Company in Philadelphia, Pennsylvania, wrote the governor of Mississippi to argue that the distribution of limbs prevented poverty. "The condition of the mutilated victims of war

Table 3. Mississippi budget and limb expenditures, 1866–70

Dates	Amount spent on prosthetic limbs ($)	Total state budget ($)
May 1866–April 1867	203.00	555,627.00
May 1867–April 1868	24,712.25	576,934.72
May 1868–April 1869	444.00	502,723.11
May 1869–April 1870	1,180.00	684,247.97
Totals	26,539.25	2,319,532.80

Source: *Journal of the Senate of the State of Mississippi*, 1866–71, MS. The senate journals detail the state budgets and are available on microfilm.

assumes, in this view, great public importance," he noted. "It becomes the wise statesman to inquire whether these unfortunate men can, in any way, be restored to usefulness." Thus, prosthetic limbs served as a prime mechanism to restore men to an honorable, self-sufficient place in southern society. If Mississippi agreed to purchase Palmer limbs "at a lower rate, *in proportion to quality*," than any other manufacturer, the veterans would at least move beyond their "impoverished and mutilated condition" and be less of a potential drain on the state's coffers. The Condell Life-Like Limb Company, headquartered in New York, took a different tack, throwing their hat in the ring with a note that their limbs had the "lightness, strength, durability and perfection of action" that was "unequaled by any others ever planned and constructed at any time, or in any country." Condell provided both a five-year warranty and a reasonable rate to fill the orders as quickly as possible. The company also offered a plethora of testimony from patients who loved their artificial limb and used it to walk over rough ground, kick above their head, and walk down several sets of stairs. Other men testified to the fact that they now performed everyday tasks with ease, including holding eating utensils, writing, and escorting two ladies to dance without one of them knowing they had "taken hold of the arm of death." The prosthetic devices returned disabled men to a place of societal normalcy and allowed them to once again master the daily functions of life required to display honorable manhood.[22]

Mississippi's governor was weighing these various proposals, just as James Orr, governor of South Carolina, commenced the arduous process of selecting a limb manufacturer for his state. Orr benefited from significant research done by medical personnel in Virginia (who had examined seventeen different companies) and Georgia (who had examined eleven different), before selecting the leg manufactured by Douglas Bly as superior. Despite this wealth of evidence favoring the Bly leg, Orr had been inundated by correspondence from E. J. Starr, an agent for the Byrd and Kolbe Company who made the case that sectionalism was more important than a superior product. "Your Excellency," Starr noted, "would prefer giving the contract for furnishing artificial legs to a native South Carolinian, rather than to a Yankee manufacturer." Orr disagreed and signed a significant contract with the Bly Company because, as he noted, "the artificial legs manufactured by you have given universal satisfaction to those supplied."[23]

Once the official prosthetic limb provider was selected, the state could begin handing out the devices. Typically an amputee had to fill out a rather extensive application to procure a prosthetic device in any of the seven southern states, needing to prove that he was a citizen of his respective state and had lost his limb in an honorable fashion fighting for the Confederacy. Amputees who exited the war in an unmanly manner, through desertion, were denied any assistance. Applicants, through their own sworn testimony and that of a few witnesses, verified their military service, chronicled the terms of their enlistment and how they mustered out, and described when and where they received their amputation. This information had to be verified with an affidavit from two medical professionals, acknowledging that the amputation had been a result of the Civil War. A county official then had to approve the statements, attesting to the fact that the physicians who provided affidavits were indeed reputable and respectable men. Once the application had been approved, the amputees traveled by rail or steamship at the expense of the state to a prescribed location (usually the state capital or a major city) in order to receive their new limb.[24]

Thousands of Confederate veterans made such journeys. Once arrived, they would undergo a proper fitting. Even so, numerous Confederate veterans complained about their chaffing, chronic pain, or difficulty in mobility that made their prosthetic experience exasperating. J. L. Cathey complained about his artificial leg: "I have worn it one time and since that time I cannot get my leg in it to try it anymore. My stump is too short for a leg of the fashion mine is." J. M. McLean, who received an artificial right arm to replace the one he lost at Gettysburg, remarked, "I can say that the arm is really of no service to me, except to fill the vacancy. It is an encumbrance and hurts me to wear it." Another veteran expressed annoyance at the fact that anyone could hear him walking from a hundred yards.[25]

John McCurdy, a member of the Twelfth Alabama who lost his right leg at Winchester, Virginia, in 1864, called his prosthetic leg "a humbug and of no use to me." Delays and a lengthy application process infuriated some applicants, including a veteran named Nesmith, who fired off an angry letter to the state auditor on July 10, 1879. After hearing nothing following two applications for aid, he inquired, "Do the lawmakers of Alabama and those charged with the execution of the laws expect our class of maimed soldiers to remain quiet without anything while another is provided for?" He threatened the auditor that unless he received his money, he would vent his grievances in the records of "the Supreme Court." With so many complaints to the state legislatures, the prosthetic programs evolved to offer veterans a one-time cash payment in lieu of a prosthetic. The shift to financial compensation left amputated men with an interesting decision: take the prosthetic device and potentially find gainful employment or take the cash payment and put it toward even more immediate needs, like food for their families. While the prosthetic limb could ensure a potentially brighter future, there were no guarantees, and many families had fallen into such dire straits that any amount of cash could get them through another grueling year.[26]

While seven former Confederate states established prosthetic limb programs, Unionist governments in the border states of Kentucky, Missouri, Delaware, and Maryland, as well as quickly reconstructed Tennessee, had little stomach for providing benefits for men they considered traitors. Florida never established a prosthetic program either, mostly because it lacked a significant number of Confederate amputees and the legislature did not find itself inundated with amputated veterans demanding financial support. Other states remained rooted in prewar notions of masculinity and refused to extend financial assistance to men who should act honorably and avoid begging for financial assistance. State legislatures in Texas and Arkansas took up prosthetic legislation, but it quickly snarled in a welter of budgetary limitations, constitutional questions, persistent Unionist sentiment, and the ideology that manhood did not have room for outside assistance.[27]

In the war's immediate aftermath, like all states across the former Confederacy, economic issues plagued the state of Texas. On August 10, 1866, the state legislature appropriated fifty thousand dollars to purchase artificial legs. Another bill floating around the Texas House appropriated twenty thousand for the purchase of cork legs. The *Houston Telegraph* praised the measure, calling veterans "casualties of war" who needed "physical repairing." The Committee on Finance disagreed, however, reporting that "our present financial embarrassments, as well as the great difficulties attending the execution of the project" prevented them from extending prosthetic devices. Legislators on the Committee on Finance did not believe that amputated men deserved to become a temporary fixture in the state budget. Representative Foster then suggested that each legislator donate one hundred dollars to buy artificial legs for the veterans, but this too was rejected by the Committee on Finance. Men in the halls of the Texas legislature could not bring themselves, through legislation or donations, to contribute to the unmanly act of disabled men relying on their government to survive. As a gesture of good faith to the class of newly returned veterans, the state appropriated only a hundred total dollars to gather information about a possible future artificial limb program, which never came to fruition.[28]

The same fate befell the Confederate amputees in Arkansas, though the state newspaper implored the legislature to take action to provide soldiers with artificial limbs. "In no state did the people respond with more alacrity to the call for help, in the hour of danger, than did the citizens of Arkansas. The courage and gallantry of our troops on the many battlefields of the war have secured for us a record of glory and renown unsurpassed on the pages of world history." Although southern women had been working to protect the graves of the dead, they had neglected to push for financial assistance for the men who survived. Thus, it may be up to the state, according to the paper, to care for and recognize "the disabled living" and "the crippled warriors." Two months later, when the Arkansas legislature had yet to act, the *Gazette* again implored action. "We do not believe that any man whose sympathies were with us in the late struggle, can contemplate with solid indifference, the possibility of one who periled his life in defense of his country, becoming an object of charity of a neighborhood or being compelled to become a common beggar, to obtain wherewith of keeping soul and body together." As other states acted on behalf of amputees, Arkansas could not remain on the sidelines and ignore the men who had formed a "bond of mutual sympathy and affection" through their military service. The *Gazette* demanded that a bill appear and concluded with a call to arms: "Prepare for action."[29]

Eventually, the Arkansas legislature passed a sweeping measure in early 1867 designed to provide artificial limbs and wide-scale relief for all widows, orphans, and wounded and disabled soldiers. The efforts of the legislature, however, were stymied by Governor Isaac Murphy, a staunch Unionist, who opposed the legislation and vetoed the bill. Although he claimed to feel "warm sympathy for the afflicted and indigent," he pointed out that the men in question fought "against the government of the United States in the late rebellion, and also against the present State government." "Honoring the enemies of the United States by conferring rewards and pensions of them," he concluded, "for services rendered as soldiers when fighting against that government [and] the armies of the union, is certainly not supporting the constitution of the United States, or the constitution of the State acting in harmony there-with."[30]

Supporters of maimed Confederate veterans were outraged at the governor's veto. The *Gazette* lashed out, reminding readers that the beneficiaries of the bill "are not enemies of the United States, but they are good and loyal citizens" and a vast majority are "women and children, and some of them were, at the time of the war, helpless infants." Providing artificial limbs also made sound economic sense because they would help transform the men from a "burden upon the community" to men who could earn "a livelihood for themselves." Echoing the governor's use of the term "reward," the editorial agreed that the veterans' benefits were at base a reward for "what they lost in responding to the call of the State of Arkansas."[31]

Responding to the furor, the Arkansas Senate overrode the governor's veto by a commanding margin of twenty to one; however, the House did not follow suit, as the members expressed Unionist sentiment or a reluctance to create an entire class of dependent citizens, and the legislation evaporated after a long and arduous debate. At an impasse, the legislature returned to a much-diminished version of a veterans' bill that focused on a limb program for amputees and some measure of support for maimed veterans, indigent widows, and children of deceased soldiers. Ten thousand dollars was appropriated for the purchase of artificial limbs, and a tax was to be put in place to help those most distressed, but a month later the Arkansas legislature adjourned with the arrival of military rule under the Reconstruction Acts, which stalled and then killed the bill, and nothing of its kind was taken up for nearly three decades.[32]

Arkansas supporters of veterans remained diligent and shifted their focus to establishing a Confederate home for disabled veterans, rather than force the state legislature to accept the premise that destitute men remained dependent on their actions for survival. This also stirred deeply mixed reactions among the public. Jacob Trieber, a prominent Republican, wrote, "It does look a little strange that a state refuses to make some provision for the support of men crippled in a cause, no matter whether right or wrong, when they simply obeyed the call of the State." Deacon Elliott Sheppard, by contrast, viewed all Confederate homes, reunions and monuments as a "standing menace to the country – a keeping alive of the war issues, and the instilling of the doctrine of secession in the minds of their children." Private charities did what they could, but Arkansas's few veterans' homes were chronically underfunded. Finally, in 1893, the legislature passed House Bill 346, appropriating thousands of dollars for the soldiers' home in Little Rock to provide medicine, a physician, furnishings, and routine maintenance.[33]

Throughout the South, the establishment of residences for indigent Confederate veterans remained a popular mechanism for legislatures to provide assistance to their most handicapped and helpless men without specifically making each veteran a dependent ward of the state. This jibed with the traditional antebellum pattern of state legislatures funding almshouses and mental hospitals for disadvantaged citizens. Limited funds created deplorable conditions in most almshouses, however, and in some states benevolent citizens helped to create a more robust and better funded system more tailed to veterans' needs. In many ways, as veteran homes sprung up across the South, state legislatures, through providing much-needed funds, took a major step forward in acquiescing that destitute and disabled men needed their help to rebuild their lives.[34]

Virginia's major home for Confederate veterans, named in honor of Robert E. Lee, opened in 1885. In 1889, the state of Tennessee turned over the Hermitage, the estate of former president Andrew Jackson, along with a ten-thousand-dollar allocation, to the Association of Confederate Soldiers, Tennessee Division in order to use the property as a home for indigent and disabled soldiers, as well as their widows and orphans. In

Louisiana, between 1883 and 1890, amputees could apply for admission to the veterans' home on Esplanade Street in New Orleans, for which the state allocated fifty-five thousand dollars. The adjutant general of Louisiana reported, "The Soldiers' Home now affords comfortable quarters, clothing and subsistence to fifty-one Confederate veterans, all disabled from injuries, wounds or loss of limbs in line of duty." The John Bell Hood Camp of the United Confederate Veterans and the Albert Sydney Johnston Chapter of the Untied Daughters of the Confederacy raised enough funds to establish a home in Austin, Texas. W. H. King, the adjutant general for Texas in 1890, admitted that the legislature could not "make direct appropriations of money to help said Home" per constitutional restrictions, but the state did give the rent collected from one state building to help the home, which ranged from fifteen hundred to two thousand dollars per year. In Kentucky, the legislature agreed after the turn of the century to appropriate up to ten thousand dollars per year to fund a new Confederate home at Pewee Valley, Kentucky. General Joseph Lewis, commander of the famed Kentucky Orphan Brigade during the Civil War, addressed the crowd. "The foundation [of the home] teaches a lesson which should not be lost on our young men. It shows that men who do their duty honestly and fearlessly are not forgotten in their old age."[35]

In addition to providing funding for the maintenance of a Confederate home, the state legislatures in Louisiana and Texas provided land grants for amputees and indigent veterans. Parcels of land reversed the emerging trend of creating a partially dependent class of veterans who relied on the state legislature to fund prosthetic limbs, cash payments, or the upkeep of a residence. Rather, the land grants encouraged disabled and indigent men to remain self-sufficient and regain independence through land maintenance and cultivation. (Of course both Louisiana and Texas had large swaths of unsettled land, and complimentary parcels could expand settlement patterns across the state.) Although the men may have been physically unable to farm the land themselves, the hope was that they could hire workers, use family members, raise just enough crops to keep themselves from needing public assistance. The veteran could also sell the land and pocket the proceeds; regardless the legislature's conscience was clean. Ultimately Louisiana provided plots of 160 acres to injured veterans under the program, while Texas offered plots of 1,280 acres to injured or disabled veterans who could not support their families.[36]

In order to receive a tract of land, veterans applying to the program had to prove that their military injury, which had been acquired in an honorable manner, prevented them from engaging in manual labor. Furthermore, the men had to admit to living in poverty without any means of supporting their families. The vast majority of the land grant applications came from men who suffered generally disabling gunshot wounds, but quite a few were amputees. John F. Hanson, who lost his leg at Yellow Bayou in Louisiana, applied for his grant on November 14, 1881, roughly seven months after the provision cleared the legislature. Private John White of the Fourth Louisiana lost his arm at Shiloh and testified in his application that he kept "his face to the enemy" during the battle. Another veteran from Louisiana had lost his right arm when a comrade's gun accidentally went off during a dress parade. As a member of the Twenty-Eighth Louisiana, Private Jeau P. Guidroz's own gun misfired at Vicksburg, resulting in the loss of three fingers on his right hand. James Williams, a veteran from the First Texas, also applied for a land grant due to the leg he lost at Knoxville in 1863. Other men in Texas complained of chronic pain owing to their arm amputations. John D. Polk, who had his finger blown away at the Battle of Pleasant Hill in Louisiana, procured land because the missing finger had damaged his entire hand. All of the men argued that they deserved their parcels for their military service and sacrifice; and all claimed to desperately need the land to make a living.[37]

The final mode of assistance extended by southern state governments emerged in the form of a pension system established to provide a quarterly cash payment to all disabled veterans for the rest of their lives. This system effectively created a permanent class of dependent men who relied on their pensions to survive. Legislation for these programs was not instituted until well after redemption. As amputated men faded from history or found themselves in a position of destitution that forced them to beg for funds, legislators started to accept the fact that they had to rebuild the men who had given so much in the war. As historian Kathleen Gorman has noted, the creed of the New South called on southerners to remember the Old South and embrace the Lost Cause. Thus, a pension program not only cared for the veterans but performed the cultural work of legitimizing the new regime. Southern state governments spent hundreds of thousands of dollars on men who, in their dwindling, had become physical embodiments of the Lost Cause. As monuments sprung up in town squares and groups gathered to reminisce, recall, and rewrite the history of the war, the spotlight appropriately turned toward the veterans whose daily lives did not mirror a triumphant Lost Cause celebration. Considering that many had been living in abject poverty and deplorable conditions, most welcomed the financial assistance, however late in coming.[38]

Although the programs varied from state to state, pension legislation shared several broad features. As they had done with their prosthetic limb applications, veterans needed to verify honorable military service, residency, and the nature and condition of their injuries that incapacitated them. Applicants again remained dependent on comrades to serve as eyewitnesses to their military service and on physicians to confirm that the disability was severe and suffered in the service of the state. In some states, like Georgia, a more severe injury resulted in a higher pension payment (see appendix C) and states usually increased the pension allocation to keep pace with inflation. Wounded veterans also had to swear before county or state officials that they held at least a small amount of property and a meager salary to prove that they were not just deadbeats. While the pension would ultimately make these men dependent on the state, they had to prove themselves worthy of such large-scale financial help. Successful applicants received their payment four times per year. In short, Confederate applicants had to prove themselves destitute and damaged but still honorable in order to receive not charity, but the recognition of a grateful state.[39]

Even solidly Democratic legislatures faced some political squabbling over these financial assistance programs. Although Florida had started their pension program in 1885, Governor Francis Fleming, who served from 1889 to 1893, objected to what he called an "evil," believing it lowered a man from a position of "honorable distinction." The governor maintained that anyone asking for a pension participated in an unmanly action. If a southern veteran, no matter his physical condition, asked for a pension, he diminished his masculine stature among his peers, according to the governor.[40]

Legislators in Tennessee quickly found that if they framed their legislation as a mechanism to support both Union and Confederate Tennessee veterans, they gained some traction among their colleagues. In 1883, Governor William B. Bate, a wounded veteran who rejected amputation, signed a law providing ten dollars a month to Confederate and Union veterans (who did not already collect a federal pension) who had lost both eyes from war-related injuries. In the case of Tennessee, it certainly helped to have a wounded veteran sitting in the governor's office who could ensure that his comrades in arms gained financial support. Pension legislation continued to evolve over the next decades, as the state agreed first to help both Confederate and Union indigent veterans who had lost various limbs in the war and finally to spend several million dollars on general veteran care.[41]

As a veritable pension fever erupted across the South, and many southern states started to piggyback off one another, Arkansas, which had seen its earlier attempts to care for Confederate veterans wilt amid political contention, took up the reigns once more in 1891. The *Gazette*, which had consistently supported the interests of disabled veterans, again called on the legislature to care for men who had "struggled through life thus far, it may be, with one limb, with health gone, or bending over the grave from age." The proposed 1891 Pension Act underwent extensive debate, as supporters rallied behind the image of the empty sleeve and detractors wondered whether true southern men would accept such financial assistance and become, in effect, dependent wards of the state. Some wondered if honor prevented a man from lowering himself to the point where he had to admit that he could not longer be self-sufficient. "Patriots do not go out and fight to be rewarded with pension and bounties," one state senator declared. "The true southern soldier is not asking for a pension. He is too proud and noble." House and Senate galleries filled to capacity with spectators, mostly women, in support of the pension measure and resoundingly cheered each time a politician extolled "the daring and heroism of the boys who wore the grey." With so much pontificating about veterans, one eyewitness commented, "One could almost imagine he heard the reveille, the clink of arms, the roar of musketry and the booming of cannon as brave men marched with steady tramp into the very jaws of death, unawed by the shower of shot and shell that mowed down their ranks like sickles wielded in a harvest field." Despite some reservations, the legislature overwhelmingly approved the pension system on April 2, 1891.[42]

Pension programs were not easy sells everywhere, however. In 1899 a major pension bill faced significant opposition in the Texas legislature. Emphatically voting in the negative, Representative Greenwood raised constitutional objections and declared himself being "everlastingly, eternally, physically, mentally, and morally opposed to pensions." He did not deny the service of the Confederate soldiers, whom he revered "for their bravery and heroic deeds in defense of our fair Southland in a cause that they believed to be just." But he believed they had more than enough resources in the Confederate Home, which was already maintained "at the expense of the State of Texas." Greenwood could not see the state legislature specifically making each veteran dependent on the state, especially if the system would inevitably "open the flood gates of fraud and corruption."[43]

Greenwood did not stand alone in his opposition. Representative Childers argued that a veteran had to be a pauper in order to draw any state aid. At the same time, he did not believe a pauper could live on eight dollars a month and should go live in the Confederate Home, rather than rely on the state for a cash payment. Representative Morrow stated, "I believe the granting of pensions is a species of class legislation, and is so subject to imposition and fraud that I think it bad public policy to embark in it on any new lines." Morrow recalled his youthful days, when he agreed with the Confederate "struggle for States' rights." But an "act of public charity" would only go awry; better for local charities and county authorities to care for their own.[44] Representative Kittrell also voted in the negative, saying, "I am unwilling to vote for a law requiring an ex-Confederate soldier to swear he is an absolute pauper before he can receive a pension." Texans had returned from the war defeated and physically broken, but now, to require a man to admit he could not provide for his family and lived in abject poverty would only further erode his masculine status in society. The sheer embarrassment should not be imposed on anyone, especially veterans who fought for the state and the Confederate nation. Kittrell concluded, "I had rather stay here until July than see such a bill passed."[45]

In the midst of the pension debate, Texas governor C. A. Culberson weighed in with his impressions on how Texas could extend aid to Confederate veterans. The governor referenced an earlier act that had provided for the veterans of the Texas Revolution and defined indigent "as that which shall not allow the ownership of property to exceed one thousand dollars." The governor then surveyed the rest of the southern states to gauge their pension obligations. He reported the data shown in table 4 for 1897.

Culberson asserted that Texas aligned closest with Georgia, as the state had over two million people, compared to Texas's population of just over three million. If the same percentage of individuals applied for a pension

Table 4. Southern state pensioners and expenditures, 1897

State	Number of pensioners	Amount allocated/spent in pension program ($)
Alabama	7,105	116,532
Arkansas	1,336	35,000
Florida	600	65,000
Georgia	10,390	609,520
Mississippi	not available	75,000
North Carolina	not available	105,000
South Carolina	4,714	100,000
Tennessee	537	59,940
Virginia	3,541	110,800

Source: *Senate Journal of Texas, 26th Legislature*, 1899, 209–10.

in Texas as they had done in Georgia, the governor estimated that over fifteen thousand applications would cost the state almost a million and a half dollars a year. If the state found that it was spending more, it would know that it had been the victim of "fraud and imposture" and could revisit the program.[46]

As the House and Senate took up debate on the new legislation, Texas swore in a new governor, Joseph D. Sayers. Sayers agreed with his predecessor on many of the legal questions, and added that anyone caught trying to defraud the pension office should be subjected to prosecution at the felony level. The new governor also demanded an extreme burden of proof on each applicant, as the state itself might not be able to locate muster rolls, hospital records, and other evidence that was now decades old. "I feel that a proper regard, not only for the taxpayers of the State, but also for the wishes of all who worthily wore the gray," he said, "demands the exercise of the utmost caution and skill in the preparation of any measure intended to carry the amendment into effect." Even with some hesitation over potential fraud, Sayers followed the overwhelming support for the measure in the legislature and signed the pension bill into law on May 12, 1899.[47]

Despite supplying the Confederacy with nearly forty thousand soldiers, Kentucky, as a border state, occupied a unique status among southern states that sought to assist its Confederate veterans. In the immediate aftermath of the war, the Commonwealth of Kentucky provided no support whatsoever to Confederate amputees because Unionists dominated the governor's mansion and legislature. Although some historians have

argued that Kentucky turned into a Confederate state after 1865, the identity shift did not go as deep as, or at least did not take the form of, legislation to care for wounded veterans. To be sure, some Kentuckians crafted
a postwar Confederate memory in the form of speeches, reunions, and
monuments, but they failed for decades to pay more than lip service to
Confederate memory, which may diminish the long-standing identity-
shift thesis.[48]

The Kentucky General Assembly did not even consider financial support for Confederates until 1910 when the state legislature passed a bill
to provide indigent veterans with twelve dollars a month. The governor,
Augustus Wilson, vetoed the bill, arguing, first, that Confederate veterans
contributed no real public service to a state that never seceded from the
Union. The argument that Confederate veterans had just done what the
state asked them to do did not work in Kentucky. Second, Wilson did not
believe that thousands of citizens who remained loyal to the Union during
the war should suddenly be forced to foot the bill for men who had fought
on the wrong side of a great national question. "There are tens of thousands of men and widows who have been just as hard worked and con-
scientious farmers, laborers, preachers, doctors and those in all other call-
ings, as the Old Confederate soldiers who are today in just as great need
or a pension," he noted. Third, the measure proposed to raise revenue for
the pension by adding one cent to the state tax of fifty cents per one hundred dollars of income. The miniscule tax would produce an additional
seventy thousand in revenue per year, but the pension program could cost
up to seven hundred thousand dollars. To meet that obligation, the governor argued that the state would need to raise the tax rate to sixty cents.[49]

The Kentucky legislature tried again in 1912 and passed another act to
grant pensions to indigent and disabled Confederate veterans and their
widows, perhaps hoping a new governor, himself a Confederate veteran,
would sign the legislation. They were right, as Governor James McCreary
approved the measure, which immediately offered aid to needy veterans
who had endured nearly fifty years of neglect. Eligible Confederate veterans had to have been a continual resident of Kentucky since January
1907 and could not also be collecting a pension from the U.S. or a foreign
government.[50]

One of Kentucky's first pension applications came from James M. Harp,
a resident of Frankfort, Kentucky. Born in Kentucky in 1844, Harp had
enlisted in 1862 and served until captured by Union forces in 1864, after

which he spent several months at Camp Morton, a military prison. In his application, Harp claimed he owned no real estate or personal property and earned around fifty dollars a year. Harp swore he avoided intoxicants, he had an eyewitness corroborate his military service, and he also provided a physician who diagnosed Harp as having a dramatically reduced ability to earn a living on account of his age, his physical condition, malnutrition, and damaged teeth. The presiding judge signed off on the application in June 1912 and it ended up in Frankfort filed as pension 188 on June 11, 1912. Harp, now sixty-nine years old, met all the requirements and eagerly awaited his first payment. Despite the approval of James M. Harp's pension application, however, the state auditor, H. M. Bosworth, denied payment on the basis of the unconstitutionality of the new pension law, citing the Kentucky Constitution Bill of Rights, section 3, which stated, "No grant of exclusive, separate, public emoluments or privileges shall be made to any man, or set of men, except in consideration of public service." How could Confederate veterans offer the appropriate public service that warranted a payment if they had fought against Kentucky, which remained loyal to the Union? In effect, the auditor had nullified the law and declared Harp a traitor, along with all of his fellows.[51]

Harp immediately sued, and the Franklin Circuit Court heard the case in the spring of 1913. On May 3, the court ruled in favor of Harp. Still Bosworth refused to authorize payment and appealed the ruling to the Kentucky Court of Appeals.[52]

When Harp's lawyers presented their arguments to the Court of Appeals, they stressed the fact that Harp (and his fellow Confederate veterans) *had* committed a public service by defending both the state *and* the federal constitution. The man most responsible for this unorthodox argument was J. H. Hazelrigg, who spent the bulk of his argument intermixing Lost Cause rhetoric with the history of secession and war that included an examination of the Kentucky Resolution in the late 1790s as a justification for secession. Walking a very taught tightrope, in front of a staunchly Unionist courtroom, Hazelrigg attempted to suggest that Confederate veterans had not been traitors but had been animated by fundamentally *American* impulses.[53]

In bolstering his case, Hazelrigg turned to legal precedents that considered military service synonymous with public service. In one Connecticut case, Jude Cooley ruled that since a government could declare and conduct war, it also had the legal right (and obligation) to "levy taxes in order to pay bounties for military services performed or promised." In a separate case in Massachusetts, a panel of justices ruled in favor of honoring Union veterans with pensions, noting that Civil War veterans deserved "recognition by the payment of sums of money, the erection of statutes or the bestowal of medals, decorations or other badges of honor." In the eyes of the Massachusetts court, the veterans had served and sacrificed for both the nation and the Commonwealth of Massachusetts and had done so for the purpose of promoting the public welfare: and, in turn, the state had to make sure that they would never "forget the great service of those who volunteer." In Hazelrigg's argument pensions emerged as a state obligation to the collective memory of its soldiers. Besides, Hazelrigg argued, the state had already created a Confederate Home funded by tax dollars; if that was not unconstitutional, neither was the pension program.[54]

Hazelrigg also crafted an unusual if innovative argument challenging the very idea that Kentucky had remained a Union state throughout the war. The attorney noted that a portion of the state had voted to secede on November 18, 1862, and elected a Confederate governor and sent members to the Confederate legislature. Obviously the state did not completely secede, but Confederate soldiers had defended a "de facto government" from the northern invading forces that had violated the state neutrality. Hazelrigg then pivoted to provide a legal history of secession, covering the Embargo Act, the Louisiana Purchase, New England Federalists who had attempted to depart the Union during the War of 1812, and the nullification controversy in South Carolina. The history lesson ended with the attorney explaining how the Civil War had emerged only after "an intense alleged moral movement swept over a large part of the north over the execution of the Border Ruffian, John Brown, altogether overlooking and condoning his effort to arouse a servile insurrection, inevitably to result in a massacre of helpless women and children." Hazelrigg even quoted prominent abolitionists who had once denounced the Union as a "covenant with death" to demonstrate the contingent nature of "loyalty," not merely in Kentucky but throughout American history.[55]

Hazelrigg closed with reconciliationist sentiment and an attempt to suggest that the best way to bury the hatchet was to treat all veterans as Americans. "The services of each soldier was for a cause he knew to be right, or so well knew, as to be ready to die for it," he noted, "and it can-

not be said that they are not public services . . . worthy of recognition."
The nation had moved beyond the Civil War, and the people emerged
cemented together "by trade, by commerce, by railways, by social and
business alliance, by common perils and sufferings in peace and in war,
by the ever growing pride in our ever growing country, by the knowledge
imparted and encouraged." The pension program was not charity; it was
a form of atonement, self-honoring, and self-forgiveness. "In the beginning [there was] neither North nor South," Hazelrigg concluded. "Let
Kentucky say–to the Union Veteran, 'You are provided for'; to the Southern Veteran, 'Your State, by its judicial as well as by its Executive and
Legislative Departments, will contribute its mite to provide for you.'"[56]

In addition to the creativity of his attorney, Harp also benefited from
the support of Captain William J. Stone, a Civil War veteran, who testified on his behalf. Stone admitted having no formal legal training, but he
decided to speak out because of the strong love he held for his comrade
and the great concern he had "for the welfare of those who are living and
the widows of those who are dead and who are now indigent, disabled,
and dependent." Stone tackled numerous issues, including the service of
Confederate soldiers, the value of a pension, and its potential financial
burden on a state and filled his entire testimony with a wealth of Lost
Cause and reconciliationist rhetoric designed to tug at the heart strings
of everyone present. He particularly noted how each and every soldier
fought for the right of every state "to manage its own local affairs in its own
way," a principle, he claimed, that North and South shared. Stone quoted
a former Union general who extended his hand in friendship to former
Confederate men and believed that they should not be considered crimi-
nals for doing what they, as men, thought was right in their own minds.[57]

Stone returned to the question of public service by arguing that if the
state decided to deny a Confederate veteran a pension on the basis of
public service, it needed to reconfigure the entire aid structure of the
state. "If that [financial] condition is good, you must open the doors of the
lunatic asylums, the feeble-minded institute, the blind asylum, the deaf
and dumb asylum, the State Normal Schools, and cease the appropriate
of money to the Children's Home Society." Each year, the state allocated
thousands of dollars in charity to groups of individuals who had failed
to provide even the semblance of public service. The individuals whom
Stone listed composed a special class, and if the court refused to recognize

veterans as a special class, a clear case of discrimination emerged "against these maimed and diseased and indigent citizens of the State because they had been Confederate soldiers." Stone drove his point home by stating, "There is no other class of citizens of our State who have sacrificed so much in defense of principle; who have risked so much; who have suffered so much; who have lost so much; and who have done so much to crown with glory and honor the character of our people and establish an honorable place for the State in the history of times."[58]

Stone also diffused concerns about the financial burden a pension would pose by examining funds the state had already allocated for the recognition of Confederate veterans. Monuments to John C. Breckenridge, John H. Morgan, the birthplace of Jefferson Davis, and the Chickamauga Battlefield had cost the state fifteen thousand dollars. The state also spent funds on the maintenance of Confederate grave sites and, in 1902, had decided to spend a hundred twenty-five for each inmate sent to the newly established Confederate Home in Kentucky.[59]

Stone shamelessly played on the emotional heartstrings of the court through a comparison to Union veterans. He noted how the federal soldiers returned home to a joyous celebration that recognized them as heroes and awarded them with pensions and veterans' homes. In contrast, Kentucky's Confederate soldiers had returned to a region they no longer recognized, to damaged homesteads and the defiled grave sites of women and children who had died during the war. Rather than wallow in failure, Confederate men acted honorably as they rebuilt their communities and women exhibited the "highest type of womanhood" through their service in the United Daughters of the Confederacy. Although men and women had successfully maneuvered through the challenges of the Civil War, they now needed assistance to survive the postwar world as a destitute and damaged class of citizens. He concluded, "These grand old heroes, though they have lost the military tread, and robust manhood, and are now bowed in form and tottering in their walk, will continue uncomplainingly to make good citizens as they pass along the road toward the dark winter of death."[60]

The Court of Appeals for the State of Kentucky issued its ruling on June 20, 1913. Chief Justice J. P. Hobson ruled that Kentucky had been neutral during the Civil War and that, therefore, both Union and Confederate veterans in Kentucky deserved pensions. The U.S. government, in

the court's opinion, had failed to recognize the "public service" of all veterans, and the judge ordered Bosworth to pay Harp his pension.[61]

For hundreds of amputees, the pension system was the culmination of
a decades-long debate over the obligations of state government to men
who had fought for their state (and against the federal government).
Furthermore, it reflected a fundamental shift in how southerners thought
about manhood, permitting a measure of dependency among men who
had tried their best to remain self-sufficient but could not overcome the
exasperating challenges of disability. All of the pension programs were
designed for men who were struggling, financially, but some men were
struggling more than others. Kentuckian James R. Williams, for instance,
had lost his left leg at Shiloh and spent time as a prisoner of war. Although
he had no wife and earned a pittance of twenty bushels of corn each
year, he at least had a home worth seven hundred dollars, nineteen acres
of land valued at five hundred fifty, and a horse and cow worth a hundred. On the other end of the spectrum, William H. Brown, a member
of the Seventh Kentucky, lost his index finger and suffered from a gunshot wound to his left shoulder. He applied for a pension after spending
his postwar years earning fifty cents a day as a farmhand. By the 1910s, his
wife had died and he had no estate.[62]

Kentucky required pensioners to prove that they were earning less than
$300 a year and had personal property worth less than $2,500. Many veterans had little idea how to measure such validations, but there are signs
that the pension boards tried to accommodate them. W. Z. Rudd, who lost
an index finger on his right finger at Shiloh, failed at farming after the war.
When he applied for a pension, he reported an estate worth $1,200 and
personal property valued at $100. However, the judge corrected his appli-
cation and reported an estate worth $505 and personal property valued at
$281, which guaranteed Rudd a pension in Kentucky. The same applies
to William J. Sullenger, a member of the Twelfth Kentucky Cavalry, who
enlisted in 1863. During the Battle of Harrisburg, Kentucky, he lost his
left leg below the knee. Following the war, he worked as a truck farmer
and earned roughly $150 a year. He possessed about twelve and a half
acres of land worth $600 and some personal property valued at $100.
When Sullenger applied for his pension in Kentucky, the judge amended
his application to reflect property worth only $182 and personal property
valued slightly higher at $180.[63]

Collectively the pension files provide a window into the inability of Confederate veterans to find extensive employment or financial stability after the war. James Wall suffered from the loss of a left arm and a wound to his left knee that made him immobile, even though he tried to work in manual labor. One elderly veteran could barely make a living, especially with his old age and missing arm, yet he still attempted to farm in Florida. William Brown struggled with only one arm and a bad case of arthritis. His physician certified that he "should not attempt to earn any part of his living by manual or any other kind of labor." Another Confederate veteran, who lost a leg at Petersburg, worked 160 acres of land in Bradford County, Florida, with eighteen cattle and a horse. Yet, his missing leg and advanced age meant that he needed a pension to survive. Joseph Tyler owned no property and had numerous medical problems, including a missing leg from the Battle at Cedar Mountain in 1862, kidney disease, faltering eyesight, and a "failing mind."[64]

Many veterans continued to deal with the pension office even after their claim had been established. Charles Burrem, who fought with the Thirty-Seventh Tennessee, lost his right leg at the hip joint at Stones River on December 31, 1862. In 1919, he requested an increase in his pension, as his old age and the missing leg continued to plague him. In a response from the Pension Board, the secretary noted that in the original pension application, Burrem listed his birthday as October 28, 1841. In the increase request, the birthday appeared as October 28, 1819. The secretary concluded that the board had to follow the first birthday listed and the request for an increase was denied. Alex Crawford, who lost a leg during the Atlanta campaign in 1864 with the Thirty-Second Tennessee, faced a dire medical situation, according to his physician, who pleaded on his behalf to the Pension Board. Crawford exhibited paralysis in his only leg, lost his right hand to cancer, and could not use his left arm. The physician requested an immediate pension increase in 1916. Initially, the Pension Board requested more information, including sworn affidavits about his medical condition and property holdings. Once the information had been sent, the board still denied the increase, due to a state law that limited the pension at ten dollars per month. Crawford also listed two different dates for his birth (as Tennessee did provide a pension increase once a veteran reached eighty years old).[65]

Confederate George Thomas, who lost his arm at Cedar Run, had a difficult time holding on to his pension after he applied for one in Tennessee in 1891. A man wrote to the secretary of the Pension Board on behalf of Thomas, asking to place the pension into the hands of a trustee. The man wrote, "When the money is paid to him the saloons get it instead of his family and they need it badly. . . . He [Thomas] is an old confederate and an honest man and will see that it is properly applied." Marion Page was denied a veteran's pension from the state of Florida, even though he lost his right leg at Sharpsburg while serving in the Fifth Florida. Page had already been collecting money from the state through a pauper pension and was barred from double-dipping into the state treasury.[66]

After surveying responses from across the states of the former Confederacy, Dr. Joseph Jones, the Surgeon General of the United Confederate Veterans, praised some of the states for "their devotion to their sons who rallied to their defense in the hour of bloody and desolating war." Jones held out hope, however, for "better, nobler and more generous assistance for the disabled and impoverished Confederate soldiers." Despite such optimism, the state legislatures and their efforts to provide for amputated Confederates produced mixed results. Several state governments found themselves ensnarled in the politics of reconciliation, rigid antebellum notions of masculinity that rejected dependency, and constitutional questions in the midst of lengthy debates on whether or not Confederate veterans deserved financial assistance. Prosthetic limbs, although they enhanced mobility and comfort and allowed some wearers to find work, were distributed by only half of the southern states and for just a brief period. While Confederate amputees welcomed the opportunity to procure a parcel of land, land grants appeared in only two states, also lasted a brief period, and appeared only several decades after the war, when many of the wounded men could no longer physically work the land. Pension programs took decades to materialize, by which time hundreds of amputated veterans had already succumbed to poverty and unemployment, and, in extreme cases, starvation and death. For the most part, the war's amputees remained dependent on the assistance of women in their households and towns and on local charities and benevolent organizations to survive. Gradually state governments did respond, but in the end that response was fairly meager, and undoubtedly prolonged the suffering that many amputated men faced in the aftermath of their injuries.[67]

EPILOGUE

> It is a sad thing to lose a limb, but it is also a sad thing to die; and what rational being, if he could have his choice, would not rather part with an extremity than with his life?
> —Dr. Samuel D. Gross, *A System of Surgery*

In the fall of 2005, I received a photograph in the mail that forever changed my thinking about military history. Within the confines of a sanitized hospital room sat Army Sergeant Bryan Anderson, who had recently returned from Baghdad as part of the American military campaign known as Operation Iraqi Freedom. Bryan, a winner of the Purple Heart, sat leaning in a chair as he painted a small ceramic dog dressed in a holiday scarf and hat. His young eyes stared attentively at the craft project as the muscular right arm, complete with a tribal arm-band tattoo, reached into a scattered pile of art supplies. That right arm rested gently on an artificial left one, easily noticeable by its bright flesh hue; a plastic sleeve seamlessly connected the manufactured limb to a remaining stump halfway up his upper arm. Although Bryan sat at a table, hiding his lower body, the description of the photograph indicated that he had suffered major injuries that resulted in the loss of both of his legs. The triple amputee found comfort in art, and the sign above his head noted that occupational therapy "makes it possible."

A year later, another photograph arrived in the mail. Sergeant David Bronson, laying on his right side, worked diligently putting together what appeared to be a model vehicle. Dressed in a plain gray tee shirt and a pair of gym shorts emblazoned with the army logo, Bronson's muscular body fills most of the photograph. In the bottom-right corner, a hand entered the photograph to lift up his left leg to display his stump; Bronson lost his leg below the knee following an injury while serving in Iraq. The backside of the photograph again indicated the joy the wounded amputee found in the simple act of constructing a model provided by generous donors.

In September 2010, a third photograph arrived in the mail from Disabled American Veterans. Bobby Lisek, a combat veteran, posed in front of a dark background, sitting with his hands embracing his infant daughter. Lisek's left leg, amputated above the knee, has been replaced by a mechanical prosthetic that terminated in a New Balance sneaker. On the back of the photograph, the soldier reflected on his injury, stating, "I knew I had to fight back. This photo says it all and why I had to fight."[1] Lisek sacrificed a leg in service to his country and remained determined not only to recover but to return home again to see his baby girl.

These images of Bobby Lisek, Sergeant Bryan Anderson, and David Bronson caused me to wonder about the plight of amputated war veterans. Since 2001, the United States has been continuously at war, in Iraq, Afghanistan, and elsewhere, and thousands of men and women have returned home, bruised, battered, mentally wounded, and physically altered. Thousands of amputated soldiers fill medical wards from Washington to Germany. Most of these wounded veterans return to their homes and their communities with little media attention and little notice beyond their families. It seems undeniable that our nation not only has neglected our military wounded, as evident from improper maintenance of the Walter Reed Medical Center, but remains largely ignorant of the plight of men and women who remain dependent on their families, their communities, and their government to recover from their plight.

During Memorial Day weekend of 2009, I spent a few hours among the war monuments scattered around the National Mall. As I slowly walked along the Vietnam Memorial, my eyes were drawn not to the names on the wall, but to the three amputees who used their functioning arms and hands to caress the names of the fallen. The veterans ranged in age and had been wounded in different wars. It was touching to see a father and son, combat veterans from Vietnam and Iraq, respectively, standing before the Vietnam Wall with a missing limb. The memorial has truly emerged as a place for male and female veterans of any combat to return and reflect on the meaning of service and sacrifice. As I returned to the steps of the Lincoln Memorial to contemplate what I had witnessed, another young military man ran by, using the warm spring afternoon to exercise among the visible memories of the war dead embodied in the monuments. My eyes, as well as those of the people sitting in my vicinity, went directly to the young man's legs, one of them a steel shaft attached to his stump, which allowed him to glide with the grace of a gazelle. One woman commented to her friend, "Now that's a real man." "Indeed," I thought. Members of the crowd, clearly impressed with his physical prowess, commented in awe before continuing their day of sightseeing and reflecting on war's impact on our nation.

In 2009, First Lieutenant Joe Guyton sat down with the *Washington Post* to describe the loss of both of his legs in Afghanistan. He kept telling himself not to look down at his legs, both when the explosion happened and during his recovery, as if to ignore the reality of his disability. However, once he received prosthetic devices, which at first felt "like stilts," he dreamed of walking and then running, and then he thought "life will be normal again." Guyton described the "sick jealousies" of seeing other military patients who had lost only one leg. As people interacted with him, Guyton realized that they saw him first and sometimes only as handicapped, and he said, "There's a huge stigma about what you can and can't do." He poignantly reflected on the realization of his leglessness: "You see people out walking around, and it seems easy enough. But what you don't see is them at home using a wheelchair or scooting around. Try being at that level for a while. It's degrading. It's like being a child again. And you know this isn't a temporary situation. It's going to be like this for the rest of your life."[2]

Our nation is currently dealing with a war that is sending legions of men and women home with amputations and other forms of physical and mental trauma. According to Pentagon records in 2012, 1,653 soldiers lost limbs in the two wars in Afghanistan and Iraq via explosions from IEDs and other devices. Five soldiers lost all four limbs. One of those men, Brendan Marrocco, looks forward to when he can be on his own. After receiving a double arm transplant, he remains optimistic. "My arms have given me a lot of hope. I hated not having my hands. You do so much with them."[3]

Amputated veterans who served in combat are all around us, and yet we rarely see stories about the damaged bodies of war; it is part of our selective memory about the dark side of our military engagements. Outside of Lieutenant Colonel Ladda Tammy Duckworth, who became the first female amputee elected to Congress in 2012, representing the Eighth

District of Illinois, amputated veterans do not dominate our collective memory of war or our halls of government, where they could advocate on behalf of their fellow wounded warriors.[4] Video footage and still photographs of soldiers usually reveal combat scenes or joyous returns, not the bloodied stumps, charred flesh, and reconstructed bodies trying to cope with their new reality. Physically and emotionally wounded men and women returning from combat remain dependent on the federal gov-ernment to provide adequate medical care, prosthetic devices, and the necessary support to transition from soldier to disabled veteran. It is my hope that the readers of this book will never forget the physical sacrifices men and women have made in combat throughout the history of our nation. The decade of my life spent researching and writing about Confederate amputees has given me a powerful sense of respect for those who soldier on with an empty sleeve. Men and women will forever return home from war physically and emotionally altered. Historians must never forget those sacrifices and should work diligently to prevent the causalties of our conflicts from fading from the pages of our history.

APPENDIX A
Amputation Statistics

Table A.1 displays a sampling of casualty figures and the number of amputations performed from select Confederate units during the course of the Civil War. All figures were obtained from Confederate States Army Casualties: Lists and Narrative Reports, 1861 to 1865, viewed at the Mississippi Department of History and Archives, Jackson. Much of the information is incomplete and inconsistent, which explains why a unit, date, and so on might be missing. The total casualty number encompasses all casualties (killed, wounded, missing) unless indicated as just the number of wounded who required medical attention. Although the sampling is rather sparse and random, the overall theme among the casualty listings is the relatively miniscule number of amputations performed.

Table A.1. Amputations performed, 1861–65 (selected data)

Date	Geographic location	Unit	Number of amputations	Total casualty number listed
July 28, 1863	Helena, Ark.	4th Brigade, Missouri Volunteers	3	354 wounded
July 28, 1864	Atlanta, Ga.	A. M. Manigault's Brigade	8	87
September 1863	Chickamauga	Eufaula Light Artillery, Alabama	1	14
September 1863	Chickamauga	19th and 24th Arkansas	2	90
September 1863	Chickamauga	9th Kentucky	2	102
August 30, 1862	Richmond, Ky.	2nd Brigade, 4th Div. Army of Ky.	12	243
Dec 24–26, 1864	Fort Fisher, N.C.	No specific units–battle total	5	62
July 1863	Gettysburg	5th North Carolina	3	143
July 1863	Gettysburg	6th North Carolina	7	174
July 1863	Gettysburg	21st North Carolina	2	113
July 1863	Gettysburg	57th North Carolina	2	63
July 1863	Gettysburg	Stonewall Brigade	6	170 wounded
July 1863	Gettysburg	Dole's Brigade	2	192
July 1863	Gettysburg	Ramseur's Brigade	8	122 wounded
September 22, 1863	Fort Johnson, S.C.		1	7
July 17, 1863	Battery Wagner, S.C.		2	34
July 31, 1863	Battery Wagner, S.C.		1	15
August 20–September 6, 1863	Morris Island		8	458
June 1864	Fort Sumter		2	not indicated
November 7, 1861	Fort Walker		1	15
December 6, 1861	Ball's Bluff		1	113 wounded
August 1862	Second Manassas	21, 33 and 41st Virginia	1	408 wounded
May 1863	Chancellorsville	3rd Alabama	2	159
May 1863	Chancellorsville	19th Georgia	1	38
May 1863	Chancellorsville	5th North Carolina	4	61 wounded
May 1863	Chancellorsville	12th North Carolina	2	119
May 1863	Chancellorsville	10th Virginia	3	109

Date	Location	Unit		Casualties
no date	Fredericksburg	Posey Brigade	1	184 wounded
no date	Fredericksburg	Pickett Division	1	60 wounded
no date	Fredericksburg	Ransom Division	13	535
December 31, 1862	Murfreesboro, Tenn.	Adam's Brigade of Hardee Corps	2	708
December 31, 1862	Murfreesboro, Tenn.	Hansen Brigade	8	372
December 31, 1862	Murfreesboro, Tenn.	Nathaniel's Brigade	4	692
May 1863	Chancellorsville	10th Alabama	2	100
May 1863	Chancellorsville	6th North Carolina	2	42 wounded
May 1863	Chancellorsville	21st North Carolina	1	73 wounded
May 1863	Chancellorsville	54th North Carolina	1	40 wounded
May 1863	Chancellorsville	57th North Carolina	5	73 wounded
January 20, 1863	Kellys Stone, Va.	R. A. Pryor Brigade	3	31 wounded
May 8, 1862	McDowell, Va.	10, 21, 37, 42, 48 Virginia	3	393 wounded
November 1863	Mine Run, Va.	James Daniel's Brigade	10	518 wounded
November 1863	Locust Hill	Stonewall Brigade	5	129 wounded
May 1863	Salem Church, Va.	11th Alabama	2	76 wounded
	Seven Days Campaign, Va.	W. Crenshaw Battery	2	9
	Seven Days Campaign, Va.	15th Georgia	1	105
June 27, 1862	Seven Days Campaign, Va.	Fourth Texas	3	205 wounded
April 1862	Baton Rouge, La.		3	16 wounded
July 9–17, 1863	Fort Jackson, La.		2	35 wounded
	Jackson, Miss.	Breckenridge Division	5	43 wounded
June 10–11, 1864	Tishimingo Creek, Miss.	Forrest Cavalry	10	493 wounded
March 23, 1862	Winchester, Va.		1	63 wounded
1864		Fourth Alabama	14	341
1864		Eighth Georgia	12	125 wounded
1864		Ninth Georgia	9	100 wounded
1864		15th and 45th Alabama	8	286
August 1863	White Sulphur Springs	Chapman's Battery	1	6
July–September 1863	First Military District	Mixed Units	14	674 wounded
April 1864	Salina River, Ark.	16th Missouri	1	40 wounded

APPENDIX B
Prosthetic Limb Programs

The following charts chronicle the prosthetic limb programs in the states of Alabama, North Carolina, Louisiana, and South Carolina. The data show the expenditure amount on prosthetic devices for the four states and the number of limbs purchased in Alabama and South Carolina.

Table B.1. Artificial leg expenditures, Alabama 1867–79

Year	Amount spent ($)	Number of limbs
1867	13,060	218
1868	630	12
1872	3,190	53
1873	4,030	65
1874	240	4
1875	3,310	57
1876	2,200	38
1877	100	2
1878	325	6
1879	n/a	132
Total	27,085	587

Source: "Auditor Records," Confederate Pension Records, Application for Artificial Limbs, AL. In 1879, when the program shifted from artificial limbs to cash payments, the auditor records no longer indicate how much each veteran received or if he received a limb over money.

Table B.2. Artificial limb expenditures, North Carolina, 1866–71

Year	Amount spent ($)
1866	22,656.29
1867	54,403.83
1868	3,470.00
1869	630.00
1870	150.00
1871	0.00
Total	81,310.12

Source: Wegner, *Phantom Pain*, 32–33.

Table B.3. Artificial limb expenditures, Louisiana, 1880–89

Year and type of allocation	Amount allocated ($)
1880 (limbs)	12,000.00
1881 (limbs)	8,000.00
1882 (limbs)	1,300.00
1882 (repairs)	1,000.00
1883 (limbs)	1,300.00
1883 (repairs)	1,071.77
1884 (limbs and repairs)	8,000.00
1885 (limbs and repairs)	8,000.00
1886 (limbs and repairs)	1,500.00
1887 (limbs and repairs)	1,500.00
1888 (limbs and repairs)	7,608.91
1889 (limbs and repairs)	9,000.00
Total (1880–89)	60,280.68

Source: "Report of Surgeon General, 1892," United Confederate Veterans Association Records, LSU.

Table B.4. Artificial limb expenditures, South Carolina, 1867–69

Date	Number of legs furnished	Cost to South Carolina ($)
July 1867	16	1,194.40
August 1867	19	1,418.35
September 1867	22	1,642.30
October 1867	17	1,560.18
November 1867	18	1,489.65
December 1867	24	1,864.50
January 1868	21	1,567.65
February 1868	1	74.65
June 1868	15	1,231.73
January 1869	3	223.95
February 1869	4	298.60
Total	160	12,565.96

Source: "Vouchers to Douglas Bly," S126097 Lists of Disabled Soldiers, 1867, SC.

APPENDIX C

Pension Programs

The following charts chronicle pension programs in Georgia, Florida, and Kentucky. The data show state expenditures on pensions and, in the case of Georgia, the amount of funds provided to each applicant based on the nature of his injury.

Table C.1. Georgia pension payments based on injury

Nature of injury	Amount paid per year in Georgia ($)
Loss of both eyes	150
Loss of one eye	30
Loss of hearing	30
Loss of entire foot or leg	100
Loss of entire hand or arm	100
Loss of both hands/arms	150
Loss of both feet/legs	150
Loss of hand/foot and arm/leg	150
Leg or arm rendered useless	50
1 finger or toe	5
2 fingers or toes	10
3 fingers or toes	15
4 fingers or toes	20
4 fingers and thumb or 5 toes	25
Other injury preventing manual avocations of life	50

Sources: *Acts of the General Assembly of the State of Georgia*, 1888–89, 1:16–18, GA; "Report of Surgeon General, 1892," United Confederate Veterans Association Records, LSU.

Table C.2. State of Georgia pension payments, 1880–1902

Year(s)	Amount spent in Georgia for Confederate pensions ($)
1880–82	70,210
1883–84	59,055
1885–89	248,100
1890	185,610
1891	183,240
1892	588,415
1893	428,600
1894	424,640
1895	425,740
1896	545,140
1897	574,960
1898	610,060
1899	653,710
1900	677,520
1901	696,727
1902	858,895
Total 1880–1902	7,230,622

Sources: Georgia pension payments in *Lost Cause* 7, no. 4 (November 1902): 53, United Daughters of the Confederacy Records, box 40, KYHS. The law approving the payment of pensions to widows can be found in *Acts of the General Assembly of the State of Georgia*, 1888–89, 2:39–40, GA.

Note: Georgia added widows in 1892 and indigent men in 1896. The state also spent $30,000 in 1886 on artificial limbs, in addition to the pension. The state utilized tobacco taxes to help fund the program.

Table C.3. State of Florida pension payments, 1885–90

Year	Number of pensioners in Florida	Amount spent by State of Florida on pensions ($)
1885	58	1,777.50
1886	100	7,653.80
1887	167	9,368.83
1888	318	32,647.76
1889	384	34,486.38
1890	218[a]	35,000.00[a]

Source: "Report of Surgeon General, 1892," United Confederate Veterans Association Records, LSU.

a. The number of pensioners declined to the 1890 number in July 1889 after the state revised the law to grade pensions according to specific disability. The financial figure for 1890 is the amount the state appropriated for pensions that year.

Table C.4. State of Kentucky pension payments, 1913–1966

Date Range	Amount of state funds spent on pensions for Confederate veterans/widows ($)
1913–19	3,079,319.11
1923–31	1,700,000.00
1930s	800,000.00+
1941–45	300,000.00+
1966	600.00

Source: Simpson, *Index of Confederate Pension Applications,* 6–7, KYHS.

NOTES

UTX   Center for American History, University of Texas at Austin
VHS   Virginia Historical Society, Richmond

Introduction. Empty Sleeves in Civil War History and Memory

1. Tapp and Klotter, *The Union, The Civil War and John W. Tuttle*, 88.
2. Haunted History tour, New Orleans, May 23, 2012.
3. *Gone with the Wind* (Los Angeles: Metro Goldwyn Mayer, 1939).
4. *The Horse Soldiers* (Los Angeles: Metro Goldwyn Mayer, 1959). Recent films, including *Cold Mountain*, contain riveting and graphic hospital sequences.
5. *Lincoln* (Los Angeles: DreamWorks, 2012), viewed on November 16, 2012.
6. Hacker, "A Census-Based Count of the Civil War Dead." Recent books that deal with death and the Civil War include Neff, *Honoring the Civil War Dead*; Faust, *This Republic of Suffering*; and Schantz, *Awaiting the Heavenly Country*. Recent titles that examine the environmental impacts of the Civil War include Nelson, *Ruin Nation* and Brady, *War upon the Land*. For more on disease and its impact on Civil War soldiers, see Meier, *Nature's Civil War*; Long, *Rehabilitating Bodies*, 113–45 and 210–37; Bell, *Mosquito Soldiers*; Humphreys, *Intensely Human*; and Downs, *Sick from Freedom*. The most recent medical history of the Civil War does spend several pages examining the Confederacy, though a majority of the book still deals with the U.S. side of the conflict and only a few pages touch on amputation. See Humphreys, *Marrow of Tragedy*, 30–33 and 184–242. Some of the few historical articles and monographs pertaining to amputation include Frick, "Soldiers with Empty Sleeves"; DeBrava, "The Offending Hand of War in *Harper's Weekly*"; Lewellen, "Limbs Made and Unmade by War"; McDaid, "With Lame Legs and No Money"; Berry, "When Metal Meets Mettle"; Wegner, *Phantom Pain*, ix; Jordan, "Living Monuments"; Marten, *Sing not War*; Rutkow, *Bleeding Blue and Gray*; Bollet, "Amputations in the Civil War," in Schmidt and Hasegawa, *Years of Change and Suffering*, 57–67; and Hasegawa, *Mending Broken Soldiers*. Historian John David Smith examined the life of William Thomas, an African American soldier who coped with the loss of his arm from the Civil War. See his work *Black Judas*, esp. 34–42. For a thorough cultural examination of Union amputee James Tanner, see Marten, *America's Corporal*. One recent article examined the ramifications of amputation on Union soldiers. See Clarke, "'Honorable Scars,'" in Cimbala and Miller, *Union Soldiers and the Northern Home Front*. For more on the experience of amputation, see Figg and Farrell-Beck, "Amputation in the Civil War." For a pertinent discussion of amputees in England following World War I, see Koven, "Remembering and Dismemberment."
7. Initially, the call for historians to examine the ramifications of the Civil War on the lives of everyday Americans came from Maris A. Vinovskis, "Have Social Historians Lost the Civil War?" See also Friedmann, *Psychological Rehabilitation of the Amputee*, 20, 32, and 43. Although his study looks at modern notions of amputation, he argues that amputees worried about how their family and friends would view them, as they faced a "loss of self-esteem, loss of completeness of body image, loss of respect for one's appearance and functional ability, and inability to relate to oneself, one's spouse and one's family, friends and employer in a normal manner."
8. Glover, *Southern Sons*, 3, 91, 97, and 101; Friend and Glover, "Rethinking

Southern Masculinity," in Friend and Glover, *Southern Manhood*, x and xi; Wyatt-Brown, *Southern Honor*, 14; Edwards, "Problem of Dependency," 315; Dailey, *Before Jim Crow*, 90–95; Berry, *All That Makes a Man*, 12 and 20–21. For an antebellum account of the origins of manhood, see McCurry, *Masters of Small Worlds*; "The Christian Soldier: The True Hero," Hamet Pinson Family Papers, LSU. For more on how the image of the whole man equated manhood, see Greenberg, *Honor and Slavery*, 3; Bederman, *Manliness and Civilization*, 5–8 and 11; Rotundo, *American Manhood*, 233–34; as well as Jarvis, *Male Body at War*, 112–18. For more on honor and southern manhood, see Wyatt-Brown, *Southern Honor*, 34–36, 133–34, 144–59, and 164–70; Cash, *Mind of the South*; Greenberg, *Masters and Statesmen*; Stowe, *Intimacy and Power in the Old South*; Freeman, *Affairs of Honor*, as well as Ayers, *Vengeance and Justice*. For more on gender notions in the antebellum and wartime South, as well as ways men defined themselves in the period, see Brown, *Good Wives, Nasty Wenches and Anxious Patriarchs*; Edwards, *Scarlett Doesn't Live Here Anymore*; Mayfield, "'The Soul of a Man!'"; Lindman, "Acting the Manly Christian"; and Jabour, "Male Friendship and Masculinity in the Early National South."

9. "The Vine and Oak," http://www.readcentral.com/chapters/Henry-Rowe-Schoolcraft/Algic-Researches-Vol-2/029 (accessed September 13, 2013); Greenberg, *Honor and Slavery*, 3 and 15; Nielsen, *Disability History of the United States*, 42, 86, and 89–91. See also Long, *Rehabilitating Bodies*.

10. Humphrey, *Peg Leg*, 27–29, 43, 55, and 56. For another example of an amputee prior to the Civil War, see the Alfred Flournoy Papers, LSU. Alfred Flournoy lost his leg in Pensacola, Florida, while fighting with Andrew Jackson in 1818. On May 22, 1826, the U.S. Congress granted him a land pension due to his missing leg. We have no records of how Flournoy thought or felt about his missing leg, other than the fact that Congress recognized his sacrifice. Some surgical manuals printed prior to 1860 contain numerous medical case studies of amputation, but they rarely reveal the reaction of the patients or how society perceived their missing appendages. For example, see Eve, *Collection of Remarkable Cases in Surgery*, 556–67. The surgical cases noted that the very first hip amputation in America took place in 1806 in Kentucky. Medical data in 1852 indicated that only a few dozen hip amputations had taken place in the United States. In addition, one anecdote from prior to the Civil War notes a man from Georgia who received the medical attention of an itinerant doctor for an ulcer on his leg. The doctor started to cut the leg but failed to apply a tourniquet and ran off. The damaged patient requested amputation from a medical professor, as he could not bare the pain associated with his injury. See Eve, *Collection of Remarkable Cases in Surgery*, 822.

11. Humphrey, *Peg Leg*, 93–94, 124–25, 246, and 248. Overall, there are a limited number of manuscript collections that convey what the loss of a limb meant prior to the Civil War. Some helpful collections include the Joseph Lyon Miller Papers, VHS, which contain a letter about a young man named Thomas who had his leg amputated in 1848. Nicholas Adam, who fought in the Seminole War in 1836 in Florida, died due to the absence of amputation of his wounded leg. For more on Adam, see the Papers of the Summer, Dreher, Efird and Mayer Families, USC. Neither collection provides any detail beyond a simple amputation performed or not performed.

12. Griffen, "Reconstructing Masculinity from the Evangelical Revival to the Waning of Progressivism," in Carnes and Griffen, *Meanings for Manhood*, 191;

Whites, *Civil War as a Crisis in Gender*, 11; Wiley, *Life of Johnny Reb*, 21–27. For more on how young Confederates perceived the war as a solidification of manhood, see Carmichael, *Last Generation*, esp. 162–64 and Wetherington, *Plain Folk's Fight*, esp. 81–111.

13. Berry, "When Metal Meets Mettle," 16.

14. Travis, *Wounded Hearts*, 38. Backwoods brawling, where both men fought to uphold their honor, had the ability to produce numerous scars, but the act of physical fighting ended up a lower-class endeavor on the eve of the Civil War. Brawls and wrestling matches emerged as the lower-class version of dueling, as commoners lacked access to the mechanisms elite men used to assert their honor. See Gorn, "Gouge and Bite."

15. Whites, *Civil War as a Crisis in Gender*, 8. Peter Carmichael argues that southern men faced public humiliation because they had failed to live up to the manly standard of winning the war. See his work, *Last Generation*, 208.

16. Friedmann, *Psychological Rehabilitation of the Amputee*, 43 and 52.

17. Nelson, *Ruin Nation*, 178; Friedmann, *Psychological Rehabilitation of the Amputee*, 43.

18. Laura F. Edwards offers a thorough discussion of gender, politics, and honor in her work, *Gendered Strife and Confusion*, 113–29. Edwards argues that men defined themselves as men through mastery of their wives, children, and household. Historian Susan-Mary Grant notes that amputation emerged as the "symbolic wound" for the Confederacy, one that could easily be seen and understood by society. See her article " Lost Boys," 233–59. For more on the definitions of manhood in the South, see Berry, *All That Makes a Man*; McCurry, *Masters of Small Worlds*; Friend and Glover, *Southern Manhood*; Greenberg, *Honor and Slavery*; Wyatt-Brown, *Shaping of Southern Culture*; and Wyatt-Brown, *Southern Honor*. For more on scars and their impact on manliness, see Gorn, "Gouge and Bite," 18–43.

19. War Department, Surgeon General's Office, "Report on Amputations at the Hip-Joint in Military Surgery," 25, box 57, Joseph Jones Papers, TU; "Description of the Last Campaign of the Civil War," box 24, Joseph Jones Papers, TU. See also U.S. War Department, *War of the Rebellion*.

20. War Department, Surgeon General's Office, *"Report on Amputations at the Hip-Joint in Military Surgery,"* 21.

21. This study focuses solely on white Confederate soldiers, surgeons, and civilians. While one can find an occasional reference to a black soldier or amputee, source materials pertaining to African Americans and disability in the Confederacy remain elusive. Just as black bodies bearing the scars of slavery contributed to antebellum southern white attitudes toward black masculinity, scarred and unscarred Native American bodies also impacted the framing of manhood. For more on black soldiers and health during the Civil War, see Long, *Rehabilitating Bodies*, 113–45 and 210–37; Bell, *Mosquito Soldiers*; Humphreys, *Intensely Human*; and Downs, *Sick from Freedom*. For more on the environmental impact on the Civil War body, particularly soldiers, see Meier, "No Place for the Sick," 176–206.

Chapter 1. The Surgeons

1. Daniel, *Recollections of a Rebel Surgeon*, 165–72.

2. *Gone with the Wind* (Los Angeles: Metro Goldwyn Mayer, 1939); "dismal fail-

ures" quoted in Parish, *American Civil War*, 147; "toxic effects" quoted in Eicher, *Longest Night*, 789; "gangrene" quoted in McPherson, *Battle Cry of Freedom*, 486; "radical and conservative" quoted in McPherson, *Ordeal by Fire*, 418; "operated in ignorance" in Dean, *Shook over Hell*, 48–53; "carelessly threw" quoted in Donald, Baker, and Holt, *Civil War and Reconstruction*, 371; "butcher shop" quoted in Guelzo, *Fateful Lightning*, 267 and 273. In addition, Charles P. Roland, *American Iliad*, 64, argues that "gore-daubed surgeons, overwhelmed by multitudes of casualties, cut and sawed and ligatured, creating ghastly mounds of severed arms and legs" after the Battle of Shiloh. He sees amputation taking place "continuously, followed in most instances by death." David Goldfield, in his recent *America Aflame*, 269, follows suit and argues that "surgeons were careless in their amputations and unmindful of even the limited sanitary knowledge of the time." In the latest book on the medical hell of the Civil War, Michael C. C. Adams argues that surgeons had to quickly remove a limb before gangrene set in. He further asserts that surgeons lacked time, tools, operating facilities, and medical knowledge. See his *Living Hell*, 68, 89–92. Not all historians have agreed with this negative assertion pertaining to surgeons. Bruce Catton, *American Heritage Picture History of the Civil War*, 360, contends that no one should be blamed for the poor medical care as both sides tried their best in an age of bad care. The same can be said for Terry L. Jones, *American Civil War*, 439, 441, and 461, who argues that medical care improved during the Civil War, as medical personnel used new techniques, devices, and clean conditions that led them down the road to medical modernity. He does not believe that surgeons deserved their poor reputation. James I. Robertson, Jr. notes that surgeons do not deserve the negative nicknames provided to them by Civil War soldiers because medical professionals worked hard and remained devoted to the care of their patients. See his *Soldiers Blue and Gray*, 158–59. See also Buell, *Warrior Generals*, 360, who notes that armies evolved during the war to move beyond medical care that had once been "primitive and haphazard."

3. Cunningham, *Doctors in Gray*, 228–30; "amputation" quoted in Schmidt, "Years of Change and Suffering," http://dartmed.dartmouth.edu/summer11/html /years_of_change.php (accessed July 17, 2013); "ingenuity" quoted in Brodman and Carrick, "American Military Medicine in the Mid-Nineteenth Century," 78; Bollet, "Amputations in the Civil War," in Schmidt and Hasegawa, *Years of Change and Suffering*, 57–67. See also Freemon, *Gangrene and Glory*, Devine, *Learning from the Wounded*, 209–10; and Bollet, *Civil War Medicine*. Finally, in her most recent book, Margaret Humphreys sees the health crisis of the Civil War as dramatically improving as the war progresses. See her work *Marrow of Tragedy*, 10, 30–33 and 184–242.

4. Letterman, *Medical Recollections of the Army of the Potomac*, 49; Keen, *Addresses and Other Papers*, 433. For more on southern doctors, see Stowe, *Doctoring the South*.

5. *Campaigns of Walker's Texas Division by a Private Soldier*, 201; Letter for Father and Mother, July 22, 1861, Charles Hutson Papers, #362, UNC; Evans, *Confederate Military History vol. V: North Carolina*, 70. See also Williams, *People's History*, 231.

6. Daniel, *Soldiering in the Army of Tennessee*, 69; Holland, *Keep All My Letters*, 53; Underwood, *Women of the Confederacy*, 164; *Hospital Life in the Army of the Tennessee by Kate Cumming*, 17, Joseph Jones Papers, TU.

7. Nelson, *Ruin Nation*, 169; Benson, *Berry Benson's Civil War Book*, 11; Daviess,

History of Mercer and Boyle Counties, 106; Lewellen, "Limbs Made and Unmade by War," 40.

8. Pitcock and Gurley, *I Acted from Principle,* 57. For a negative impression of a Fayetteville, Arkansas, hospital, see Letter from Fred, Ira Russell Papers, ARK.

9. Freemon, *Gangrene and Glory,* 48; Jones, *American Civil War,* 446.

10. Wegner, *Phantom Pain,* 13–14; Berry, *All That Makes a Man,* 223; Theodore Livingston letter to sisters Helen and Scotia, October 25, 1863, Livingston Letters, MOC; Wiley, *Life of Johnny Reb,* 267.

11. Pitcock and Gurley, *I Acted from Principle,* 363.

12. Koonce, *Doctor to the Front,* 43; Adams, *Doctors in Blue,* 9; *Civil War Letters, Volume I, West Tennessee,* 12 and 63; Bollet, *Civil War Medicine,* 27–28; Cunningham, *Doctors in Gray,* 21–22 and 218. Cunningham also extensively traces the rise of the medical profession across the South in the antebellum period and notes the readily available surgical manuals for future surgeons. In 1861, the Confederate Congress created a medical department that contained a Surgeon General, four surgeons, and six assistant surgeons. Additional legislation noted that a surgeon and assistant surgeon could be appointed by the president for each regiment once they enlisted for service. Several other men worked in the role of contract surgeon outside of the department, although that number is unknown. See also *Civil War Letters, Volume II, East Tennessee,* 99 and Humphreys, *Marrow of Tragedy,* 233.

13. McMullen, *Surgeon with Stonewall Jackson,* 16–17; Chisolm, *Manual of Military Surgery* (1864), 119; Bollet, *Civil War Medicine,* 148.

14. Nelson, *Ruin Nation,* 163 and 165–66.

15. "Every Kind of Wound and Disease," 12, MOC; *Southern Bivouac,* September 1882–August 1883, 363a–64a; Brinsfield, *Spirit Divided,* 160–61.

16. See Warren, *Epitome of Practical Surgery for Field and Hospital,* 137–68; Bernard and Huette, *Illustrated Manual of Operative Surgery and Surgical Anatomy,* 54–96; Carnochan, *Comparative Merits of the Partial Amputations of the Foot,* SCH. Many Confederate surgeons did not have extensive experience in surgical practices. In medical school, surgical classes were optional, and potential doctors routinely merely listened to lectures and gained very little hands-on experience in school, as many states barred dissection. Most physicians learned through serving as an apprentice to another physician. For more, see Stowe, *Doctoring the South.*

17. Tripler and Blackman, *Handbook for the Military Surgeon,* 53–60; Gross, *Manual of Military Surgery or Hints on the Emergencies of Field Camp and Hospital Practice,* 11; Samuel Gross Confederate Pamphlet-Manual of Military Surgery, 11, 34–37, DUKE; "Instructions for Amputation from the Manual for Military Surgery prepared for the use of the Confederate States Army, 1863," 14, MOC; *CSA Medical and Surgical Journal* 2, no. 1 (January 1865): 3. The authors of surgical manuals referenced some European cases, which revealed that if amputation was exercised appropriately and with caution, the surgical procedure preserved life and diminished suffering. Timing was everything, as a surgeon had to perform the operation on the field within the first forty-eight to sixty hours in order to guarantee survival

18. Gross, *System of Surgery,* 548–49; Daniel, *Recollections of a Rebel Surgeon,* 249–50; Cuttino, *Saddle Bag and Spinning Wheel,* 54.

19. Chisolm, *Manual of Military Surgery* (1862), 409 and 422, VHS; Chisolm, *Manual of Military Surgery* (1864), 172, 410, 414, and 417–18, UAB.

20. Warren, *Epitome of Practical Surgery for Field and Hospital,* 81, 87 and 93; Chisolm, *Manual of Military Surgery* (1862), 423.

21. MED, pt. 3, vol. 2, 412.

22. Abraham Watkins Venable Scrapbook, 1851–65, UAB; Thompson, *History of the Orphan Brigade,* 165.

23. "Every Kind of Wound and Disease," 12, MOC; Chisolm, *Manual of Military Surgery* (1862), 433; *Southern Bivouac,* September 1883–August 1884, 500–501; Hall T. McGee Diary, Eighteenth S.C. Heavy Artillery, May 16, 1864, SCH.

24. Chisolm, *Manual of Military Surgery* (1862), 426; Welsh, *Medical Histories of Confederate Generals,* 24–26. Brandon, aged sixty, returned to military service. However, his prosthetic device created problems for him and his crutches scared his horse. He spent the rest of the war in the Reserve Corps and lived until 1890 on his former plantation.

25. Chisolm, *Manual of Military Surgery* (1864), 426–27; Formento, *Notes and Observations on Army Surgery,* 24; Bollet, *Civil War Medicine,* 80; Cunningham, *Doctors in Gray,* 226–27.

26. Williams, *People's History,* 231; Bollet, *Civil War Medicine,* 1–2; Robson, *How a One-Legged Rebel Lives,* 35–36; Daniel, *Recollections of a Rebel Surgeon,* 213; Bollet, "Amputations in the Civil War," in Schmidt and Hasegawa, *Years of Change and Suffering,* 58.

27. Warren, *Epitome of Practical Surgery for Field and Hospital,* 97–99; Chisolm, *Manual of Military Surgery* (1862), 434–35.

28. Chisolm, *Manual of Military Surgery* (1862), 409–10 and 424.

29. Chisolm, *Manual of Military Surgery* (1862), 426; Pitcock and Gurley, *I Acted from Principle,* 363.

30. Chisolm, *Manual of Military Surgery* (1862), 420–21 and 427–28.

31. Warren, *Epitome of Practical Surgery for Field and Hospital,* 103–8; Bollet, *Civil War Medicine,* 151. For more on the differences between circular and flap methods, see Gross, *System of Surgery,* 541–46 and Devine, *Learning from the Wounded,* 173–214.

32. Chisolm, *Manual of Military Surgery* (1862), 425–28.

33. Bollet, *Civil War Medicine,* 292 and 382.

34. Ibid., 210. In addition, Shauna Devine recently argued that some surgeons sought to understand the disease process in their patients. See her *Learning from the Wounded,* 62. For cases of historians who argue that Civil War physicians did not understand the spread of disease and can be described as ignorant and inept, see McPherson, *Battle Cry of Freedom,* 486–87 and *Ordeal by Fire,* 417–18; Dean, *Shook over Hell,* 50–55; Williams, *People's History,* 208–10; Wells, *House Divided,* 178; Eicher, *Longest Night,* 787–88; and Goldfield, *America Aflame,* 242–43 and 268–73.

35. Breeden, *Joseph Jones,* 160 and 211–12. Williams, *People's History,* 235, argued that the only way to stop gangrene was with amputation. For a recent thorough examination of gangrene, see Devine, *Learning from the Wounded,* 94–131.

36. Bollet, *Civil War Medicine,* 203.

37. Welsh, *Two Confederate Hospitals and Their Patients,* 18–20. By 1864, the United States Sanitary Commission recommended speedy amputations in order to save a life and cautioned against the presence of mutilated patients in a hospital, which created a negative atmosphere or a "perfectly unendurable" situation.

See Hammond, *Military Medical and Surgical Essays Prepared for the United States Sanitary Commission*, 459–62 and 479. Samuel Stout ordered some hospital facilities to put their patients to work. See Samuel Stout Correspondence, Medical and Hospital Series, box 1, MOC and Schroeder-Lein, *Confederate Hospitals on the Move*.

38. Rules of the Third Georgia Hospital, UTX. Historian Jonathan Daniel Wells admitted that hospital workers eventually understood the importance of washing with soap and water. See Wells, *House Divided*, 178.

39. Welsh, *Two Confederate Hospitals and Their Patients*, 20–21.

40. Theodore Livingston, letter to sisters Helen and Scotia, October 25, 1863, Livingston Letters, MOC; Watkins, *Co. Aytch*, 186–87; Governor Brown Petition, MS 1170, Telamon Cuyler Collection, UGA.

41. Davis, *Battle at Bull Run*, 253; Wilson, *Brief History of the Cruelties and Atrocities of the Rebellion*, 14–19; "Report of the American Sanitary Commission," *British Medical News*, August 31, 1861; *Report of the Joint Committee on the Conduct of the War: Rebel Barbarities*, 3:452 and 463–67.

42. Daniel, *Shiloh*, 305; *An Impressed New Yorker*, 177–78. The horror of Shiloh is revealed in some battlefield records indicating an 80 percent mortality rate among some soldiers who underwent amputation. See Cunningham, *Doctors in Gray*, 229.

43. Chisolm, *Manual of Military Surgery* (1864), 172, 370, 409, and 417–18; Gross, *System of Surgery*, 509.

44. Chisolm, *Manual of Military Surgery (*1864), 409; Gross, *System of Surgery*, 509.

45. Daniel, *Recollections of a Rebel Surgeon*, 250–52; *Confederate States Medical and Surgical Journal* 1, no. 9 (1864): 129–31; Alexander Hoff to Alden March, February 18, 1863, Hoff Papers, History of Medicine Division's Modern Manuscripts Sections, National Library of Medicine, Bethesda, Md. See also *CSA Medical and Surgical Journal* 1, no. 8 (1864): 128. For further examples of problematic descriptions of surgeons, see McMullen, *Surgeon with Stonewall Jackson*, 15; Chisolm, *Manual of Military Surgery* (1864), 172, 370, 409, and 417–18; and Bollet, *Civil War Medicine*, 436.

46. Wegner, *Phantom Pain*, ix; Johnson, *Muskets and Medicine*, 255. The Union number does not account for amputations on officers performed in private homes or by family physicians. At the same time, the Union number also does not include amputations performed after the war, so undoubtedly the number should increase significantly. See MED, pt. 3, vol. 2, 877. In her recent work, Margaret Humphreys estimated the total number of Union amputations at sixty thousand. See *Marrow of Tragedy*, 292. Lisa Marie Herschbach estimated that twenty thousand Confederate soldiers underwent amputation during the Civil War in "Fragmentation and Reunion," 96–97, 232. Dixon Wecter offered an estimate of twenty-five thousand Confederate amputees in his work *When Johnny Comes Marching Home*, 209.

47. Reports on Amputation Cases, Howard's Grove General Hospital, Richmond, Va., 1862, NARA. First Mississippi Hospital at Jackson, 1863–65. The six men are A. D. Saddler (Twenty-First Miss.), Jonathan Green (Forty-Fourth Ala.), J. A. McGowan (Forty-First Miss.), John Bini, F. Kepler (Thirtieth La.), and Wyatt Feflin (Ninth La.); Cunningham, *Doctors in Gray*, 222. Medical and Hospital Series, box 2, Winder Hospital, MOC; Breeden, *Joseph Jones*, 222. Among the numbers of amputees at Winder, forty-one lost their legs, twenty-two lost some portion of

their arms, ten lost a finger, nine lost a foot or ankle, and four lost a hand or wrist. Cunningham also listed amputations performed in Constantinople in 1855 and discovered a comparable number of amputations with a slightly higher mortality rate (46 percent compared to the 42 percent around Richmond). The Crimean War had a mortality rate of nearly 62 percent for amputations. At Chimborazo Hospital in Richmond, surgeon E. H. Smith reported on thirteen different cases of compound fracture of the femur in 1862 and 1863. Among the cases, the surgeon performed six amputations, leading to two patient deaths (one from tetanus, which could develop on a stump that had a continual amount of discharge). Seven patients received conservative surgery, utilizing splints, of whom two died. Following the Battle at Chickamauga in September 1863, Carlyle Terry, the chief surgeon for a field hospital within Hindman's Division, Army of Tennessee, reported the details of forty-nine different surgical cases. The medical staff performed twenty amputations and three resections. Fourteen of the amputees fully recovered, as did all the patients who underwent resection. The death of only six patients after amputation prompted the surgeon to declare "the great success of his operations." See *Confederate States Medical and Surgical Journal* 1, no. 2 (February 1864): 24–25 and *Confederate States Medical and Surgical Journal* 1, no. 5 (May 1864): 75–77.

48. Medical and Hospital Series, Isaac S. Tanner Collection, box 2, MOC. The twenty-six amputations at Cold Harbor include twelve fingers, eight arms, five toes, and a hand. The Plymouth, N.C., amputations include fifteen fingers, thirteen legs, three arms, two toes, and a foot. At Drewry's Bluff, physicians treated 534 gunshot wounds and performed only eight finger amputations, five arms, four legs, and a foot. The N.C. 1865 amputations included eight arms, four legs, and two fingers. At Chester Station on May 18–21, 1864, 211 soldiers suffered gunshot wounds and only eight underwent amputation, including four fingers, three arms, and a leg.

49. Duffy, *Rudolph Matas History of Medicine in Louisiana*, 306–7; Welsh, *Two Confederate Hospitals and Their Patients*, 119, 135, and 150. Amputees at Fairgrounds Hospital 1 in Atlanta included Pvt. Lewis Crouch (Nineteenth S.C., finger), Simon Morse (Nineteenth S.C., thumb), Sgt. C. T. Ezell (Fifty-Fourth Ala., leg), G. B. Gordon (Second Ky., hand), George Lee (Twenty-Seventh Tenn., arm), Second Lt. Jesse A. Shelton (Fiftieth Tenn., leg), and Alex Warren (Fifty-Fourth Ala., finger). Among the amputees, one soldier returned to duty, six were furloughed, three were sent to another hospital, one was discharged from service, and the other remained unreported. More information can be found in Welsh, *Two Confederate Hospitals and Their Patients*, appendix C on CD-ROM, Fairgrounds Hospital 1 Listing, 66, 88, 205, 265, 200, 253, and 294. Amputees at Fairgrounds Hospital 2 included S. Anderson (Twenty-Second Ala., leg), F. Grassit (right thigh), J. S. Gray (left leg), Wiley Knight (arm), Z. P. Lee (right leg), H. D. McCrory (left leg), J. L. Potillo (right arm), Pvt. A. V. Carlile (Fortieth Ala., left thigh), Sgt. D. A. Crow (finger), L. M. Durine (Seventh Ark., leg), J. N. Fox (leg), Lt. S. G. Corchoran (Thirty-Third Tenn., leg), and Jacob Fritz (arm). Among these amputees, two died from their amputation and another three were discharged from military service due to the operation. The lack of precise data may rest in the fact that the number of gunshot-wounded victims swelled around the time of the battles at Murfreesboro, Chickamauga, and Atlanta, when several of the hospital beds still had patients.

The name listing is available in Welsh, *Two Confederate Hospitals and Their Patients*, appendix C on CD-ROM, Fairgrounds Hospital 2 Listing, 4, 31, 41, 45, 55, 65, 67, 75, 112, 227, 129, and 158.

50. Hospital Records, Louisiana Military Commission Collection, LSU. In all the survey hospitals, 480 amputations and 51 resections took place. Among the amputations, leg and thigh amputations accounted for the most (195), followed by arms (146), fingers (118), and toes (21). Marshall Hospital in Columbus, Georgia, performed zero amputations from September 1864 through February 1865. Over the same time span, Walker Hospital, also in Columbus, performed twenty-five amputations. The following hospitals were surveyed as part of the collection to determine amputation numbers for July to September 1864: First Ark. Fort Gaines, Ga.; First Fla. Fort Gaines, Ga.; Twenty-Second Ga. Augusta Ga.; Twenty-Third Miss. Atlanta Ga.; Second Ga. Hosp., Augusta, Ga.; Third Ga. Augusta Ga.; Academy, Forsyth, Ga.; Asylum Augusta Ga.; Athens, Ga.; Atlanta, Ga.; Augusta, Ga.; Augusta Arsenal; Bainesville, Ga.; Barnesville Ga.; Bell Greensboro, Ga.; Blacks Hosp, Augusta, Ga.; Blind School, Macon, Ga.; Bragg Americus, Ga.; Brown Milledgeville, Ga.; Buckner Hosp, Newman Ga.; Cannon La Grange, Ga.; Catoosa, Griffin, Ga.; City Hall, Macon, Ga.; Clayton, Forsyth, Ga.; Concert Hall Montgomery, Ala.; Convalescent, Macon, Ga.; Dawson Greensboro, Ga.; Depot Macon, Ga.; Direction Griffin, Ga.; Erwin Barnesville, Ga.; FG #2, Vineville, Ga.; FG#1 Vineville, Ga.; Floyd House Macon, Ga.; Foard Americus, Ga.; Foard Hospital, Forsyth, Ga.; Foard Newman, Ga.; Forsyth, Ga.; Fort Gaines Ga.; Gamble Newman, Ga.; General Columbus, Ga.; General Covington, Ga.; General Eufaula, Ala.; General Notasulga, Ala.; Georgia Hosp Augusta, Ga.; Gilmer Hosp, Forsyth, Ga.; Grant Hospital, Vineville, Ga.; Greensburg, Ga.; Griffin Ga.; Hardee Hosp, Forsyth, Ga.; Hill Cuthbert, Ga.; Hood Cuthbert, Ga.; Institute, Macon, Ga.; Johnston Hosp, Forsyth, Ga.; Kingston Barnesville Ga.; Ladus Montgomery, Ala.; LaGrange, Ga.; Law LaGrange, Ga.; Lee Hospital, Columbus, Ga.; Lewellen Barnesville, Ga.; Lumpkin Cuthbert, Ga.; Macon, Ga.; Madison, Montgomery, Ala.; Marshall Hosp, Columbus, Ga.; Medical College, Wilmer Ga.; Montgomery, Ala.; New Atlanta, Ga.; Newsom Thomaston, Ga.; Ocmulgee Macon, Ga.; Officers Augusta, Ga.; Polk, Vineville, Ga.; Quintard, Griffin, Ga.; Reid West Point, Ga.; SP Moore, Griffin, Ga.; St Mary La Grange, Ga.; St. Mary Montgomery, Ala.; Stonewall Montgomery, Ala.; Stout Macon, Ga.; Stout Madison, Ga.; Stout Milledgeville, Ga.; Texas Hosp, Auburn, Ala.; Thomaston Ga.; Union Springs, Ala.; Vineville, Ga.; Walker Columbus, Ga.; Watts Montgomery, Ala., Columbus, Ga. Hospital Records and Columbus, Miss., Hospital Records, 2.325/AA35 Samuel Hollingsworth Stout Papers, UTX.

51. Hospital Records, Ocmulgee Hospital, Macon, Ga., EMY. During the six months, the surgeons treated 376 gunshot wounds and performed seventy-six amputations and thirty-one resections. MS 218 Mays Confederate Hospital Records, UGA. Surgeons at Mays Confederate Hospital, created on July 2, 1864, performed a few amputations over the course of its existence. The dilapidated records for the hospital indicated a wide variety of amputations performed, including a thigh, a right arm at the shoulder, a middle finger on the left hand, and a right thumb. H. Thomasson, W. Dickson, H. Lewis, and R. M. Jackson each lost their right arm, while Lt. E. Parker and John Berryhill lost their left arms. M. Parker, of the Thirty-

Fifth Georgia, lost his left leg and L. B. Lightfoot, a member of the Third Georgia, lost his middle finger on his left hand. In addition to Georgia patients, J. H. Taylor, from South Carolina, had his left thigh amputated. The total numbers of amputations are not precise, but surgeons did indicate they performed seventeen amputations between August 10 and 13, 1864. For additional surgeon cases, see Medical Case History Journal by Dr. Henry Dye, Arkansas History Commission; Fatout, *Letters of a Civil War Surgeon*, 108 and 110.

52. Koonce, *Doctor to the Front*, 78–79. Historian David Williams argued that soldiers described doctors as callous, especially when they made medical diagnosis. See Williams, *People's History*, 210.

53. Beers, *Memories*, 215; March 24, 1865, letter to parents, Livingston Letters, MOC; January 19, 1863, letter to Lizzie, Thomas Henry Pitts Papers, EMY; MED, pt. 3, vol. 2, 95–96.

54. April 6, 1862, entry, Lemuel A. Scarbrough Diary, Manuscript, EMY; *Memphis Press-Scimitar*, August 15, 1959. The soldier survived the war, worked in the cotton business in Memphis, fathered fourteen children with two different wives, and lived to the age of eighty-one with both of his feet intact. Welsh, *Medical Histories of Confederate Generals*, 216–18. Although Trimble avoided his first amputation, he got shot in the leg at Gettysburg and lost the lower half of his left leg. Trimble recovered in a federal hospital in Baltimore, received an artificial leg that assisted him in walking with his crutches, and spent the duration of the war as a Union prisoner at Johnson Island. Welsh, *Medical Histories of Confederate Generals*, 223–24. The soldier who had his arm damaged survived the war, worked as a farmer and lawyer, and won election to Congress and as lieutenant governor of Virginia. For other examples of limbs being saved, see Yeary, *Reminiscences of the Boys in Gray*, 824.

55. Cimbala, *Soldiers North and South*, 176; Johnson, *Muskets and Medicine*, 257–58.

56. MED, pt. 3, vol. 2, 30; Barnes, *Medical and Surgical History of the Civil War*, 388; "May 31, 1863" and "June 11, 1863," Dr. B. W. Allen Civil War Journal, UAB; MED, pt. 2, vol. 2, 171; Welsh, *Medical Histories of Confederate Generals*, 92–93. Other examples can be found in Bollet, *Civil War Medicine*, 157; "Funeral Eulogy," Watson and Morris Family Papers #5150-z, UNC; "July 1862 letter to mother," Hatrick Family Scrapbook #4365, UNC; Robert Franklin Account, Ocmulgee Hospital, Macon, Ga. EMY.

57. Koonce, *Doctor to the Front*, 123; OR ser. 1, vol. 24, 423; *South Carolina Women in the Confederacy*, 108.

58. Pitcock and Gurley, *I Acted from Principle*, 42–43, 51–52, 138–41, 150–52, 224, 228, and 230. See also Wiley, *Life of Johnny Reb*, 267–69.

59. Medical Personnel Collection, Medical and Hospital Series, box 2, MOC.

60. MED, pt. 1, vol. 1, appendix, 7; Bollet, *Civil War Medicine*, 440–41; Hagerman, *Dearest of Captains*, 32.

61. Brig. Gen. Samuel W. Ferguson Memoirs, 20, SCH; Thompson, *History of the Orphan Brigade*, 299–300. Additional examples of reminiscences of surgeons can be found in Robson, *How a One-Legged Rebel Lives*, 149; Cimbala, *Soldiers North and South*, 177; "July 1, 1862," James Richmond Boulware Diary, USC; Hartman and Coles, *Biographical Rosters of Florida's Confederate and Union Soldiers*, 1:139–40.

62. Poem to Drs. Watson and Long, MS 2345 E. Merton Coulter Papers, box 12, UGA.

63. Styple, *Writing and Fighting the Confederate War*, 26 and 108.

64. Houck, *Confederate Surgeon*, 79.

65. Cunningham, *Doctors in Gray*, 269.

Chapter 2. The Patients

1. Formento, *Notes and Observations on Army Surgery*, 51–53.

2. Meier, "No Place for the Sick," 184 and 196; Gorn, "Gouge and Bite," 39–40. Gorn notes that southern men expected to undergo pain and suffering, as both elements were part of a man's fate. For more, see Meier, *Nature's Civil War*.

3. *Confederate Veteran Magazine* 13 (November 1905): 516; Gammage, *The Camp, the Bivouac, and the Battlefield*, 73; Lee Barfield to Wife, May 14, 1863, GA. Other dangerous circumstances could manifest if a soldier never found the field hospital. Before the engagement at Antietam in 1862, C. B. Deishler, a soldier from Virginia, found himself shot in the arm. A few comrades tied a sling around his arm and he traveled to the field hospital. A group of surgeons examined the damaged arm and instructed him to travel to the division hospital to undergo amputation. Deishler never found the hospital and traveled home, without ever undergoing an operation. See Yeary, *Reminiscences of the Boys in Gray*, 182–83.

4. Friedmann, *Psychological Rehabilitation of the Amputee*, 24; Mary Jane Vaughn Clark letter, May 7, 1862, MOS.

5. Cunningham, *Doctors in Gray*, 227; Friedmann, *Psychological Rehabilitation of the Amputee*, 24; Rable, *God's Almost Chosen Peoples*, 171–72; Yeary, *Reminiscences of the Boys in Gray*, 9–10 and 106–7. Rable presents several examples of soldiers (mostly Union) who interpreted the loss of their limb as a religious sacrifice. The men would rather enter heaven as an amputee than hell as a physically complete specimen. Some soldiers tended to view their empty sleeve as a marker of both sacrifice for the nation and sacrifice for their Savior, Jesus Christ. For more on the role of religion in shaping the lives of Confederate soldiers, see Berry, *All That Makes a Man*, 91–94 and Wiley, *Life of Johnny Reb*, 174–91 and 264–69.

6. *Confederate Veteran Magazine* 2 (October 1894): 283. Hickey survived the war, but his marriage to a religious woman prompted him to join a church, and he continually asked his fellow parishioners to pray for him.

7. Eugene Ferris Collection, box 2, folder 1, UM. For more on altered courage due to recovery from an illness, see Linderman, *Embattled Courage*, 116–17 and 130–33.

8. Marshall, *Life of William B. Bate*, 54; Freemon, *Gangrene and Glory*, 157; *Confederate Veteran Magazine* 2 (November 1894): 337; Welsh, *Medical Histories of Confederate Generals*, 15. Bate survived until March 9, 1905, and enjoyed a lengthy postwar political career, serving as a senator and governor of Tennessee.

9. Fletcher, *Rebel Private*, 102–3.

10. Ibid., 104–6.

11. Elliott, *Doctor Quintard*, 79.

12. Hacker, Hilde, and Jones, " Effect of the Civil War on Southern Marriage Patterns," 49–50; Harwell, *Journal of Kate Cumming*, 273.

13. Underwood, *Women of the Confederacy*, 116–17. Although we have no way of knowing how this relationship turned out, it seems plausible that his fiancée accepted him back, especially since the soldier later expressed concern over the lack of communication, rather than his physically altering injury.

14. "Walter Lenoir Diary, 23," Lenoir Family Papers #426, UNC. See also "September 21, 1862 Letter to Mother," "January 12, 1863 letter to brother," "February 25, 1863 letter to brother," "April 26, 1863 letter to brother," "Walter Lenoir Diary, 28," Lenoir Family Papers #426, UNC.

15. "Letter to Sister Sarah Joyce Lenoir, 27 March 1864," Lenoir Family Papers #426, UNC.

16. M. D. L. Stephens Manuscript, UM.

17. For more on reputation and honor among southern men, see Wyatt-Brown, *Southern Honor*; Greenberg, *Honor and Slavery*; Friend and Glover, *Southern Manhood*; and Berry, *All That Makes a Man*.

18. Marlow, *Matt W. Ransom*, 99–100; Dorsey, *Recollections of Henry Watkins Allen*, 12–13, 74, and 144–45. Other examples of men waiting for death can be found in Welsh, *Medical Histories of Confederate Generals*, 4, 5, 16, and 182; Letter to Major A. J. Foard, November 30, 1861, Samuel Hollingsworth Stout Papers, EMY. Ransom survived the war with a deformed limb. He spent twenty-three years in the United States and served as U.S. ambassador to Mexico. For more on the notion of the honorable and courageous death, see Linderman, *Embattled Courage*, 12 and 124–28 and Berry, *All That Makes a Man*, 163–92. Other examples can be located in January 20, 1865 letter to parents, Livingston Letters, MOC; #00044, John C. Parker, #00013, J. J. Howard, #01224, Alexander Nation, Confederate pension applications, Texas Comptroller's Office Claims Records, TX.

19. Eugene Ferris Collection, UM. For more on a desire to command soldiers until the bitter end, see McWhiney and Jamieson, *Attack and Die*.

20. Welsh, *Medical Histories of Confederate Generals*, 2–3; *Confederate Veteran Magazine* 32 (1924): 59–60.

21. Evans, *Confederate Military History vol. V: North Carolina*, 314–17; Evans, *Confederate Military History vol. VIII: Alabama*, 395–97. Grimes survived the war intact and also survived an assassination attempt on August 14, 1880. Bulger had served in the Alabama legislature before the war and initially opposed secession. Upon his wounding at Gettysburg, a member of a Union medical staff nursed him back to health. Bulger spent some time in a prison camp at Johnson Island and then returned to Alabama, where voters sent him back to the legislature. In another example, Capt. J. Frederick Cooper, an officer from Georgia, arrived on an operating table with a smashed knee. Although the physician recommended immediate amputation, Cooper cried, "Stop, doctor. Can't you save my leg?" The physician, Dr. Miller, responded, "No, it is impossible. It must come off, I tell you." Cooper rephrased his entreaty, "Doctor, is there a possible chance for me to save this leg?" The surgeon paused and then said, "Perhaps, one chance in a hundred, but I warn you now that if it is not speedily cut off you will be a dead man in two weeks." "Doctor, I will take that chance," replied Cooper. The physician called for the next patient. Cooper perished seven weeks later because he resisted amputation. See *Hospital Life in the Army of the Tennessee by Kate Cumming*, 25–26, Joseph Jones Papers, TU; Wilkinson and Woodworth, *Scythe of Fire*, 90–91. In addition, other

examples of bravado and death can be located in Mays, *Let Us Meet in Heaven*, 241–47, 251–53, 256–59.

22. Evans, *Confederate Military History vol. VIII: Alabama*, 409–11. Fry recovered and spent some time at Johnson Island. After the war, he lived in Cuba for three years and returned to the United States in 1868, taking up work in the cotton industry.

23. Brinsfield, *Spirit Divided*, 89; Warren, *Epitome of Practical Surgery for Field and Hospital*, 83–84.

24. *Lost Cause* 7, no. 5 (December 1902): 74, accessed in United Daughters of the Confederacy Records, KYHS. For more on the experiences of battle, see Wiley, *Life of Johnny Reb*, 28–35 and 80–89. Other wounded officers can be found in Welsh, *Medical Histories of Confederate Generals*, 1–2 and 12.

25. *An Impressed New Yorker*, 179–80; *Hospital Life in the Army of the Tennessee by Kate Cumming*, 25–26, Joseph Jones Papers, TU; Wilkinson and Woodworth, *Scythe of Fire*, 90–91.

26. Freemon, *Gangrene and Glory*, 81–82.

27. Arnold, *Early Life and Letters of General Thomas J. Jackson*, 349–50; Hunter McGuire, MD, "Last Wound of the Late General Stonewall Jackson: The Amputation of the Arm and His Last Moments and Death," *Richmond Medical Journal*, May 1866, UAB; "May 7, 1863 letter," William Davis Cotton and Family Papers, LSU.

28. Arnold, *Early Life and Letters of General Thomas J. Jackson*, 350–55.

29. Sears, *Chancellorsville*, 447. For more on Jackson's death, see Arnold, *Early Life and Letters of General Thomas J. Jackson*, 356–59; *Confederate Veteran Magazine* 13 (May 1905): 230; Blanton, *Medicine in Virginia in the Nineteenth Century*, 314.

30. Dabney, *Life and Campaign of Lieutenant General Thomas J. Jackson*, 730–31.

31. Undated newspaper clipping, William Davis Cotton and Family Papers, LSU; Fahs, *Imagined Civil War*, 88–89. See also Hettle, *Inventing Stonewall Jackson*.

32. Pfanz, *Richard S. Ewell*, 257–59; MED, pt. 3, vol. 2, 242; Welsh, *Medical Histories of Confederate Generals*, 64; Blanton, *Medicine in Virginia in the Nineteenth Century*, 315; Jones, *American Civil War*, 439.

33. Pfanz, *Richard S. Ewell*, 271 and 279; Pfanz, *Letters of General Richard S. Ewell*, 235, 238, and 250; MED, pt. 3, vol. 2, 242. Ewell used a prosthetic leg, but the poor fit led to the ulceration of the stump of his damaged leg and his removal from command in the fall of 1863.

34. "October 21, 1863 letter," John Thompson Darby Papers, USC; Lewellen, "Limbs Made and Unmade by War," 45. See also Miller, *John Bell Hood*.

35. For more cases of Confederate officers who lost limbs during the war, see Welsh, *Medical Histories of Confederate Generals*, 60, 184, 193–94, and 219–22; Owen, *History of Alabama and Dictionary of Alabama Biography*, 3:180; http://www.archives.alabama.gov/reference/flags/062.html (accessed July 26, 2010); Douglas, *Douglas's Texas Battery*, 89; *Confederate States Medical and Surgical Journal* 1, no. 9 (September 1864): 13; Jernigan Furlough Application, 2G385 Samuel Hollingsworth Stout Papers, UTX.

36. May 13, 1864, and May 28, 1864 entries, James William Howard Journal, AUB; Nelson, *Ruin Nation*, 188.

37. Thompson, *History of the Orphan Brigade*, 551, 559, 1016, and 1022; Thompson, *History of the First Kentucky Brigade*, 584, 607, 639, 686, 692, 741, 753, 756–57,

763, 774, 840, 853, 880, 884, 907, 912, 915, and 924; MED, pt. 3, vol. 2, 132; War Department, Surgeon General's Office, "*Report on Amputations at the Hip-Joint in Military Surgery,*" 43.

38. Douglas, *Douglas's Texas Battery,* 187; Bollet, *Civil War Medicine,* 268; Hartman and Coles, *Biographical Rosters of Florida's Confederate and Union Soldiers,* 1:251.

39. Evans, *Confederate Military History vol. VI: South Carolina,* 755–56; War Department, Surgeon General's Office, "*Report on Amputations at the Hip-Joint in Military Surgery,*" 50.

40. Evans, *Confederate Military History vol. VIII: Alabama,* 798–99. For additional examples of Confederate soldiers who lost an arm, see Yeary, *Reminiscences of the Boys in Gray,* 449; Wetherington, *Plain Folk's Fight,* 118 and 120; Evans, *Confederate Military History vol. VI: South Carolina,* 810–11. See also MED, pt. 2, vol. 2, 214 and 912; Yeary, *Reminiscences of the Boys in Gray,* 369–70; and Evans, *Confederate Military History vol. VIII: Alabama,* 595–98.

41. Medical Personnel Collection, Medical and Hospital Series, box 2, MOC; Wegner, *Phantom Pain,* 14.

42. Formento, *Notes and Observations on Army Surgery,* 55–56.

43. Surgeon B. A. Pope remarks, 2G381 Samuel Hollingsworth Stout Papers, UTX; T. B. Williams remarks on Hoffman, 2G381 Samuel Hollingsworth Stout Papers, UTX; Hartman and Coles, *Biographical Rosters of Florida's Confederate and Union Soldiers,* 3:961; OR ser. 1, vol. 33, 8; OR ser. 1, vol. 34, 841; Nelson, *Ruin Nation,* 178; "October 31, 1863" and "November 12, 1863," Dr. B. W. Allen Civil War Journal, UAB. For other instances of the removal of a finger, toe, foot, or hand from a Confederate private, see "Letter to Mary, October 12, 1862," Confederate Papers Collection #172, UNC; Hartman and Coles, *Biographical Rosters of Florida's Confederate and Union Soldiers,* 1:185; Welsh, *Medical Histories of Confederate Generals,* 223.

44. Clegham furlough application, 2G384 Samuel Hollingsworth Stout Papers, UTX; "July 22, 1863" and "July 29, 1863," Dr. B. W. Allen Civil War Journal, UAB.

45. Daniel, *Recollections of a Rebel Surgeon,* 86.

46. Wecter, *When Johnny Comes Marching Home,* 188; Berry, *All That Makes a Man,* 11–12.

47. MED, pt. 3, vol. 2, 132; *Lost Cause* 1, no. 5 (October 1898): 1–2, United Daughters of the Confederacy Records, box 40, KYHS

48. Nelson, *Ruin Nation,* 181; *Macon Daily Telegraph,* May 2, 1862; Yeary, *Reminiscences of the Boys in Gray,* 664.

49. *CSA Medical Journal* 2, no. 2 (February 1865): 29; Hartman and Coles, *Biographical Rosters of Florida's Confederate and Union Soldiers,* 2:644. See also Berry, *All That Makes a Man,* 42–44.

50. Brinsfield, *Spirit Divided,* 88–89.

51. Hagerman, *Dearest of Captains,* 49–50.

52. Freemon, *Gangrene and Glory,* 157; Welsh, *Medical Histories of Confederate Generals,* 15–16; McPherson, *For Cause and Comrades,* 80; Gorn, "Gouge and Bite," 40. See also Bynum, *Unruly Women,* 141 and Wiley, *Life of Johnny Reb,* 80–89. For more on honor and desertion, see Rubin, *Shattered Nation,* 78–79.

53. Yeary, *Reminiscences of the Boys in Gray,* 9–10 and 106–7; Evans, *Confeder-*

ate Military History vol. XI: Kentucky, 441–42. For additional examples of remarks about officers and the loss of their limbs, see Evans, *Confederate Military History vol. V: North Carolina*, 289–91 and 334–37 and William Trousdale Papers, box 8, folder 2 and box 3, folder 3, TN; Gross, *System of Surgery*, 564–65; OR ser. 1, vol. 28, 441; OR ser. 1, vol. 22, 204; OR ser. 1, vol. 20, 725–26.

54. Jones, *Southern Historical Society Papers* 8 (1880): 445–46; Yeary, *Reminiscences of the Boys in Gray*, 3–4 and 549; *Confederate Veteran Magazine* 17 (February 1909): 78.

55. *Southern Bivouac*, September 1882–August 1883 (Wilmington, N.C.: Broadfoot, 1992), 26–27. For more on the notion of courage in battle, see Linderman, *Embattled Courage*, 21, 73–79, and 128–30.

56. Freemon, *Gangrene and Glory*, 31; Rutkow, *Bleeding Blue and Gray*, 29–30.

57. MED, pt. 1, vol. 2, 412; Harry Lewis to Mrs. John Lewis, July 20, 1862, Harry Lewis Papers, #1222-z, UNC; "Olustee Description, Charles A. Hentz Memoir," Hentz Family Papers #332, UNC.

58. *Confederate States Medical and Surgical Journal* 1, no. 9 (September 1864): 132; Brock, *Southern Historical Society Papers* 25 (1897): 168; MED, pt. 2, vol. 2, 443; Yeary, *Reminiscences of the Boys in Gray*, 501, 710–11, and 815–16. For more examples of Confederate soldiers who underwent amputation but did not survive, see Bolling Hall Family Papers, 1785–1923, AL; Hartman and Coles, *Biographical Rosters of Florida's Confederate and Union Soldiers*, 1:450; Jones, "Five Confederates," 182; MS 658 Col. Samuel P. Lumpkin Papers, UGA; Welsh, *Medical Histories of Confederate Generals*, 81; http://www.archives.alabama.gov/marschall/J-Walker.html (accessed July 26, 2010); Henry Adicks Papers, USC; "Quitman, MS Texas General Hospital," Adjutant General Civil War Records, Texas State Troop Records, TX.

59. Civil War in Kentucky Scrapbook, KYHS.

60. Freemon, *Gangrene and Glory*, 157; *Confederate Veteran Magazine* 1, no. 4 (April 1893): 118.

61. OR ser. 2, vol. 4, 35; Yeary, *Reminiscences of the Boys in Gray*, 398–99, 582, and 783. For additional information on captured Union soldiers facing medical care from Confederate officials, see Letter from John Chisolm to Carolina Agatha Dabney, August 18, 1861, Sanders Family Papers, sec. 50, VHS.

62. Thompson, *History of the First Kentucky Brigade*, 789; OR ser. 2, vol. 6, 854; Wiggins, *Georgia's Confederate Sons*, 83; Hartman and Coles, *Biographical Rosters of Florida's Confederate and Union Soldiers*, 2:540. See also Thompson, *History of the First Kentucky Brigade*, 651, 767, 829, and 839.

63. Evans, *Confederate Military History vol. VI: South Carolina*, 561–62.

64. *Confederate Veteran Magazine* 12 (1904): 68.

65. March 8, 1865 letter from Edward Johnson, Pattie Burnley Papers, KYHS; Evans, *Confederate Military History vol. XVI: Florida*, 328–29 and 352–53; January 20, 1865, letter to family from Archie Livingston, Livingston Letters, MOC; *Confederate Veteran Magazine* 21 (1913): 28–29. See also Bohannon, "Wounded and Captured at Gettysburg," 14–15.

66. "A Bill to Amend an Act Entitled 'An Act to Provide an Invalid Corps,' approved 17 February, 1864," Confederate Pamphlets #36, DUKE; William Mooney, http://

www.history-sites.com/cgi-bin/bbs62x/nccwmb/webbs_config.pl?md=read
;id=2472 (accessed January 17, 2013); Cimbala, *Soldiers North and South*, 53; Cunningham, *Doctors in Gray*, 42–43. Cunningham indicated that records show at least
1,063 officers (231 of them "totally disqualified") and 5,139 soldiers (2,061 "totally
disqualified") served in the Invalid Corps. The record remains incomplete, making an accurate count nearly impossible. More information on the Union Invalid
Corps can be found in Nielsen, *Disability History of the United States*, 80–83.

67. Welsh, *Medical Histories of Confederate Generals*, 14–15 and 241; Wetherington,
Plain Folk's Fight, 150; OR ser. 4, vol. 2, 399. For additional examples of Confederate soldiers who survived amputation and lived for several decades, see Formento, *Notes and Observations on Army Surgery*, 20–21; *Confederate Veteran Magazine*
22 (1914): 568; *Confederate Veteran Magazine* 25 (1917): 175, 275, and 326–27.

68. Welsh, *Medical Histories of Confederate Generals*, 114–15; Underwood, *Women
of the Confederacy*, 237; Ozark Folk Encyclopedia, vol. A2, ARK.

69. MS 2642 R. D. Harris Papers, UGA; Breeden, *Joseph Jones*, 171–72; Martin,
Southern Hero Matthew Galbraith Butler, 77; Welsh, *Medical Histories of Confederate
Generals*, 32. Butler survived the war and worked as a lawyer, president of a min-
ing company, and U.S. senator.

Chapter 3. The Women

1. Letter from Evangeline to Will dated January 22, 1862, *Crutcher-Shannon
Papers*, UTX. For more on antebellum notions of dependency, see McCurry, *Masters of Small Worlds*.

2. Jabour, *Scarlett's Sisters*, 189 and 263; Ott, *Confederate Daughters*, 4, 10 and 11;
Glover, *Southern Sons*, 4; Gorn, "Gouge and Bite," 40. Laura Edwards argues that
men needed a wife and a home in order to feel complete. See Edwards, *Gendered
Strife and Confusion*, 127–29. Modern psychological professionals use the term
"devotees," who are individuals who are sexually attracted to individuals with disabilities. See Schweik, *Ugly Laws*, 321. For more on the experience of Confeder-
ate women during and after the war, see Rubin, *Shattered Nation*, 54–77; Goldfield,
Still Fighting the Civil War, 89–120; Censer, *Reconstruction of White Southern Womanhood*; Drago, *Confederate Phoenix*; Dailey, *Before Jim Crow*; Edwards, *Scarlett Doesn't
Live Here Anymore*; Farman, *Women of the American South*; Faust, *Mothers of Invention*;
Long, *Great Southern Babylon*; Whites, *Gender Matters*; and Berry, *All That Makes a
Man*, 95–111.

3. Hilde, *Worth a Dozen Men*, 11.

4. Jabour, *Scarlett's Sisters*, 256; Faust, *Mothers of Invention*, 92; Underwood,
Women of the Confederacy, 274; Schurr, "It Is Heart-Breaking to Hear Them Groan."
For more on the various roles of women during the Civil War, see McCurry, *Con-
federate Reckoning*; Berkin, *Civil War Wives*; Whites and Long, *Occupied Women*; and
Taylor, *Divided Family in Civil War America*, 130–33.

5. *Charleston Courier*, July 22, 1863; *Charleston Courier*, July 23, 1863. The reporter anticipated another day of amputations, as "Yankee blood leaks out by
the basket full." The Union blockade of the city prevented the arrival of reme-
dial supplies for the medical staff in Charleston needed to even care for their own

wounded soldiers, let alone the Union invaders. Thus, many of the Union amputees suffered a great deal as Charleston's citizens felt compelled to care for the enemy.

6. W. L. Kennon, "A Tribute to the Womanhood of the Confederacy, 1934," UM; Janie Smith, http://ncgenweb.us/cumberland/cumberland.htm (accessed July 14, 2009).

7. Gillespie, *Lady with the Milk White Hands*, 20; Hagerman, *Dearest of Captains*, 39; Faust, *Mothers of Invention*, 106.

8. Underwood, *Women of the Confederacy*, 84–85.

9. Daniel, *Recollections of a Rebel Surgeon*, 68–69; Beers, *Memories*, 135, 136, 144, and 158.

10. Faust, *Mothers of Invention*, 238–44. For more on the burdens of nursing, see Faust, *Mothers of Invention*, 92–113; Long, *Rehabilitating Bodies*, 180–209; Hilde, *Worth a Dozen Men*; and Schultz, *Women at the Front.*

11. Berlin, *Confederate Nurse*, 135–36 and 140–41.

12. July 1864 letter and May 9, 1864 letter, Lucas Ashley Family Papers, DUKE; Josephine Crump Papers, ARK; Whites, *Civil War as a Crisis in Gender*, 92.

13. Wiley, *Southern Woman's Story*, 106–8.

14. Ibid.

15. *Hospital Life in the Army of the Tennessee by Kate Cumming*, 14–15, 19 and 20, Joseph Jones Papers, TU.

16. Harwell, *Journal of Kate Cumming*, 141 and 155; *Hospital Life in the Army of the Tennessee by Kate Cumming*, 23–24, Joseph Jones Papers, TU

17. Tuesday July 19 diary entry, William Beavens 3244Z, UNC; Swank, *Confederate Letters and Diaries*, 76; Benson, *Berry Benson's Civil War Book*, 42.

18. Nelson, *Ruin Nation*, 185; Letter from Miss L.D. Lewis to Mrs. Hopkins, June 11, 1861, Alabama Hospitals in Richmond, Administrative Files, AL.

19. June 19, 1862, June 30, 1862, and August 23, 1862 letters from Mrs. Joseph S. McGruder, Asa T. Martin Papers, AUB; Letter to William Battle, October 16, 1862, in Battle Family Papers #3223, UNC.

20. Hilde, *Worth a Dozen Men*, 107–8. See also Whites, *Civil War as a Crisis in Gender*, and Faust, *Mothers of Invention.*

21. Greenville Ladies Association Minutes, 1861–65, DUKE; *Jacob Mordecai Papers*, DUKE.

22. Ott, *Confederate Daughters*, 48; July 26, 1861, in Margaret Ann Mata Morris Grimball Diary, 1860–66 #975-z, UNC; Sketch of the Soldiers Relief Association of Charleston, SCH; February 1864 article and November 11, 1864 article, Mary Snowden Papers, USC. In Augusta, Georgia, women pushed for the development of a wayside hospital at a local rail stop in order to care for wounded and diseased soldiers. See Whites, *Civil War as a Crisis in Gender*, 57–59 and 91.

23. Jabour, *Scarlett's Sisters*, 274; Taylor, *Divided Family in Civil War America*, 187–88; Hacker, Hilde, and Jones, " Effect of the Civil War on Southern Marriage Patterns," 39–70; McClurken, *Take Care of the Living*, 55–57. McClurken notes that southern society expected women to remarry in order to rejoin the patriarchal fold. However, the large number of dead white men limited marriage access for many women. Death statistics on the American Civil War are still evolving past the traditional number of 620,000 total battle deaths, especially with Hacker's

"A Census-Based Count of the Civil War Dead," 307–48. Hacker hypothesizes that the death toll could be increased up to at least another 150,000. At minimum, 20 percent of the draft-age southern white male population died in the war, though Hacker's revised data would increase that percentage. Death statistics also neglect the Confederate soldiers who may have died from wounds acquired from the war shortly after they returned home. For more on the marriage of southern women, see Berry, *All That Makes a Man*, 108–9; Censer, *Reconstruction of White Southern Womanhood*, 32; and Faust, *Mothers of Invention*, 139–52. For other cases of difficulty with marriage prospects, see Port Royal Diary Entries, May 5, 1864 and August 5, 1864, Sue Richardson Collection, EMY.

24. "The Homespun Dress Song," in Mobile, AL UCV Program, May 18, 1905, United Confederate Veterans Association Records, LSU; Loula Kendall Rogers Journal, September 28, 1860, August 1 and October 26, 1861, Loula Kendall Rogers Papers, EMY; C. Alice Ready Diary, March 6, 1862, UNC; See also Ott, *Confederate Daughters*, 114. Ott argues that some women warned other women about marrying any soldier rather quickly, especially those who simply wanted to have the baby of a soldier away at war.

25. Crist, *Papers of Jefferson Davis*, 62; Wetherington, *Plain Folk's Fight*, 155.

26. "Blighted Hopes," in Annie Jeter Carmouche Papers, TU; Underwood, *Women of the Confederacy*, 64–65; Whites, "'Stand by Your Man,'" in Farman, *Women of the American South*, 133–49. In gender theory, the image of the "sturdy oak" represents men and their ability to handle impossible tasks with confidence and control. For more on the sturdy oak, see Lindsey, *Gender Roles*, 227.

27. "The Empty Sleeve," M. J. Solomons Scrapbook, DUKE.

28. *New Orleans Daily Picayune*, January 15, 1871.

29. Samuel A. Bird, Twelfth S.C. Volunteers, accessed at fold3.com on January 11, 2012. Asylum information provided via email dated Friday December 16, 2011, from Diane Miller Sommerville; Jabour, *Scarlett's Sisters*, 271; Sutherland, *Very Violent Rebel*, 122. For more, see Faust, "Altars of Sacrifice," in Clinton and Silber, *Divided Houses*, 175; Bynum, *Unruly Women*, 132; Rable, "'Missing in Action,'" in Clinton and Silber, *Divided Houses*, 139.

30. Beers, *Memories*, 205–6.

31. Woodward, *Mary Chesnut's Civil War*, 443, 492, and 547.

32. Ibid., 430–31, 505, 510, 560; Woodworth, *Jefferson Davis and His Generals*, 269–70.

33. Woodward, *Mary Chesnut's Civil War*, 565, 570, 588–89, 622, and 647. Hood married Anna Marie Hennen, and the couple had eleven children in the span of a decade.

34. Underwood, *Women of the Confederacy*, 64. There are other cases of women being called to the bedside of their love interest right after an amputation, which can be located in June 14, 1864 letter and June 16, 1864 letter, James Michael Barr Papers, 1862–64, USC.

35. King, *War Time Journal of a Georgia Girl*, 120; Ott, *Confederate Daughters*, 116 and 120; Reid, *After the War*, 138 and 155; Smith and Cooper, *Window on the War*, 34.

36. Faust, *Mothers of Invention*, 16–17; Benson, *Berry Benson's Civil War Book*, 43; July 9 letter to Flax, July 9 letter to Mrs. Little, July 20 letter to Flax, November 25 letter to Flax, in Benjamin Franklin Little Papers #3954, UNC.

37. Underwood, *Women of the Confederacy*, 64. There are numerous examples in the historical literature of southern women marrying Confederate amputees and living a long and healthy life with several children. Some specific examples can be located in Evans, *Confederate Military History vol. XV: Texas*, 402, 464, 536–37, 586, and 696–98; "Eulogy," in Watson and Morris Family Papers #5150-z, UNC; Evans, *Confederate Military History vol. X: Tennessee*, 746–47 and 789–91; Evans, *Confederate Military History vol. VIII: Alabama*, 505–6, 528–29, 693–94, 730, and 764–65; Evans, *Confederate Military History vol. XIV: Arkansas*, 481–82; Evans, *Confederate Military History vol. VI: South Carolina*, 546–47.

38. Mary C. Berry Papers, ARK.

39. Ibid.; Eulogy from member of the Benton Bar Association, James C. Berry Collection, ARK.

40. Faust, *Mothers of Invention*, 59, 63, 78–79, 147, and 251; Nelson, *Ruin Nation*, 196. See also McCurry, *Confederate Reckoning*, 26–29, 86, and 93–100; Giesberg, "The Fortieth Congress," in Whites and Long, *Occupied Women*, 185–93; and Whites, *Civil War as a Crisis in Gender*, 15–40 and 132–59.

41. Pfanz, *Richard S. Ewell*, 260–64.

42. Ibid., 264–65.

43. Evans, *Confederate Military History vol. V: North Carolina*, 431, 647–48, 692–93, and 784.

44. #450 and #2697 Confederate Pension Files, KY.

45. "Report of Surgeon General, 1892," United Confederate Veterans Association Records, LSU. Historian Jeffrey W. McClurken finds a host of widows in Virginia who relied on the Baptist church for survival due to their impoverished state. For more, see his work *Take Care of the Living*, 55–57, 80–81, and 150–69. For more on the Union pension system, see Marten, *Sing Not War*, 199–243. For additional information on the plight of southern women, see Hamburger, "We Take Care of Our Women," in Green, *Before the New Deal*, 61–77, and Gross, "Good Angels."

46. "Beneficiary Land Warrant," in Abstracts Land Sales, Claims, Misc. Records, LA; Louisiana Legislative Acts #96, 1884, LA; "Emilie Verret," Soldiers Proof as Beneficiary under Act #55 of 1896, LA. Louisiana added pensions for widows a decade later, which can be found in Louisiana Legislative Acts, #125, 1898 and #169, 1902, LA. Information on the Texas land grant program can be located in *Senate Journal of Texas, 17th Legislature 1881*, 78, 119–20, 187, and 301–2; *House Journal of Texas, 17th Legislature 1881*, 287; Confederate Scrip Voucher, Archives and Records Division, Texas General Land Office. Texas paid eligible widows eight dollars a month beginning in 1899. Information on Texas can be located in *House Journal of Texas, 26th Legislature 1899*, 1250–53 and *House Journal of Texas, 26th Legislature 1899*, 816–17 and 1252. Tennessee added widows to the pension program in 1905; they received six dollars a month, and the program continued until 1969. See *Acts of Tennessee*, 1905, 425–26, TN; *Acts of Tennessee*, 1907, 15, TN; *Acts of Tennessee*, 1909, 38–39, TN; *Acts of Tennessee*, 1911, 24, TN; *Acts of Tennessee*, 1915, 105–6, TN *Acts of Tennessee*, 1889, 342–44, TN; *Acts of Tennessee*, 1891, 150–52, TN. The state also allocated another $17,000 for the home at the Hermitage in 1895. See *Acts of Tennessee*, 1895, 67 and 313, TN. Alabama started a pension program for widows of amputees in 1886 and expanded to all widows of veterans in 1899. Information on Alabama can be located in "Surviving Confederate Pen-

sioners," *Alabama Historical Quarterly* 2, no. 2 (Summer 1940): 209–13, AL; Owen, *History of Alabama and Dictionary of Alabama Biography*, 1:340; "Auditor Records," Confederate Pension Records, Application for Artificial Limbs, AL; *Alabama Acts*, no. 421 (1898–99): 226–35, AL; "Surviving Confederate Pensioners," 216; *Alabama Acts*, no. 779 (1915): 886–896, AL. Arkansas, in 1891, offered $25 per year, which increased to $100 a year in 1915. For Arkansas and widow pensions, see *Arkansas Gazette*, January 14, 1891; January 25, 1891; March 26, 1891; March 27, 1891; Arkansas Confederate Pension Records, Arkansas History Commission. Florida women garnered $150 per year. Florida information can be located in "Report of Surgeon General, 1892," United Confederate Veterans Association Records, LSU. Initially, Kentucky women received $40 a year, which increased to $120 during the Great Depression and got as high as $200 per year. One Confederate widow collected her pension until the 1970s. Information on Kentucky can be located in "An Act Granting Pension to indigent and disabled Confederate soldiers, and the widows of Confederate Soldiers" in *Acts of the General Assembly of the Commonwealth of Kentucky* (1912), KY; Simpson, *Index of Confederate Pension Applications*, 1–5, courtesy of KYHS. Although Missouri granted widows a pension, they did not increase the financial allocation. See *Journal of the Senate of the Forty-Fifth General Assembly of the State of Missouri* (1909), 195, MO; *Laws of Missouri Passed at the Session of the Forty-Seventh General Assembly* (1913), 88–90, MO; *Laws of Missouri Passed at the Session of the Forty-Eighth General Assembly* (1915), 24, MO. South Carolina started a pension program for widows in 1887. For more, see McCawley, *Artificial Limbs for Confederate Soldiers*, 4.

47. #379, #518, #2447 and #2782 Confederate Pension Files, KY; McClurken, *Take Care of the Living*, 146–47 and 167; McDaid, "With Lame Legs and No Money," 19.

48. Hartman and Coles, *Biographical Rosters of Florida's Confederate and Union Soldiers*, 2:474; A12311 Mrs. M. J. Dowless Widow's Pension Application, Florida Confederate Pension Application Files, FL; A12484 Hannah Rawls Widow Application, Florida Confederate Pension Application Files, FL.

49. A02705 James Robarts, Florida Confederate Pension Application Files, FL.

50. John B. Lightfoot, Jr. address, December 13, 1910, Medical and Hospital Series, box 1, MOC.

51. John B. Lightfoot, Jr. address, June 3, 1925, Medical and Hospital Series, box 1, MOC.

Chapter 4. The Return

1. Daniel, *Recollections of a Rebel Surgeon*, 32–33; Sommerville, "'Will They Ever Be Able to Forget?,'" in Berry, *Weirding the War*, 321–39; *Columbia (Mo.) Herald*, November 29, 1872; *Charleston News and Courier*, June 24, 1883.

2. Toalson, *No Soap, No Pay, Diarrhea, Dysentery and Desertion*, 371; Smith, *Black Judas*, 271. Caroline Janney argues that "whereas in the North at least some Union veterans were treated with disdain or simply forgotten, almost all Confederate veterans were welcomed back into their communities as heroes." However, as this chapter reveals, it is not so clear-cut when it comes to physically damaged men. See her work, *Remembering the Civil War*, 139.

3. Nielsen, *Disability History of the United States,* 83–84.

4. Koven, "Remembering and Dismemberment," 1188–91. Koven argues that amputated veterans from World War I found themselves tied to the politics of remembering the war.

5. Wetherington, *Plain Folk's Fight,* 234–35; Pfanz, *Richard S. Ewell,* 420. For more on pain in the nineteenth century, see Abruzzo, *Polemical Pain,* 2. According to Abruzzo, some argued that individuals' pain, like that of Job in the Bible, was simply God's punishment for the sins they committed or specific life choices they made.

6. #00110 G. W. L. Randle, #00810 James Dyer, #01113 David W. Russell, #01127 Jerome N. Cornwell, #01159 Charles Frank Pascoe, #32270 R. W. Murray, Confederate pension applications, Texas Comptroller's Office Claims Records, TX. See also Long, *Rehabilitating Bodies,* 36.

7. "Phantom Limb and Causalgia," http://unitproj.library.ucla.edu/biomed/his /painexhibit/panel4.htm (accessed April 22, 2011).

8. Brinsfield, *Spirit Divided,* 89; Benson, *Berry Benson's Civil War Book,* 42–43.

9. Nielsen, *Disability History of the United States,* 87; Wecter, *When Johnny Comes Marching Home,* 188, 208–9 and 215; Schweik, *Ugly Laws,* 29, 150 and 258; *Baltimore Sun,* May 25, 1865. Schweik also tells the story of one Union amputee in San Francisco who raised hundreds of dollars telling those he encountered how he lost his leg at Fredericksburg. In reality, he had never served in the war and had lost his leg due to a disease. In another instance, a man who lost his limbs working on the railroad pretended to be a Union veteran to solicit donations. The U.S. army instructed wounded Union veterans to make up what they lost in body through hard work, energy, decision, and mental vigor. Reformers followed this call, creating left-handed writing seminars to assist those who lost their dominant hand during the war. As the soldiers successfully mastered a new mechanism of penmanship, they chanted, "Your left hand you must teach to write—It's all the one you've got; Come join our class in penmanship, for it is not for naught." One Union veteran referred to his amputation as necessary to make him "a perfect man," while another saw his scars as "richer ornaments" than pure gold. For more on how Union soldiers recalled the empty sleeve, see Jordan, "Living Monuments."

10. Wetherington, *Plain Folk's Fight,* 234.

11. Rotundo, *American Manhood,* 223; Whites, *Civil War as a Crisis in Gender,* 133–59; Whites, *Gender Matters,* 174–75. For more on manhood and defeat in the postwar period, see Rubin, *Shattered Nation,* 170, 173, and 208–39.

12. *Macon Daily Telegraph,* April 20, 1865.

13. Reminiscences of Mrs. Charles C. Rainwater, DUKE.

14. March 31, 1863, Kim Rowland Diary, MOC.

15. *Confederate Veteran Magazine,* February 1899; Nelson, *Ruin Nation,* 176.

16. Reid, *After the War,* 155; Wecter, *When Johnny Comes Marching Home,* 213.

17. *South Carolina Women in the Confederacy,* 145.

18. Pfanz, *Richard S. Ewell,* 420.

19. Blackford, *Letters from Lee's Army;* Rosenburg, "Empty Sleeves and Wooden Pegs," in Gerber, *Disabled Veterans in History,* 223; "A Sketch of the Life and Travels

of David Crocket Stuart, a Confederate Soldier," W. S. Hoole Special Collections Library, University of Alabama.

20. Pfanz, *Richard S. Ewell*, 421.

21. See Gorn, "Gouge and Bite."

22. Brinsfield, *Spirit Divided*, 89; "A Sketch of the Life and Travels of David Crocket Stuart, a Confederate Soldier," W. S. Hoole Special Collections Library, University of Alabama; Glover, *Southern Sons*, 23.

23. Meriwether, *The Ku Klux Klan*, 25–28. Historian Lisa Long notes how some Civil War–era writers referred to the South as an infected appendage on the U.S. body that ended up severed through the process of secession and war. However, the appendage, once cured of the disease of slavery and war, ended up reattached (or at least in an altered form, i.e., as a prosthetic). See Long, *Rehabilitating Bodies*, 20.

24. Meriwether, *Ku Klux Klan*, 28, 29, 35, 37, 46, and 51.

25. For more on the idea of reconciliation, see Silber, *Romance of Reunion*; Blight, *Race and Reunion*; Neff, *Honoring the Civil War Dead*; and Janney, *Remembering the Civil War*.

26. Clark and Kirwan, *The South Since Appomattox*, 82; Wiggins, *Georgia's Confederate Sons*, 71; Evans, *Confederate Military History vol. XV: Texas*, 464; Evans, *Confederate Military History vol. V: North Carolina*, 687–89, "June 14, 1862," Lucy Muse Walton Fletcher Papers, DUKE; Wecter, *When Johnny Comes Marching Home*, 210.

27. Blight, *Race and Reunion*, 140–70; Robson, *How a One-Legged Rebel Lives*, 3.

28. Lewellen, "Limbs Made and Unmade by War," 40; *Acts of the General Assembly of the State of Georgia*, 1866–67, 1:143–44, GA; OR ser. 1, vol. 37, 89; Owen, *History of Alabama and Dictionary of Alabama Biography*, 4:1296. The educational endeavor cost the state $100,000, and injured veterans could attend Mercer University, Emory College, Oglethorpe University, Bowdon College, and the University of Georgia. Soldiers had to be under the age of thirty, and the program lasted for a few years until a Republican-controlled legislature ended the program and returned the state to a simple pension system. Virginia also had a program to provide schooling to children of amputated men. See McClurken, *Take Care of the Living*, 87–90.

29. Wetherington, *Plain Folk's Fight*, 235–37.

30. Evans, *Confederate Military History vol. XV: Texas*, 372–73, 464, and 696–97; Evans, *Confederate Military History vol. XIV: Arkansas*, 557–59; Wiggins, *Georgia's Confederate Sons*, 92, 116, 121, and 154.

31. "Collection overview," "June 21, 1877 and January 14, 1881 letters from Wheeler Carriage Company," McGalliard (William M. and Family) Papers, LSU.

32. "H. M. Miller letters to McGalliard, September 10, 1877 and December 4, 1877," "A. C. McDermott letters to McGalliard, February 4, 1878, December 29, 1878, April 10, 1880, April 20, 1880 and August 30, 1884," McGalliard (William M. and Family) Papers, LSU. McGalliard purchased a new iron chair in 1877 that allowed the doctor to properly examine any handicapped patients. He also continued to work on behalf of other amputated men by helping some of his friends garner an artificial limb. For more, see "August 27, 1877 receipt from Wilson Adjustable Iron Chair Company," McGalliard (William M. and Family)

Papers, LSU; "J. L. Laxton letter to McGalliard, November 2, 1884," McGalliard (William M. and Family) Papers, LSU.

33. Fairclough, "'Scalawags,'" 807–8.

34. Editorial, *New York Tribune*, September 2, 1868; *New Orleans Times*, September 4, 1868. For other examples of northern amputees used in political debates, see *Harper's Weekly*, October 2, 1862 and *Harper's Weekly*, August 5, 1865. Also see Friedmann, *Psychological Rehabilitation of the Amputee*, 20, 32, and 43. Although his study looks at modern notions of amputation, Friedmann argues that amputees worried about societal perceptions and dealt with a host of self-esteem and competency issues.

35. Charles Brown Monroe, a former second lieutenant in the Ninth Florida, lost his attempt to garner the gubernatorial nomination in 1904, even though he emphasized the four Yankee bullets in his foot. See Hartman and Coles, *Biographical Rosters of Florida's Confederate and Union Soldiers*, 1:181.

36. Blair, *Cities of the Dead*, 127; Welsh, *Medical Histories of Confederate Generals*, 160–61; Jones, *American Civil War*, 447; Evans, *Confederate Military History vol. VI: South Carolina*, 386–87 and 498–500; Welsh, *Medical Histories of Confederate Generals*, 125–26; *Arkansas Gazette*, February 9, 1913; Letter from Frank Stern, James Henderson Berry Collection, ARK; Unknown author of eulogy, James Henderson Berry Collection, ARK. See also *Atlanta Constitution*, May 21, 1903.

37. Hartman and Coles, *Biographical Rosters of Florida's Confederate and Union Soldiers*, 1:251; Wiggins, *Remembering Georgia's Confederates*, 48; http://www.archives .alabama.gov/conoff/carmichael_j1.html (accessed July 26, 2010); Evans, *Confederate Military History vol. X: Tennessee*, 610–12, 624–26, and 789–91; "Funeral Notices," Harbison Family Papers #5285, UNC; Scribner, "A Short History of Brewton," 32.

38. Evans, *Confederate Military History vol. VIII: Alabama*, 724–28.

39. Blair, *Cities of the Dead*, 131.

40. Nielsen, *Disability History of the United States*, 81; Wetherington, *Plain Folk's Fight*, 235; Wyatt-Brown, *Shaping of Southern Culture*, 252; Friedmann, *Psychological Rehabilitation of the Amputee*, 32; McDaid, "With Lame Legs and No Money," 24–25; Lewellen, "Limbs Made and Unmade by War," 40; Marten, *Sing Not War*, 250–51; C. P. Boozer letter, 26160 Miscellaneous Papers, Artificial Limbs, SC.

41. Rosenburg, "Empty Sleeves and Wooden Pegs," in Gerber, *Disabled Veterans in History*, 204–5 and 211; Rosenburg, "Southern Poor Boys," in Logue and Barton, *Civil War Veteran*, 96–97; McDaid, "With Lame Legs and No Money," 23–24.

42. McDaid, "With Lame Legs and No Money," 23–24; Daniel, *Recollections of a Rebel Surgeon*, 165–67 and 171; Wegner, *Phantom Pain*, 21 and 25; Long, *Wages and Earnings in the United States*.

43. Schweik, *Ugly Laws*, 32–34, 149 and 292; *Acts of the General Assembly of the State of Georgia*, 1882, 1:64, GA.

44. Rosenburg, "Southern Poor Boys," in Logue and Barton, *Civil War Veteran*, 96.

45. Record Book, Soldiers Home Hospital and Association for the Relief of Maimed Soldiers, Richmond, Virginia, 1862–65, 241, NARA; Rosenburg, "Empty Sleeves and Wooden Pegs," in Gerber, *Disabled Veterans in History*, 207. For more on ARMS, see Hasegawa, *Mending Broken Soldiers*, 46–69. Historian Megan Kate Nelson observed that prosthetic limb programs not only served as "moral pro-

grams that rewarded men for their sacrifices," but also "bolstered the Empty Sleeve image of brave and patriotic amputees" that intended "to gather up their disarticulated parts and make them whole again—to rebuild the ruins of men." The process of constructing and fitting a prosthetic device to the amputee actually "restored the individuality of each veteran amputee," as each patient received a uniquely constructed device to fit the specific dimensions of his damaged limb. A prosthetic limb could serve as a mechanism to elevate an amputee's self-status of worth and help him overcome and accept the reality of his missing limb. See Nelson, *Ruin Nation*, 211 and 226; Nelson, "Worthy Substitute for Nature."

46. Record Book, Soldiers Home Hospital and Association for the Relief of Maimed Soldiers, Richmond, Virginia, 1862–65, 35–36, NARA; Record Book, Soldiers Home Hospital and Association for the Relief of Maimed Soldiers, Richmond, Virginia, 1862–65, 37 and 43, NARA. ARMS continued to receive various reports about the effectiveness of prosthetic devices. They examined the Palmer leg, which had some unique features, including a hinge further back, which made the leg easier to maneuver. Metallic springs used in the device held up well against adverse weather conditions. The Palmer manufacturers also selected tough and light wood in order to construct the device.

47. Nelson, *Ruin Nation*, 210; "Affidavit," Record Book, Soldiers Home Hospital and Association for the Relief of Maimed Soldiers, Richmond, Virginia, 1862–65, NARA.

48. United Daughters of the Confederacy Goals, United Daughters of the Confederacy Records, box 34, KYHS; H. A. Sommers speech, United Daughters of the Confederacy Records, box 34, KYHS; B.S. Grannis speech, United Daughters of the Confederacy Records, box 35, KYHS. For more on veteran organizations after the Civil War, see Blight, *Race and Reunion*; Goldfield, *Still Fighting the Civil War*; Ayers, *Promise of the New South*, 332–36; and Brundage, *Southern Past*. For a solid exploration of the UDC, see Cox, *Dixie's Daughters*.

49. "1893 UCV Report," Joseph Jones Papers, LSU; "UCV Constitution, 1894," United Confederate Veterans Association Records, LSU; UCV program in United Daughters of the Confederacy Records, box 42, KYHS; Nielsen, *Disability History of the United States*, 85. For more on the UCV, see Ayers, *Promise of the New South*, 334–36; Brundage, *Southern Past*; Blight, *Race and Reunion*; and Foster, *Ghosts of the Confederacy*.

50. April 26, 1880, speech and April 26, 1881, speech, MS1066 Charles Colcock Jones Papers, UGA.

51. *Charleston News and Courier*, May 14, 1879; "Decoration Day, no date," Mary Snowden Papers, USC; Bowman, *Civil War Almanac*, 103. The Charleston paper reported on a Decoration Day ceremony in 1879 where a black Confederate amputee watched "with interest" and worked with "the arrangements and decorations of the graves." The *Civil War Almanac* reveals that at Secessionville, the Confederates suffered 144 wounded, which included the unnamed black Confederate soldier.

52. Amputees from Confederate Home Roster, TX. For more on the veteran homes, see Rosenberg, *Living Monuments* and Williams, *My Old Confederate Home*.

53. Hospital Register, Kentucky Confederate Home, Pewee Valley, KY; Confederate Soldiers Home, Reference Book B, KY; #1133 Thomas B. Cheatham, Confederate Pension Files, KY.

Chapter 5. The State

1. Gold, "'Fighting It Over Again,'" 310. For more on the failures of Reconciliation after the Civil War, see Janney, *Remembering the Civil War*.

2. *Raleigh Daily North Carolina Standard*, November 22, 1865.

3. *Nashville Daily American*, March 16, 1889.

4. Wecter, *When Johnny Comes Marching Home*, 213–14; Lewellen, "Limbs Made and Unmade by War," 42; McClintock, "Civil War Pensions and the Reconstruction of Union Families," 456–80. Civil War veterans were entitled to receive a new limb every five years, and the allowance eventually increased to $100 for the foot or arm and $125 for the leg.

5. Williams, *My Old Confederate Home*, 9–10; Rosenburg, "Empty Sleeves and Wooden Pegs," in Gerber, *Disabled Veterans in History*, 206; "Proceedings of the Second Confederate Congress, November 7–December 14, 1864," in Vandiver, *Southern Historical Society Papers* 51 (1959): 326–27; "Proceedings of the Second Confederate Congress, December 15, 1864–March 18, 1865," in Vandiver, *Southern Historical Society Papers* 52 (1959): 488–89. For more on the debate in the U.S. Congress over extending aid to Confederates, see Brock, *Southern Historical Society Papers* 26 (1898): 313–15; Linker, *War's Waste*, 17.

6. The Civil War, as historian Paul Escott noted, fundamentally shifted how white southerners thought about the role of the state government in providing financial assistance. The war created a heightened level of insolvency that forced white southerners to remain dependent on the Confederate and state governments to provide help to assist those left impecunious by the war. See his article "'Cry of the Sufferers,'" 230–31. In addition, as historian Stephanie McCurry pointed out, the Civil War forged a new social contract between the state governments and the men who enlisted to protect that government. See McCurry, *Confederate Reckoning*, 133–34. James Marten, though, sees smooth sailing for Confederate pensions and that the debates surrounding them never ended up "as deeply embroiled in partisan politics." See Marten, *Sing Not War*, 203–4. Caroline Janney echoes this sentiment, as she states, "Confederate veterans did not find themselves embroiled in the partisan wrangling over pensions and federal solders' homes as did Union veterans." See *Remembering the Civil War*, 139.

7. Wisner, *Social Welfare in the South*, 10, 23, 34, 42, 47–52, 110, 117, and 123; Green, *Before the New Deal*, xiv–xvi.

8. Marten, *Sing Not War*, 91; Rosenburg, "Empty Sleeves and Wooden Pegs," in Gerber, *Disabled Veterans in History*, 207; Carroll, "'The Living Souls, the Bodies' Tragedies'"; Wecter, *When Johnny Comes Marching Home*, 213. Shoe swaps appeared across the South, allowing amputated men to trade in an unneeded shoe due to their missing appendage.

9. Lewellen, "Limbs Made and Unmade by War," 43–44; McDaid, "With Lame Legs and No Money," 16.

10. *Illustrated Catalogue of the Celebrated Bly Artificial Limbs Manufactured by George R. Fuller*, 34, 57 and 68–69, UAB. For additional information on some of the difficulties artificial limb manufacturers faced, see William Trousdale Papers, box 4, folder 4, TN.

11. "Application for Orders and Measures, 1867," Confederate Pension Appli-

cations, Application for Artificial Limbs, AL; "Artificial Limb Correspondence," Confederate Pension Applications, Application for Artificial Limbs, AL; Owen, *History of Alabama and Dictionary of Alabama Biography*, 1:340.

12. Robson, *How a One-Legged Rebel Lives*, 187.

13. "New Market, Va., February 1, 1864 Notice," Henry Kagey Papers, DUKE.

14. Owen, *History of Alabama and Dictionary of Alabama Biography*, 1:340; Chickasaw, Calhoun and Lafayette County, box 340; Copiah County, box 349; Hinds and Holmes County, box 339; Attala County, box 8279; Noxubee County, box 8372, all in Indigent and Disabled Soldiers and Dependents, 1863–68, MS; *Journal of the Senate of the State of Mississippi*, 1866–67, 132–60, MS; Wegner, *Phantom Pain*, 33. The records are rather incomplete, as some counties returned no data or just a list of names with no reference to the specific injury. A perusal of all the county records revealed the names of at least 140 confirmed Confederate amputees in Mississippi, which comes from counting amputees off of the county lists in boxes 340, 8237, 339, 8279, 17056, 12051, 12052, and 8372 as part of the Indigent and Disabled Soldiers and Dependents, 1863–68, MS. Counties that actually listed the names of amputated Confederate veterans include Chickasaw, Calhoun, Lafayette, Lowndes, Holmes, Covington, Hinds, Attala, Copiah, Franklin, Madison, Marion, Neshoba, Harrison, Lawrence, Marshall, DeSoto, Tishomingo, Tippah, Warren, Newton, Noxubee, and Oktibbeha. Leake County listed 22 disabled men and Copiah listed 11 with no clear indication as to what defined their disability (number not included in the 107 count). Samuel Doolittle, William Wilson, and Joseph D. Read all requested seventy-four dollars to pay for the artificial leg they purchased, while W. C. Evans needed financial assistance due to a fleshy stump that did not allow for the proper fitting of an artificial leg nine inches from his hip. James Barsfield, who lost a leg during the war, lived destitute with four children and no corn. Copiah County reported eleven destitute and disabled men. In Noxubee County, B. F. Upton lived in a destitute condition with a missing leg and eight children. Glen Phillips, who lost an arm, had three children to support. John Dew, who lost a leg during the war, also lived destitute. In Lafayette County, nine men reported losing a leg during the Civil War and four missing an arm. Out of the fourteen in the county, five reported large families of at least five members and several indicated destitution.

15. Wegner, *Phantom Pain*, 21; S126097 Lists of Disabled Soldiers, 1867, SC.

16. "N.C. Ratified Law January 23, 1866," S126160 Miscellaneous Papers, Artificial Limbs, SC; Wegner, *Phantom Pain*, 20–21. South Carolina included the North Carolina resolution among their papers as evidence of other states acting on behalf of their amputated veterans. Wegner points out that the North Carolina legislature debated giving artificial limbs to women but later tabled the measure. The debate is a historical curiosity, considering no recorded women lost a limb while fighting for the Confederacy. Considering, though, a few hundred women fought in the Civil War disguised as men, the legislature might have considered the measure because they were aware of a local female veteran.

17. Lewellen, "Limbs Made and Unmade by War," 40. The state legislature in North Carolina remained active in selecting other avenues for support of amputated men, in addition to prosthetic limbs. In February 1867, the legislature debated a new bill that provided a liquor license to any veteran who lost a leg or

arm during the Civil War. If the sale of alcohol was less than a quart, the veteran did not need to pay any state or county taxes on the sale. Although some legislators supported the measure, it failed to materialize as a law. Historian Ansley Wegner wondered whether the legislature failed to pass the bill because of their disdain for alcohol or a nagging suspicion that amputated veterans would overindulge in their new business. See Wegner, *Phantom Pain*, 32.

18. The state of Georgia in March 1866 appropriated $20,000 to furnish legs and arms to Confederate amputees and another $30,000 nine months later. By January 12, 1869, the state had exhausted the entire initial amount and had roughly $18,000 left from the second appropriation. If an applicant for an artificial limb had a remaining stump that did not allow the prosthetic to fit properly, the veteran could instead draw a cash payment in the amount of the artificial limb. See *Acts of the General Assembly of the State of Georgia*, 1865–66, 1:224, GA; *Acts of the General Assembly of the State of Georgia*, 1866–67, 1:145, GA; "Report of Surgeon General, 1892," United Confederate Veterans Association Records, LSU. Georgia exempted amputated men from paying poll taxes. See *Acts of the General Assembly of the State of Georgia*, 1882–83, 1:120, GA. Virginia set aside $20,000 to purchase artificial limbs in January 1867, and the program evolved to both include African American Confederate amputees and allow veterans to exchange their limbs for a cash payment, which was designed to silence the criticism of Confederates who hated their devices. See McDaid, "With Lame Legs and No Money," 18–19; McClurken, *Take Care of the Living*, 145–47. Virginia added black veterans and the cash payment program in 1872. Historian Jeff McClurken noted that Virginia spent $343,000 on the prosthetic limb program from its beginnings through 1886. Otto J. Whitlock hated his prosthetic leg that "broke down as a worthless thing," and William H. Tolley, who had gained weight, wanted a new leg with stronger irons. Sidney Turner, who lost a leg at Gettysburg, simply wore his leg out from all of his traveling as part of his employment, which prompted Virginia to provide him with a new leg. The limb programs required the state to locate another $20,000 in funds in 1873 to continue paying for the program. The cash payments set off a flurry of complaints from some veterans who found the inequity of payments appalling. James W. Bolton received only $30 out of the possible $60. His neighbor, W. A. B. McComb, heard rumors in the county of men who "lost part of one finger" getting the full amount, as opposed to men who "who had their hands so maimed that they cannot grip anything except one or two fingers" getting the smaller amount. Alabama's legislature authorized $30,000 to provide artificial legs or a one-time cash payment of $100 if the veteran could not use an artificial device. In 1876, the legislature appropriated another $5,000, and maimed veterans received either a new limb or a payment of $75. The following year, after a decade of addressing prosthetics for legs, the state allocated an additional $5,000 for the purchase of artificial arms, prompting twenty veterans to apply for the limb or comparable cash payment. See "Surviving Confederate Pensioners," 213–14; *Alabama Acts*, no. 643 (1866–67): 695–98, AL; Owen, *History of Alabama and Dictionary of Alabama Biography*, 1:340; "Application for Orders and Measures, 1867," Confederate Pension Applications, Application for Artificial Limbs, AL; "Artificial Limb Correspondence," Confederate Pension Applications, Application for Artificial Limbs, AL. Among the first 215 applications for a prosthetic limb received by

the manufacturer, 108 sought a limb for above the knee and 107 for a limb below the knee. See "Application for Orders and Measures, 1867," Confederate Pension Applications, Application for Artificial Limbs, AL. The occupations of the Confederate veterans who applied for prosthetic legs varied quite a bit. An absent leg failed to deter many veterans from returning to the farm or their skilled craft positions. Among the first 237 applications for an artificial leg, a majority worked as farmers, with a few dozen self-identified as shoemakers. Other applicants worked as teachers, clerks, merchants, printers, carpenters, and engineers. A few amputees listed their occupation as student. Still others served as tax collectors or sheriffs or worked as millers, merchants, blacksmiths, bookbinders, and butchers. In 1872, with another round of limbs going to the maimed, Alabama veterans indicated their occupations as dentist, harness maker, agriculturalist, bookkeeper, tax assessor, plasterer, shoemaker, clerk, and, of course, farmer. One amputee collected tolls at a bridge. The occupations can be found at "Auditor Records," Confederate Pension Records, Application for Artificial Limbs, AL. "Surviving Confederate Pensioners," 214–15; Owen, *History of Alabama and Dictionary of Alabama Biography,* 1:340.

19. "Trescott and Logan letter to the Senate," S126160 Miscellaneous Papers, Artificial Limbs, SC; S165087 *Journals of the House of Representatives, Early State Records* (1863–66), SC. In addition to offering an eloquent argument as to why South Carolina had to act, the men suggested an aggressive limb program may cost the state between $50,000 and $175,000. South Carolina allocated $20,000 to pay for artificial legs.

20. Prior to the legislation, handicapped men relied on the Ladies Benevolent Association to initially garner a device. Over the course of three years, the state allocated $22,300 to purchase and later repair broken artificial limbs or provide the amputee with a cash payment in lieu of an artificial device. Louisiana Legislative Acts #69, 1880; 1882, 94, LA; Louisiana Legislative Acts #69, 1880, LA; "Report of Surgeon General, 1892," United Confederate Veterans Association Records, LSU; Rosenburg, "Empty Sleeves and Wooden Pegs," in Gerber, *Disabled Veterans in History,* 208–11. The state allowed $80 for a leg, $65 for an arm, $65 for loss of sight in an eye, $20 for the loss of hearing, $80 for those who lost the ability to speak, and $65 for any other disability. The legislature followed suit in 1883 and again allocated $1,300 for limbs and $1,071.77 for repairs. A. McDermott, headquartered in New Orleans, agreed to bill the state $80 for each leg and $65 for each arm. For repairs to an artificial leg, McDermott charged the city $25 and $15 for repairs to the artificial arms. The state of Louisiana started caring for indigent families during the Civil War when the state legislature passed several bills that appropriated over $9 million in aid to displaced and indigent soldiers, wives, and children. See Zornow, "State Aid for Indigent Soldiers and Their Families in Louisiana," 375–80. For more on the political chaos in Louisiana during Reconstruction, see Hogue, *Uncivil War,* esp. 1–13.

21. Foote, *Civil War,* 3:1041. Historian Eric Foner wrote that "Mississippi expended 20% of its revenue in 1865 on artificial limbs for Confederate veterans." See his work *Reconstruction,* 125. Foner cites William Harris's work on Reconstruction. Yet, Harris writes, "A bill was passed and approved by Governor Humphreys which provided that 20 per cent of the revenue of the state, but not more

than sixty thousand dollars, was to be reserved annually by the state treasurer" to mostly care for widows and children over amputated men. The fund was not specifically designed for providing prosthetics. County boards had been instructed to take a census to determine who deserved the funds, but 25 percent of the counties failed to submit a report by 1867, which displeased the state treasurer, who had refused to distribute any money until the entire census had been completed. The legislature ordered the money dispersed to 13,630 individuals who had been identified as indigent (which had been capped at $60,000, resulting in payments of just a few dollars). J. L. Power, the superintendent of Army records in Mississippi, recommended that the state legislature appropriate $30,000 to buy three hundred legs. The legislature agreed and passed the bill in the fall of 1866. The state also noted that maimed veterans or the children of deceased or disabled soldiers were allowed a free education at any state university. Then, the state of Mississippi shut off all economic support to maimed veterans until the Pension Act of 1889. See Harris, *Presidential Reconstruction in Mississippi*, 164–65; *Journal of the Senate of the State of Mississippi*, 1866–67, 132–60, MS; *Journal of the Senate of the State of Mississippi*, 1870, 107; *Journal of the Senate of the State of Mississippi*, 1871, 263, MS. The statistic has been repeated in countless textbooks and other prominent writings on the Civil War, including Carter, *Angry Scar*, 43, which does not provide a footnote for the assertion. See also Jones, *American Civil War*, 447. The myth of state expenditure on artificial limbs in Mississippi continues (and even has grown). For example, see http://www.collectorsweekly.com/articles/war-and-prosthetics (accessed January 14, 2014), where the author notes that Mississippi spent half of its state budget on prosthetic limbs in 1866. The newly exaggerated statistic even appears in Adams, *Living Hell*, 200, where the author incorrectly notes that Mississippi spent half of its budget on artificial limbs.

22. Wegner, *Phantom Pain*, 25–27; "Palmer Letter," Indigent and Disabled Soldiers and Dependents, 1863–68, MS; "Condell Statement," Indigent and Disabled Soldiers and Dependents, 1863–68, MS; "Condell Letter, February 15, 1866," Indigent and Disabled Soldiers and Dependents, 1863–68, MS. A. A. Marks, who had an artificial limb company in New York City, offered Mississippi artificial legs for seventy-five dollars each and artificial arms at sixty dollars above and forty dollars below the elbow. Marks proudly touted the fact that his limbs won a gold medal at the Fair of the American Institute in 1865. Richard Clement, a manufacturer of artificial limbs in Philadelphia, offered his limbs at seventy-five dollars each (which was the same rate quoted to the U.S. government). He took great pride in his twenty years of experience in manufacturing prosthetic legs and proudly listed the names of several veterans who could attest to the value of the limbs, including Richard Ewell. Clement, when he did not hear back, even offered a price reduction, which clearly reflected the competitive nature of garnering an artificial limb contract. Residents in Vicksburg, Mississippi, turned to Charles M. Evans, who manufactured limbs of the "best quality," according to a newspaper advertisement. Evans claimed to have slashed prices on the prosthetic devices and guaranteed that each and every limb would provide total satisfaction to the purchaser. See *Jackson Mississippi Weekly Clarion*, February 16, 1879; "Letter from A. A. Marks, April 19, 1866," Indigent and Disabled Soldiers and Dependents, 1863–68, MS; "Clement letters to Powers, September 15, 1866 and October 12, 1866," Indigent and Disabled Soldiers and Dependents, 1863–68, MS.

23. "Limb Contract Correspondence," S126160 Miscellaneous Papers, Artificial Limbs, SC; "Trescott Letter," S126160 Miscellaneous Papers, Artificial Limbs, SC; McCawley, *Artificial Limbs for Confederate Soldiers*, 1; "Bly Monthly Reports," S126160 Miscellaneous Papers, Artificial Limbs, SC; *Illustrated Catalogue of the Celebrated Bly Artificial Limbs Manufactured by George R. Fuller*, 23–26 and 71–72, UAB. Bly offered two different legs: an Anatomical Patent Leg ($150) and an army and navy leg ($74.65). The state agreed on a contract signed March 27, 1867, to furnish each amputee with enough funds to secure the army and navy leg. Veterans who wanted the more expensive model were responsible for paying the difference. Through the first eleven months of the program, Bly distributed 157 army and navy or ball and socket legs and only 17 anatomical patented legs at the additional cost to the veteran. The devices held up well under all conditions and needed only to be toweled off if they got wet. Recipients needed to oil and clean their limbs roughly once a month in order to keep them in good working order. Of note, the governor also received offers to sign a contract from F. Olin Dannelly, who admitted his company was not financially stable. Richard Clement, from Philadelphia, also tried to secure the contract by offering ample testimony from his patients and newspaper endorsements, which claimed the limbs allowed for superior mobility and the opportunity to earn a living that would end destitution. The *Pittsburg Evening Chronicle* endorsed the Clement leg: "When, however, in the checkered changes of life the dread misfortune comes, and the faithful limb succumbs to the surgeon's knife and saw, it is a great consolation to the mutilated patient to know that human art has prepared an artificial substitute." See "Clement and Dannelly correspondence," S126160 Miscellaneous Papers, Artificial Limbs, SC; *Pittsburgh Evening Chronicle*, October 11, 1866.

24. "Report of Surgeon General, 1892," United Confederate Veterans Association Records, LSU; *Acts of the General Assembly of the State of Georgia*, 1886–87, 2:27, GA; *Acts of the General Assembly of the State of Georgia*, 1888–89, 1:16, GA; Confederate Pension Application, GA. See also Wegner, *Phantom Pain*, 25–27 and 32–33 and Rosenburg, "Empty Sleeves and Wooden Pegs," in Gerber, *Disabled Veterans in History*, 208–10. In North Carolina, the state paid for the amputees to travel to Raleigh and gave them free housing during the fitting process. The amputees had to bring only their documentation, a blanket, and some bread and dried meat for sustenance. Veterans who wanted the cash payment over the limb still had to travel to Raleigh and undergo a medical examination by surgeon E. Burke Haywood. In Georgia, any applicants found guilty of trying to fraudulently acquire a limb could receive up to three years in prison and a fine of one hundred dollars. For more on pensions and retirement in Georgia, see Short, "Confederate Veteran Pensions," 75–101. In South Carolina, the SC RR offered free transportation for amputated men to Charleston, where they received their prosthetic device. However, the railroad company was a bit cautious, as it did not want to just issue free rail vouchers to anyone who took "upon himself the character of a maimed Confederate." Thus, every passenger needed to provide documentation that expressed the sole purpose of his travel. Once veterans arrived at Bly's office at 188 King Street in Charleston, they presented Bly with documentation signed by the governor and the amputees. After having received the leg, amputees signed off that the limb was fitted to their stump. See "Railroad Offer," S126160 Miscellaneous Papers, Artificial Limbs, SC; "Vouchers and Bly Documents," S1*26096 Comptrol-*

ler General, Pension Department, Artificial Limb Vouchers, 1867–69, SC. Any applicant in Alabama who lied about his injury, military service, or residency could be convicted of committing perjury. The auditor records are unclear as to whether the state prosecuted any individuals for perjury; however, two applicants were turned down for purportedly possessing two healthy and intact legs. See "Auditor Records," Confederate Pension Records, Application for Artificial Limbs, AL. For more on assistance to Confederate veterans as an honorable process, see Gorman, "Confederate Pensions as Social Welfare," in Green, *Before the New Deal*, 36–37.

25. Wegner, *Phantom Pain*, 29. See also *Illustrated Catalogue of the Celebrated Bly Artificial Limbs Manufactured by George R. Fuller*, 1 and 6, UAB.

26. "Auditor Records," Confederate Pension Records, Application for Artificial Limbs, AL. In 1878, the state started to phase out the artificial limb program and provided a cash payment of $75 in lieu of a prosthetic device for any individual deemed a cripple. In 1879, Alabama added blind veterans to the rolls of eligible wounded men and paid them $150 if they lost their sight during their war service. According to auditor records, sixty-seven men applied for either a prosthetic arm or the cash payment of $75. The steady demand for devices or compensation prompted the state to appropriate more funds each year, from $10,000 in 1879 to $15,000 two years later, and then reaching $25,000 in 1885. The state relied on monies from the General Fund, and then levied a tax on February 13, 1891, to raise thousands of dollars. For additional information on the legislation, see "Surviving Confederate Pensioners," 209–13; Owen, *History of Alabama and Dictionary of Alabama Biography*, 1:340; "Auditor Records," Confederate Pension Records, Application for Artificial Limbs, AL. Some men preferred the money because either the injury did not allow them to properly wear the artificial limb or the prosthesis would not benefit their quality of life. William H. Wilds, who lost his right arm between the wrist and elbow at Kennesaw Mountain, could not wear an artificial arm and opted for disbursement. Sledge Robertson, a poor farmer who lost his left arm above the elbow at Corinth, Mississippi, in October 1862, also wanted the money instead of a limb because he believed he was simply too maimed to wear a prosthetic. Jesse Shivers, a lawyer who lost his left arm above the elbow, also requested the money. However, William Malone, a farmer wounded at Antietam, wanted the prosthetic arm to attach to his stump right near the shoulder on his right arm. See Confederate Pension Records, Application for Artificial Limbs, AL; "Surviving Confederate Pensioners," 209–13; "Arm Records," Confederate Pension Records, Application for Artificial Limbs, AL. There are several cases, particularly in South Carolina, of veterans complaining about the devices and asking for cash or new limbs. S. S. Bearden wore out two prosthetic legs and asked for funds to cover the replacement leg he acquired on his own accord. Another veteran broke his first artificial leg and demanded a replacement. See "Application," S1*26092* Comptroller General, Pension Department, Artificial Limb Applications for Confederate Service, 1880–1887, per Act of 1879, SC; "Foster and Stickle Correspondence," S126160 Miscellaneous Papers, Artificial Limbs, SC; "Limb Applications," S126092 Comptroller General, Pension Department, Artificial Limb Applications for Confederate Service, 1880–1887, per Act of 1879, SC; Various letters, *S126172 Comptroller General Letters Concerning Artificial Limbs*, SC; McCawley, *Artificial Limbs for Confederate Soldiers*, 3. The state allocated another $20,000

to furnish both artificial legs and arms to Confederate veterans or cash payments to amputated men if they had no need for the prosthetic. A few men asked for a prosthetic device over the cash payment, including W. R. Ford, who asked for a prosthetic arm to replace the one he lost at Petersburg. Both W. H. Watson and David Taylor requested a prosthetic arm that enabled them to plow their fields. If not possible, Taylor wanted the money. J. G. Brown requested a double payment because he had lost both legs as a member of the Second Cavalry in Virginia in July 1862. The flurry of applications and cash payments depleted the original allocation that forced the legislature to add another $7,000 in December 1880. In the following year, the veterans again depleted the fund, which prompted the legislature to provide more funds and to extend benefits to those who did not lose a limb but rather had a nonfunctioning arm or leg. The legislature continued to tinker with the definitions of disabled veterans in South Carolina to eventually include any slaves who fought for the Confederacy and lost a limb, those who had worn out their prosthetic limb, and new residents who had been in South Carolina for at least a decade. The state also equated the loss of fingers with the loss of a hand, for which veterans received a cash payment. W. L. Duke, who lost a finger at Petersburg with the Eighteenth South Carolina, had a witness testify that the loss of a finger destroyed the entire motion of the remaining appendages on Duke's hand. Thus, he received a cash payment as if he had lost his entire hand during the war. T. A. James, a member of the Seventh South Carolina, had a bullet pass through his left eye, jaw, and left shoulder at Harpers Ferry in 1862. While the missing eye failed to garner any financial compensation, the useless arm qualified. See "Limb Applications," S126092 Comptroller General, Pension Department, Artificial Limb Applications for Confederate Service, 1880–1887, per Act of 1879, SC. By 1886, the state had paid out over $46,000 to their Confederate veterans.

27. Maryland and Delaware never provided any financial assistance for Confederate veterans. Oklahoma created a pension program for any Confederate veterans residing in the state in 1915.

28. *Houston Telegraph,* September 11, 1886; State of Texas, *Journal of the House of Representatives of the Eleventh Legislature* (Austin: State Gazette, 1866), 29, 338, 728 and 785, TX.

29. *Arkansas Gazette,* September 18, 1866; *Weekly Arkansas Gazette,* November 20, 1866.

30. *Weekly Arkansas Gazette,* January 29, 1867.

31. Ibid.

32. *Weekly Arkansas Gazette,* December 25, 1866; State of Arkansas, *Acts of the General Assembly of the State of Arkansas* (Little Rock: Woodruff and Blocher, 1867), 90 and 95, ARKH.

33. *Daily Arkansas Gazette,* June 23, 1885; *Arkansas Gazette,* June 30, 1889; *Arkansas Gazette,* April 9, 1893. James Marten notes that by 1916, the head of the Arkansas home had to defend the institution against the perception of it being a "humiliating place" for the poor. See Marten, *Sing Not War,* 165–66.

34. For more on the nineteenth-century southern state governments and their funding of almshouses and mental hospitals, see Wisner, *Social Welfare in the South,* 42–47 and 53–66.

35. Lewellen, "Limbs Made and Unmade by War," 40; "Report of Surgeon

General, 1892," United Confederate Veterans Association Records, LSU; Mc-Clurken, *Take Care of the Living*, 155–56; *Acts of Tennessee*, 1889, 342–44, TN; Thomas Osborne Scrapbook, KYHS; Cynthia J. Beeman, "Texas Confederate Home," *Handbook of Texas Online*, http://www.tshaonline.org/handbook/online/articles/ynt05 (accessed November 18, 2010); "Report of Surgeon General, 1892," United Confederate Veterans Association Records, LSU; Williams, *My Old Confederate Home*, 62–63, 83, and 130–31. James McDonald, the adjutant general of Virginia, indicated in 1891 that the home cared for 130 inmates at the cost of $10,000 a year for maintenance and upkeep. The state's contribution skyrocketed to $90,000 in 1918, but declined as more veterans passed away. Furthermore, some legislators found a loophole and provided funding for maintaining the buildings and routine maintenance. Between the years of 1893 and 1895, the state appropriated $75,000 for the Confederate home in Texas, but also limited the amount that could be spent at $100,000. The home in Texas quickly grew, in terms of patient rolls. In 1894, 53 veterans resided at the home; this figure jumped to 280 patients in 1902 and 340 in 1915. The legislature continued to funnel occasional money into the home in order to routinely update the buildings, construct a new hospital, and provide for day-to-day maintenance. Over the course of sixty-six years, the home cared for over 2,000 patients. In Kentucky, the legislature raised the annual appropriation for the home and opened the door to the possible admission of wives to join their wounded husbands.

36. Louisiana provided 160 acres of land under a legislative act in 1884, and the handicapped men had eight years to file the necessary paperwork to procure a parcel of land. In all, 664 veterans received a land grant, of whom at least 163 lost a limb during the Civil War. In 1881 Texas started their program, which lasted two years but provided 2,068 land grants to disabled veterans and their widows. "Beneficiary Land Warrant," in Abstracts Land Sales, Claims, Misc. Records, LA; Louisiana Legislative Acts #96, 1884; #116, 1886; #122, 1888; and #55, 1896, "Report of Surgeon General, 1892," United Confederate Veterans Association Records, LSU; *Senate Journal of Texas, 17th Legislature 1881*, 78, 119–20, 187, and 301–2; *House Journal of Texas, 17th Legislature 1881*, 287; Confederate Scrip Voucher, Archives and Records Division, Texas General Land Office. The number of amputees in Louisiana comes from an extensive perusal of Soldiers Proof as Beneficiary under Act No. 55 of 1896, under Act 96, and under Act 116 of 1886, LA. In February 1881, Senator Lightfoot introduced an amendment to an 1879 measure that granted 640 acres of land for any indigent veterans of the Texas War for Independence. The new amendment increased the acreage to 1,280 for Texas veterans. The movement to aid Texas War for Independence veterans led to caring for Confederate amputees.

37. "John White," "Thomas Moore," and "Jeau P. Guidroz," Soldiers Proof as Beneficiary under Act #116 of 1886, LA; John F. Hanson, #001348; James Williams, #001626; T. L. Hallmark, #000551; Reuben Phares, #000550; J. K. Smith, #000606; George T. Long, #000638; W. N. B. Lewis, #000724; John W. Allen, #000222; John D. Polk, #000099, Confederate Scrip Voucher, TXL. For more examples of Confederate amputees in Texas who gained land, see L. M. Head, #000071; A. J. Nevill, #001010; J. D. McCaughan, #001137; T. H. Griffin, #000169; W. H. Woodson, #000143; Sterling Fisher, #001048; Sam H. Larremore, #000844,

Confederate Scrip Voucher, TXL. My examination of the Texas General Land Office records uncovered sixteen applications from amputees and eighty-four applications from men who faced permanent disability from a gunshot wound that never healed. Thirty-nine had an injury to the arm/hand/shoulder, fifty-two had an injury to the leg/foot/hip, and six suffered from both an arm and a leg injury. Three did not provide a specific injury, and one additional applicant claimed an amputation of his jaw.

38. Gorman, "Confederate Pensions as Social Welfare," in Green, *Before the New Deal,* 24–27.

39. Ibid., 36–37. North Carolina established the first program in 1879 that provided $60 a year to amputees, and the state later doubled the amount in 1907. Georgia provided $100 for those who lost a leg above the knee and $75 for those whose loss was below the knee. For arm amputations above the elbow, the applicant received $60, as opposed to an amputation below the elbow, for which he received $40. See Rosenburg, "Empty Sleeves and Wooden Pegs," in Gerber, *Disabled Veterans in History*, 218–19; *Acts of the General Assembly of the State of Georgia,* 1882–83, 1:120, GA; *Acts of the General Assembly of the State of Georgia,* 1884–85, 1:32 and 138; "Indigent Pension Application," Confederate Pension Applications, GA. Only a handful of amputees applied for aid as indigent veterans in the 1900s. Joshua Coffee, who lost a hand, supported a wife and seven children on a pension of $25. Larry Hobbs tried to get a pension at this late date, but state officials did not believe his damaged limb was a result of a wartime injury. See "Joshua Coffee and Larry Hobbs Applications," Confederate Pension Applications, GA. As of 1891, the state of Missouri, which remained loyal to the Union during the war, had not felt compelled to extend any financial assistance to Confederate amputees and the state legislature had not debated any legislation extending aid to former Confederates. In 1891, the state did offer to pay transportation expenses for ex-Confederate soldiers and their wives, widows, and children en route to the soldiers' home in Higginsville. The state did not contribute any funds to the home, as it remained in operation, caring for wounded and indigent Confederate veterans, through the kindness of private donors. The Senate did issue a resolution of gratitude to the private citizens "for the unselfish and devoted assistance to this worthy charity." Senator Arthur Oliver introduced a bill that followed a compromise that gave both Union and Confederate indigent and disabled veterans a pension. Although Oliver introduced the bill in 1909, it took four years for the legislation to become law. Veterans received $10 a month after the state initially appropriated $30,000 for payment of pensions. However, in 1915, the authorization increased up to $200,000 for the payment of pensions. *Journal of the Senate of Missouri of the Thirty-Sixth General Assembly, 1891,* 405 and 479, MO; "Report of Surgeon General, 1892," *United Confederate Veterans Association Records,* LSU; *Journal of the Senate of Missouri of the Thirty-Seventh General Assembly, 1893,* 626, MO; *Journal of the Senate of Missouri of the Thirty-Eighth General Assembly, 1895,* 566, MO; *Journal of the Senate of Missouri of the Thirty-Ninth General Assembly, 1897,* 84, 140, 160, 352, and 381, MO; *Appendix to the Senate and House Journals of the Fortieth General Assembly, 1899,* 36 and 142–45, MO; *Journal of the Senate of the Forty-Fifth General Assembly of the State of Missouri, 1909,* 195, MO; *Laws of Missouri passed at the Session of the Forty-Seventh General Assembly, 1913,* 88–90, MO; *Laws of Missouri passed*

at the Session of the Forty-Eighth General Assembly, 1915, 24, MO. State governmental records in Missouri are a bit limited due to a lightning strike and subsequent fire in the capitol in 1911. Former Confederate soldiers in Kansas City petitioned the state in 1895 to provide more resources to ensure the success and vitality of the Confederate Home. Two years later, Senator Charles Vandiver introduced a bill that allowed the state to maintain the residency for indigent Confederate veterans and their dependents for twenty years. The bill cleared the state legislature in 1897, and Governor Lon Stephens signed it into law. In its first two years of running the Confederate Home, the state spent $26,400 and cared for an average of 147 people. With attendance growing and maintenance issues on the rise, a state report projected a need for more than $60,000. Missouri also proposed allowing former Union and Confederate soldiers the ability to sell or canvass for goods not prohibited by law in any part of the state, which failed to muster enough support. See *Journal of the Senate of Missouri of the Fortieth General Assembly, 1899*, 59, MO. According to United Daughters of the Confederacy Records, the Confederate Home received $15,237.86 in 1896, raised via donations at the School District Elections. See "The Confederate Home of Missouri" in Robert L. Hawkins Collection, box 116, MO. The pension bill went through a series of legislative tweaks and passed April 23, 1913. Confederate veterans who served at least six months and received an honorable discharge could apply for a pension if their war wounds or the effects of old age rendered them financially destitute. Veterans had to reside in the state for at least two years before 1913. State records indicate that 4,173 men applied for a pension in Missouri. In 1898, the state of Louisiana started a pension program through which indigent veterans received $8 a month. Four years later, the state removed $5,000 from the pension fund in order to purchase another round of prosthetic limbs (or cash payments) to amputees. The state agreed to resupply limbs and cash payments to surviving veterans every four years. See Louisiana Legislative Acts, #125, 1898; #169, 1902, LA; *Alabama Acts*, no. 421 (1898–99): 226–35, AL. In 1908, the state legislature passed Act 71, which called for a census of all ex-Confederate soldiers still living in Louisiana. The enumeration, which commenced in 1911, recorded name, age, occupation, physical infirmity, military service details, and the estimated worth of the individual (income and property value). The census tabulated thirty-two amputees living in Louisiana (thirteen who lost legs, fourteen who lost arms, three who lost fingers, and two who lost feet). The men ranged in age from sixty-four (A. C. Broussard, who lost a finger) to eighty-seven (W. B. Rourk, who lost a leg). While a majority of the men farmed, a few worked as physicians, bankers, lawyers, or justices of the peace. Some of the men held no jobs and did not report any economic worth in the census. The economic values reported ranged from $40 (a farmer who lost an arm) to $4,760 (a banker who lost a leg). See Louisiana Legislative Acts #71, 1908, LA; 1911 Census of Confederate Veterans or Their Widows Pursuant to Act 71 of 1908, LA. By 1929, Louisiana still had 755 soldiers receiving a pension of $30 a month. A group of veterans had petitioned the General Assembly and governor to increase the monthly allotment from $8. The petition requested the rate increase for all soldiers and sailors who could prove their military service and residency. See "To the Governor and Members of the General Assembly of the State of Louisiana," United Confederate Veterans Association Records, LSU. In

1899, Alabama established a pension program to care for all veterans, provided they earn a miniscule income and did not hold a significant amount of property. The state of Alabama would eventually drop the property qualification in 1923. Alabama performed a census of southeastern Alabama in 1907 and ascertained that nineteen amputees still survived (twelve arms and six legs, and one who lost two fingers). By 1940, the amputees had vanished and the state only had forty-five total veterans remaining on the pension rolls. "Surviving Confederate Pensioners," 216; *Alabama Acts*, no. 779 (1915): 886–96, AL. The census tabulated veterans in Bullock, Butler, Coffee, Covington, Crenshaw, Dale, Geneva, Henry, Houston, and Pike Counties. See Jones, *Census of Confederate Veterans Residing in Southeast Alabama in 1907.*

40. Florida's program, which started in 1885, was formed to help the 15,000 soldiers who served the state on behalf of the Confederacy and returned home permanently wounded or disabled. South Carolina started their program in 1887, after receiving numerous complaints from citizens who could barely survive without additional help. Mississippi and Virginia both started their programs in 1888. See "An Act to Provide an Annuity for Disabled Soldiers and Sailors of the State of Florida, February 16, 1885" located in Florida Confederate Pension Files, FL; "Report of Surgeon General, 1892," United Confederate Veterans Association Records, LSU; Rosenburg, "Southern Poor Boys," in Logue and Barton, *Civil War Veteran*, 96; "Application and Correspondence," S 126095 Comptroller General, Claims for Disability, 1886; McCawley, *Artificial Limbs for Confederate Soldiers*, 4–6; S126098 Register of Artificial Limb Applications, 1884–88, 1893–94, SC; S126093 Applications for Artificial Limbs (Act of 1902); "A. L. Peters Contract," S126160 Miscellaneous Papers, Artificial Limbs, SC; S126094 Applications for Artificial Limbs (Act of 1907), SC; McDaid, "With Lame Legs and No Money," 20; McClurken, *Take Care of the Living*, 148–51. Florida garnered some funds for the pension system through the convict leasing system. Veterans who applied for a pension and could prove their military service and injury received $5 a month if they had been "rendered unfit to perform manual labor by reason of wounds received in line of duty." In 1887, the legislature bumped up the amount to $8 a month and then amended the legislation three years later to specifically assist amputated men. Wounded men received $150 for the total loss of sight, $30 for a missing eye, and $30 for the loss of hearing. Amputees received $100 and $150 if they lost either both arms/hands or both legs/feet. If an injury in battle caused an arm or leg to now be rendered useless, the veteran got $90. Veterans who had been inflicted with a disease or other injury that hampered their ability to "perform ordinary manual avocations of life" received $96. South Carolina provided veterans $21 for a leg missing above the knee and $35 for a leg below the knee. In terms of missing arms, veterans got $10 for an empty sleeve above the elbow and $7 for one below. In 1892, the state added missing eyes to the cash payment qualifications, and veterans received $47.50 for the empty socket. The legislature continued to add thousands of dollars to the program to pay the veterans another round of payments in the 1890s for their missing limbs. In February 1902, the state appropriated another $2,000 to repair broken prosthetic devices acquired under previous rounds of legislation ($25 for each repair). South Carolina added more funds in 1907, and the state's extensive financial program benefited nearly a

thousand amputees over the span of fifty years. Virginia's program provided $30 a year to amputees and $60 a month to double amputees or anyone blinded. The state increased the amount for two limbs to $100 in 1900 and to $150 in 1912. For one missing limb, the state raised the payment amount to $50 in 1900 and to $65 in 1912. Disabilities not associated with amputation earned a veteran $60 a year for complete disability and $15 for partial disability. Total disability rates declined to $30 in 1900 and increased to $36 in 1912, while partial disability remained steady at $15 until 1912, when the state allocated $24. However, a veteran had to attest to an abject state of poverty, earning less than $300 a year and possessing property valued at under $1,000. From 1888 to 1927, Virginia spent millions on their Confederate veterans, funded by a five-cent tax on every $1,000 of property.

41. The first major pension bill in Tennessee, in 1887, extended a generous pension of $25 per month to any Union or Confederate soldiers who lost both of their arms or legs during the Civil War. By 1891, veterans who had lost one limb received $8.33 per month, while double amputees got $10 a month, which the state paid four times per year. The state appropriated up to $200,000 per year for the payment of pensions, which steadily rose to $300,000 in 1907 and $350,000 in 1909 and topped out at $900,000 per year in 1915. See *Senate Journal Tennessee*, 1881, 198 and 210; *Senate Journal Tennessee*, 1883, 683; *Acts of Tennessee*, 1883, 323–24; *Senate Journal Tennessee*, 1885, 294–96, TN; *Acts of Tennessee*, 1887, 105–6, TN, all items at the Tennessee State Library and Archives. Nine men received the pension for blindness. Senator J. M. Simerly proposed to increase the pension rate for blind soldiers to $30 a month. J. H. McDowell proposed that senators consider providing a pension to soldiers who lost a leg, while J. P. Rogers proposed extending a pension of $10 a month to soldiers who lost an arm. Thirty-seven double amputees received the pension. See *Acts of Tennessee*, 1889, 342–44, TN; *Acts of Tennessee*, 1891, 150–52, TN; Tennessee Board of Pension Examiners Records, record group 3, box 1, folder 18, TN. *Acts of Tennessee*, 1899, 988–89, TN; *Acts of Tennessee*, 1901, 42, TN; *Acts of Tennessee*, 1903, 557–60, TN; *Acts of Tennessee*, 1905, 425–26, TN; *Acts of Tennessee*, 1907, 15, TN; *Acts of Tennessee*, 1909, 38–39, TN; *Acts of Tennessee*, 1911, 24, TN; *Acts of Tennessee*, 1915, 105–6, TN. In 1895, a soldier could have lost one eye during the war and another since the war and could receive the maximum payment for two missing eyes. The state also allocated another $17,000 for the soldier home at the Hermitage in 1895. See *Acts of Tennessee*, 1895, 67 and 313, TN. If veterans lied on their application, they could be punished with prison time and a fine of up to $500. In 1899, the Tennessee legislature drastically altered the pension law. First, they decreased the payment amounts from $25 to $15 for a veteran missing two arms or two legs. The secretary of the Pension Board also had the right to visit the residence of an applicant to ascertain whether he had been honest about the condition of both his body and his finances. However, two years later, the legislature had a change of heart and decided to return the rate for double amputees back to the original $25 per month. The legislature also added another class of pensioners in 1903: veterans who now faced disability due to the effects of advanced age. The veterans received $5 per month. The pension program remained active in Tennessee until the last Confederate veteran died in 1947.

42. *Arkansas Gazette*, January 14, 1891, January 25, 1891, March 26, 1891, and March 27, 1891; Arkansas Confederate Pension Records, Arkansas History Com-

mission. The allowance constituted $100 for a missing foot, leg, hand, or arm, $150 for missing both feet or legs, and $75 for a useless limb. Veterans also received $125 for the loss of sight, $25 for the loss of an eye, and $30 for the loss of hearing. The pension program provided for nearly 45,000 individuals over the course of forty years.

43. *House Journal of Texas, 26th Legislature 1899*, 816–17 and 1252; *House Journal of Texas, 26th Legislature 1899*, 1250–53; *House Journal of Texas, 26th Legislature 1899*, 868–69. The Texas bill would provide indigent veterans eight dollars a month through massive appropriations of $100,000 for the first year and an additional $150,000 for the second year of the program.

44. *House Journal of Texas, 26th Legislature 1899*, 1255.

45. Ibid. The vote to approve the pension legislation was 101 to 6, with 19 legislators absent.

46. *Senate Journal of Texas, 26th Legislature 1899*, 27–28 and 209.

47. Ibid., 209–10.

48. Coulter, *Civil War and Readjustment in Kentucky*, 439; Webb, *Kentucky in the Reconstruction Era*, 92–93; Marshall, *Creating a Confederate Kentucky*, 1–7.

49. Confederate Home Messenger, March 1910, United Daughters of the Confederacy Records, box 41, KYHS. In 1880, William M. Parks, who fought with a Kentucky regiment during the Civil War, applied for an artificial arm in Georgia. Parks lost his right arm above the elbow at the Battle of Fort Donelson on February 15, 1862. He moved to Georgia and applied for a limb because he had never purchased one on his own accord and Kentucky did not grant artificial limbs. Parks needed the secretary of state in Kentucky to validate his military service in order to secure an arm in Georgia. He received his limb after a doctor in Kentucky and the secretary of state backed up his claim, including the fact that he lost his arm when he had been shot by one of his comrades at Donelson. See Williams, *My Old Confederate Home*, 3; "William M. Parks Pension Application," Office of the Governor, Luke P. Blackburn, Militia Correspondence, 1879–1880, KY.

50. "An Act Granting Pension to Indigent and Disabled Confederate Soldiers, and the Widows of Confederate Soldiers," in *Acts of the General Assembly of the Commonwealth of Kentucky* (1912), KY; Simpson, *Index of Confederate Pension Applications*, 1–2, courtesy of KYHS. Kentucky placed strict parameters on its pension program tied to need and a demonstration of moral character. An applicant could not have an annual income of more than $300 or property valued at over $2,500. If the injured veteran remained dependent on his wife for survival and her estate or income topped the above figures, the pension was denied. When applicants were ready to apply for the pension, they traveled to the county clerk, stood before a judge, and provided two witnesses and a physician's written validation of the specific injury. Veterans also had to answer whether or not they used any intoxicants, which harkened to the strong temperance culture and movement in Kentucky that had been in existence since the antebellum era. If the applicants submitted an incomplete application or failed to meet the burden of proof on their income, property value, nature of injury, or length of residency or service, the pension application was rejected and the applicants had one additional chance to apply. If a later investigation unearthed any falsehoods, the state had the right to pull the application with thirty days' written notice. Applicants could send in any required infor-

mation to buttress their application and alleviate any concerns or questions in the minds of the pension officials. See Soldier's Application for Pension, Confederate Pension Files, KY.

51. No. 188 Soldier's Application for Pension, Confederate Pension Files, KY; "James M. Harp v. H. M. Bosworth, 1913," *Franklin Circuit Court Order Book, 1912–1916*, KY; Simpson, *Index of Confederate Pension Applications*, 3, KYHS.

52. "James M. Harp v. H. M. Bosworth, 1913," *Franklin Circuit Court Order Book, 1912–1916*, KY.

53. Brief for Appellee, Case #41834, Henry M. Bosworth, Auditor v. James M. Harp, Court of Appeals, State of Kentucky, KY.

54. Ibid.

55. Ibid.

56. Ibid. Historian David W. Blight, in *Race and Reunion*, noted the development of the reconciliationist vision of Civil War memory as Americans dealt with the dead from the war. As reconciliation evolved, the Lost Cause transformed the terms of reunion to give southerners a larger stake in shaping the dominant memory of the Civil War. See also Janney, *Remembering the Civil War*.

57. Brief for Appellee, Case #41834, Henry M. Bosworth, Auditor v. James M. Harp, Court of Appeals, State of Kentucky, KY. The extensive historiography pertaining to the Lost Cause contains numerous titles that are very useful in understanding how southerners constructed a particular postwar memory. Charles Reagan Wilson, who views the Lost Cause as more of a religious movement, lays out his argument in *Baptized in Blood*; Gaines Foster views the Lost Cause as more of a social and cultural phenomenon than a religious movement in his helpful work, *Ghosts of the Confederacy*. Other useful works include Silber, *Romance of Reunion*; Connelly and Bellows, *God and General Longstreet*; Blight, *Race and Reunion*; Gallagher and Nolan, *Myth of the Lost Cause*.

58. Brief for Appellee, Case #41834, Henry M. Bosworth, Auditor v. James M. Harp, Court of Appeals, State of Kentucky, KY.

59. Ibid.

60. Ibid.

61. Ibid.; Simpson, *Index of Confederate Pension Applications*, 3, KYHS. Although the final legal decision put to rest the constitutionality question of the Confederate pension law, the state assembly continued to tweak it. Revisions gradually increased the quarterly pension payment to $12 in 1918 and to $20 in 1928. Kentucky Confederates who swore a loyalty oath to the Union under duress in the final months of the war could not be denied a pension. The allocation gradually increased over the next few decades. See Simpson, *Index of Confederate Pension Applications*, 4–5, KYHS. Since the establishment of the Fourteenth Amendment to the U.S. Constitution in 1868, numerous court cases had questioned or challenged the equal protection and due process clauses, including *Bradwell v. State of Illinois* (1873) and the *Slaughter-House Cases* (1873) at the U.S. Supreme Court. The federal courts saw a clear distinction between federal and state citizenship rights, and the state had the ability to pass their own regulations and rules that applied exclusively to the citizens residing within their borders. Thus, because the justices in Kentucky saw ex-Confederate soldiers as citizens of the state, they could not be denied a pension. The case in Kentucky established a legal precedent to guar-

antee former Confederates the financial benefits of a pension system within their own state. For more on the *Slaughter-House Cases*, see Labhé and Lurie, *Slaughterhouse Cases*.

62. James R. Williams pension application, Graves County, Kentucky Confederate Pension Applications, KYHS; William H. Brown pension application, Ballard County, Kentucky Confederate Pension Applications, KYHS. Other examples of suffering can be located in #00988, Thomas B. Price; #01013, D. H. Smith; #01188, Christopher Koonce; and #01390, L. H. Taylor, Confederate Pension Applications, Texas Comptroller's Office Claims Records, TX.

63. W. Z. Rudd and William J. Sullenger pension applications, Carlisle County, Kentucky Confederate Pension Applications, KYHS.

64. A01731, James Wall, Florida Confederate Pension Application Files, FL; A05255, Jacob Link, Florida Confederate Pension Application Files, FL; A05242 William Brown, Florida Confederate Pension Application Files, FL; A02540, John W. Addison, Florida Confederate Pension Application Files, FL; A11032 Joseph Tyler, Florida Confederate Pension Application Files, FL;

65. Confederate Pension Applications, #28, TN; Confederate Pension Applications, #31, TN.

66. Confederate Pension Applications, #2, TN; Hartman and Coles, *Biographical Rosters of Florida's Confederate and Union Soldiers*, 2:496.

67. "Report of Surgeon General, 1892," United Confederate Veterans Association Records, LSU.

Epilogue

1. Photograph of Bobby Lisek, Disabled American Veterans Mailing, September 2010, author's personal collection. Following the horrific attack at the finish line of the Boston Marathon in April 2013, several wounded individuals underwent amputation at local hospitals throughout Boston. For more information on the trauma surgeons who performed various amputations that day, see "For Trauma Surgeons, Saving Lives, if Not Legs, with No Time to Fret," *New York Times*, April 16, 2013.

2. *Washington Post*, March 21, 2010, www.washingtonpost.com/wp-dyn/content /story/2010/03/20/ST2010032001715.html?sid=ST2010032001715 (accessed January 15, 2013).

3. http://www.huffingtonpost.com/2012/07/26/ied-afghanistan-war-veterans_n _1705397.html (accessed July 26, 2012); USA Today, January 30, 2013, 5D. The article notes that nearly fifty thousand soldiers have suffered wounds from both wars, including sixteen thousand who have been catastrophically wounded.

4. Duckworth lost both of her legs in combat while serving as a helicopter pilot in Iraq. She was the first female double amputee of the war. Currently, the U.S. Congress (2013–15) has sixteen members who served in Iraq or Afghanistan, of whom Duckworth is the only amputee. The conflicts in Iraq and Afghanistan mark the first time in U.S. history that a large number of women have faced prolonged combat exposure. For more on female veterans who have lost limbs, see http:// usatoday30.usatoday.com/news/nation/2005-04-28-female-amputees-combat_x .htm (accessed February 8, 2014).

BIBLIOGRAPHY

Primary Sources

MANUSCRIPTS

Alabama Department of Archives and History
ALABAMA HOSPITALS IN RICHMOND, ADMINISTRATIVE FILES

ALABAMA LEGISLATIVE ACTS
> 1866–67, no. 643
> 1867, no. 149
> 1898–1899, no. 421
> 1915, no. 779
> 1919, no. 409
> 1936–37, no. 172
> 1939, no. 483
> 1959, no. 402

BOLLING HALL FAMILY PAPERS
> Confederate Pension Records, Application for Artificial Limbs

APPLICATION FOR ORDERS AND MEASURES, 1867
> Arms Applications
> Artificial Limb-Correspondence
> Auditor Records
> HB 734, An Act for the Relief of Maimed Soldiers
> "Surviving Confederate Pensioners" in *Alabama Historical Quarterly*
> Clyde Wilson Report on Artificial Limbs

Arkansas History Commission, Little Rock, Arkansas
ACTS OF THE GENERAL ASSEMBLY OF THE STATE OF ARKANSAS
> Arkansas Confederate Pension Records
> Medical Case History Journal by Dr. Henry Dye

Auburn University Archives
JAMES WILLIAM HOWARD JOURNAL
> Asa T. Martin Papers

Eleanor S. Brockenbrough Library, the Museum of the Confederacy
KIND OF WOUND AND DISEASE: HOSPITAL LIFE WITHIN THE CONFEDERATE MEDICAL DEPARTMENT
> Instructions for Amputation from the Manual for Military Surgery Prepared for the Use of the Confederate States Army, 1863
> John B. Lightfoot, Jr. Address
> Livingston Letters
> Medical and Hospital Series

MEDICAL PERSONNEL COLLECTION
    Miscellaneous Papers
    Robertson Hospital
    Winder Hospital
KIM ROWLAND DIARY
    Isaac S. Tanner Collection

Center for American History, University of Texas at Austin
CRUTCHER-SHANNON PAPERS
    Rules of the Third Georgia Hospital
    Samuel Hollingsworth Stout Papers

Georgia Archives, Morrow, Ga.
ACTS OF THE GENERAL ASSEMBLY OF THE STATE OF GEORGIA
    Confederate Pension Applications
    Lee Barfield Letters

Hargrett Rare Book and Manuscript Library, University of Georgia
MS 218 MAYS CONFEDERATE HOSPITAL
    MS 1066 Charles Colcock Jones Papers
    MS 1170 Telamon Cuyler Collection
    MS 2345 E. Merton Coulter Papers
    MS 2642 R. D. Harris Papers
    MS 3264 Eberhart Family Papers

Historic New Orleans Collection
LETTERS OF A CONFEDERATE SURGEON, JUNIUS NEWPORT BRAGG, ELEVENTH ARKANSAS

W. S. Hoole Special Collections Library, University of Alabama
CONFEDERATE SOLDIERS, CO. G, ELEVENTH ALABAMA
    Confederate Soldiers, Co. K, Forty-Third Alabama
    A Sketch of the Life and Travels of David Crocket Stuart

Howard-Tilton Memorial Library, Special Collections, Tulane University
ANNIE JETER CARMOUCHE PAPERS
    Horace Chapin Diary
    Chicago Medical Examiner
    Charles Woodward Hutson Family Papers
    Joseph Jones Papers
    War Department, Surgeon General's Office, "A Report on Amputations at the Hip-Joint in Military Surgery"

James G. Kenan Research Center, Atlanta History Center
HANDBOOK FOR THE MILITARY SURGEON
    Tatum Family Papers

Kentucky Department for Libraries and Archives
ACTS OF THE GENERAL ASSEMBLY OF THE COMMONWEALTH OF KENTUCKY
    Confederate Soldiers Home, Reference Book B
    Confederate Pension Files, Commonwealth of Kentucky

Court of Appeals, State of Kentucky Case #41834
Franklin Circuit Court Order Book, 1912–16
Hospital Register, Ky. Confederate Home, Pewee Valley, Ky.
Office of the Governor, Luke P. Blackburn, Militia Correspondence, 1879–80

Kentucky Historical Society
BALLARD COUNTY, KENTUCKY, CONFEDERATE PENSION APPLICATIONS
Pattie Burnley Papers
Boyd-Wherritt-Wilson Papers
Carlisle County Kentucky Confederate Pension Applications
Civil War in Kentucky Scrapbook
Graves County, Kentucky Confederate Pension Applications
Graves County, Kentucky Miscellaneous Court Records
Thomas Osborne Scrapbook
United Daughters of the Confederacy Records

Louisiana State Archives, Baton Rouge, La.
ABSTRACTS LAND SALES, CLAIMS, MISC RECORDS
BENEFICIARY LAND WARRANT
LOUISIANA LEGISLATIVE ACTS: 1880, 1882, 1884, 1886, 1888, 1896, 1898, 1902, 1908
1911 Census of Confederate Veterans or Their Widows Pursuant to Act 71 of 1908
Soldiers Proof as Beneficiary under Act #96 of 1884
Soldiers Proof as Beneficiary under Act #116 of 1886
Soldiers Proof as Beneficiary under Act #55 of 1896

Manuscripts, Archives and Rare Book Library, Emory University
JOHN SAMUEL MERIWETHER PAPERS
Ocmulgee Hospital, Macon, Ga.
Thomas Henry Pitts Papers
Sue Richardson Papers
Loula Kendall Rogers Papers
Lemuel A. Scarbrough Diary
Samuel Hollingsworth Stout Papers

Mississippi Department of Archives and History
CONFEDERATE SOLDIERS AND SAILORS AND WIDOWS PENSION APPLICATIONS
Confederate States Army Casualties
First Mississippi Hospital at Jackson
Indigent and Disabled Soldiers and Dependents, 1863–68
Journal of the Senate of the State of Mississippi

Missouri State Archives
ROBERT L. HAWKINS COLLECTION
Journal of the House
Journal of the Senate
Laws of Missouri

Missouri State Historical Society
MARY JANE VAUGHN CLARK PAPERS

National Archives and Records Administration
RECORD BOOK, SOLDIERS HOME HOSPITAL AND ASSOCIATION FOR THE
RELIEF OF MAIMED SOLDIERS, RICHMOND, VA., 1862–65
> Reports on Amputation Cases, Howard's Grove Hospital, Richmond, Va., 1862

National Library of Medicine, Bethesda, Md.
HOFF PAPERS

Reynolds Historical Library, University of Alabama at Birmingham
ARTHUR G. DIETHELM AMERICAN CIVIL WAR MEDICAL COLLECTION
> DR. B. W. ALLEN CIVIL WAR JOURNAL
> Illustrated Catalogue of the Celebrated Bly Artificial Limbs
> *Richmond Medical Journal,* May 1866
> Abraham Watkins Venable Scrapbook, 1851–65

South Carolina Department of History and Archives
APPLICATIONS FOR ARTIFICIAL LIMBS (ACT OF 1902)
> Applications for Artificial Limbs (Act of 1907)
> Comptroller General, Claims for Disability, 1886
> Comptroller General, Letters Concerning Artificial Limbs
> Comptroller General, Pension Department, Artificial Limb Applications for Confederate Service, 1880–87
> Comptroller General, Pension Department, Artificial Limb Vouchers, 1867–69
> Journals of the House of Representatives, Early State Records, 1863–66
> Lists of Disabled Soldiers, 1867
> Miscellaneous Papers, Artificial Limbs
> Register of Artificial Limb Applications, 1884–88, 1893–94

South Carolina Historical Society
COMPARATIVE MERITS OF THE PARTIAL AMPUTATION OF THE FOOT
> Brig. Gen. Samuel W. Ferguson Memoirs
> Hall T. McGee Diary, Eighteenth S.C. Heavy Artillery
> Sketch of the Soldiers Relief Association of Charleston

South Caroliniana Library, University of South Carolina Libraries
HENRY ADICKS PAPERS
> James Michael Barr Papers
> James Richmond Boulware Diary
> John Thompson Darby Papers
> Papers of the Summer, Dreher, Efird and Mayer Families
> Mary Snowden Papers

Southern Historical Collection, Wilson Library, University of North Carolina at Chapel Hill
BATTLE FAMILY PAPERS
> William Beavens
> Confederate Papers Collection
> Margaret Ann Mata Morris Grimball Diary, 1860–66

Harbison Family Papers
Hatrick Family Scrapbook
Hentz Family Papers
Charles Hutson Papers
Lenoir Family Papers
Benjamin Franklin Little Papers
C. Alice Ready Diary

Special Collections, Louisiana State University Libraries
WILLIAM DAVIS COTTON AND FAMILY PAPERS
Alfred Flournoy Papers
Hamet Pinson Family Papers
Joseph Jones Papers
Louisiana Military Commission Collection
McGalliard (William M. and Family) Papers
United Confederate Veterans Association Papers

Special Collections, Perkins Library, Duke University
LUCAS ASHLEY FAMILY PAPERS
Harriet Branham Diary
George Briggs Papers
William Carrington Papers
Confederate Pamphlets
Lucy Muse Walton Fletcher Papers
Greenville Ladies Association Minutes, 1861–65
Samuel Gross Confederate Pamphlet-Manual of Military Surgery
Henry Kagey Papers
Jacob Mordecai Papers
Reminiscences of Mrs. Charles C. Rainwater
M. J. Solomons Scrapbook
Samuel Hollingsworth Stout Papers
Samuel Walkup Papers

Special Collections, University of Arkansas Libraries
JAMES BERRY COLLECTION
Mary C. Berry Papers
Josephine Crump Papers
L. H. Graves Diary
Ozark Folk Encyclopedia
Samuel Pickney Pittman Papers
Ira Russell Papers

State Archives of Florida
FLORIDA CONFEDERATE PENSION APPLICATION FILES

Tennessee State Library and Archives
BROWN-EWELL PAPERS
House Journals of Tennessee
Legislative Acts of Tennessee
Senate Journals of Tennessee

Simerly Family Papers
Tennessee Board of Pension Examiners Records, Record Group 3
William Trousdale Papers

Texas General Land Office
CONFEDERATE SCRIP VOUCHER

Texas State Library and Archives
ADJUTANT GENERAL CIVIL WAR RECORDS–TEXAS STATE TROOP RECORDS
Amputees from Confederate Home Roster
Comptroller Confederate Pension Applications
Confederate Pension Applications
Journal of the House of Representatives of the Eleventh Legislature 1866
Journal of the House of Representatives of the Twenty-Sixth Legislature 1899
Journal of the Senate of the Twenty-Sixth Legislature 1899

Virginia Historical Society
A MANUAL OF MILITARY SURGERY FOR THE USE OF SURGEONS IN THE CS ARMY
Joseph Lyon Miller Papers
Sanders Family Papers

J.D. Williams Library and Special Collections, University of Mississippi
EUGENE FERRIS COLLECTION
W. L. Kennon, "A Tribute to the Womanhood of the Confederacy, 1934,"
M. D. L. Stephens Manuscript

ONLINE SOURCES
http://www.archives.alabama.gov/conoff/carmichael_j1.html
http://www.archives.alabama.gov/marschall/J_Walker.html
http://www.archives.alabama.gov/referenc/flags/062.html
http://www.readcentral.com/chapters/Henry-Rowe-Schoolcraft/Algic-Researches
-Vol-2/029

PRINTED SOURCES
Appia, P. L. *The Ambulance Surgeon or Practical Observations on Gunshot Wounds.* Edinburgh: Adam and Charles Black, 1862.
Arnold, Thomas Jackson. *Early Life and Letters of General Thomas J. Jackson.* Chicago: Fleming H. Revell, 1916.
Barnes, Joseph K., ed. *The Medical and Surgical History of the Civil War.* Vol. 11. Wilmington, N.C.: Broadfoot, 1991.
Beers, Fannie A. *Memories: A Record of Personal Experience and Adventure during Four Years of War.* Philadelphia: J. B. Lippincott, 1888.
Benson, Susan Williams, ed. *Berry Benson's Civil War Book: Memoirs of a Confederate Scout and Sharpshooter.* Athens: University of Georgia Press, 1962.
Berlin, Jean V., ed. *A Confederate Nurse: The Diary of Ada W. Bacot, 1860–1863.* Columbia: University of South Carolina Press, 1994.
Bernard, Claude, and Charles Huette. *Illustrated Manual of Operative Surgery and Surgical Anatomy.* New York: Bailliere Brothers, 1861.
Blackford, Susan Leigh. *Letters from Lee's Army or Memoirs of Life In and Out of the Army of Northern Virginia during the War between the States.* New York: Scribner, 1947.

Bohannon, Keith, ed. "Wounded and Captured at Gettysburg: Reminiscence by Sergeant William Jones, 50th Georgia Infantry." *Military Images* 9, no. 6 (1988).

Brinsfield, John Wesley, Jr. *The Spirit Divided: Memoirs of Civil War Chaplains, The Confederacy.* Mercer, Ga.: Mercer University Press, 2006.

Brumgardt, John R., ed. *Civil War Nurse: The Diary and Letters of Hannah Ropes.* Knoxville: University of Tennessee Press, 1980.

The Campaigns of Walker's Texas Division by a Private Soldier. New York: Lane, Little and Company, 1875.

Camp-Fire Chats of the Civil War. Chicago: A.B. Gehmana, 1886.

Chisolm, J. Julian. *A Manual of Military Surgery for the Use of Surgeons in the Confederate States Army.* Richmond: West and Johnston, 1862.

———. *A Manual of Military Surgery for the Use of Surgeons in the Confederate States Army.* 3rd ed. Columbia, S.C.: Evans and Cogswell, 1864.

Civil War Letters, Volume I, West Tennessee. Melber, Ky.: Simmons Historical Publications, 1995.

Civil War Letters, Volume II, East Tennessee. Melber, Ky.: Simmons Historical Publications, 1996.

Crist, Lynda Lasswell, ed. *The Papers of Jefferson Davis: Volume 11, September 1864–May 1865.* Baton Rouge: Louisiana State University Press, 2003.

Cuttino, George Peddy, ed. *Saddle Bag and Spinning Wheel Being the Civil War Letters of George W. Peddy, M.D. and His Wife Kate Featherson Peddy.* Macon, Ga.: Mercer University Press, 1981.

Daniel, F. E., M.D. *Recollections of a Rebel Surgeon (and Other Sketches); or, In the Doctor's Sappy Days.* Austin: Von Boeckmann, Schutze and Co., 1899. Reprint, Chicago: Clinci, 1901.

Davis, William C., ed. *Diary of a Confederate Soldier: John S. Jackman of the Orphan Brigade.* Columbia: University of South Carolina Press, 1990.

Dorsey, Sarah A. *Recollections of Henry Watkins Allen.* New Orleans: M. Doolady, 1866.

Douglas, Lucia Rutherford, ed. *Douglas's Texas Battery, CSA.* Tyler, Tex.: Smith County Historical Society, 1966.

Dunglison, Robley. *General Therapeutics and Materia Medica: Adapted for a Medical Text Book with Indexes of Remedies and of Diseases and Their Remedies.* Philadelphia: Blanchard and Lea, 1857.

Elliott, Sam Davis, ed. *Doctor Quintard, Chaplain C.S.A. and Second Bishop of Tennessee: The Memoir and Civil War Diary of Charles Todd Quintard.* Baton Rouge: Louisiana State University Press, 2003.

Esmarch, Friedrich. *Resection in Gunshot Injuries.* Philadelphia: J. B. Lippincott, 1862.

Evans, Gen. Clement A., ed. *Confederate Military History vol. V: North Carolina.* New York: Broadfoot, 1987.

———, ed. *Confederate Military History vol. VI: South Carolina.* New York: Broadfoot, 1987.

———, ed. *Confederate Military History vol. VIII: Alabama.* New York: Broadfoot, 1987.

———, ed. *Confederate Military History vol. X: Tennessee.* New York: Broadfoot, 1987.

———, ed. *Confederate Military History vol. XI: Kentucky.* New York: Broadfoot, 1987.

———, ed. *Confederate Military History vol. XIV: Arkansas.* New York: Broadfoot, 1988.

———, ed. *Confederate Military History vol. XV: Texas.* New York: Broadfoot, 1989.

———, ed. *Confederate Military History vol. XVI: Florida.* New York: Broadfoot, 1989.

Eve, Paul F. *A Collection of Remarkable Cases in Surgery.* Philadelphia: J. B. Lippincott, 1857.

Everson, Guy R., and Edward H. Simpson, Jr., eds. *Far, Far from Home: The Wartime Letters of Dick and Tally Simpson, 3rd South Carolina Volunteers.* New York: Oxford University Press, 1994.

Fatout, Paul, ed. *Letters of a Civil War Surgeon.* West Lafayette, Ind.: Purdue University Press, 1996.

Fletcher, William A. *Rebel Private: Front and Rear, Memoirs of a Confederate Soldier.* New York: Meridian, 1997.

Formento, Felix, Jr. *Notes and Observations on Army Surgery.* New Orleans: L. E. Marchand, 1863.

Frazier, Donald S., and Andrew Hillhouse, eds. *Love and War: The Civil War Letters and Medicinal Book of Augustus V. Ball.* Buffalo Gap, Tex.: State House Press, 2010.

Grace, William. *The Army Surgeon's Manual, for the Use of Medical Officers, Cadets, Chaplains, and Hospital Stewards.* New York: Bailliere Brothers, 1864.

Greenleaf, Charles R. *A Manual for the Medical Officers of the United States Army.* Philadelphia: J. B. Lippincott, 1864.

Gross, Samuel D. *A Manual of Military Surgery or Hints on the Emergencies of Field Camp and Hospital Practice.* Augusta, Ga.: Steam Power Press Chronicle and Sentinel, 1861.

——. *A System of Surgery: Pathological, Diagnostic, Therapeutic and Operative.* Vols. 1–2. Philadelphia: Blanchard and Lea, 1862.

Hammond, William A., M.D., ed. *Military Medical and Surgical Essays Prepared for the United States Sanitary Commission.* Philadelphia: J. B. Lippincott, 1864.

Harwell, Richard, ed. *The Journal of Kate Cumming, a Confederate Nurse, 1862–1865.* Savannah, Ga.: Beehive Press, 1975.

Holland, Katherine S., ed. *Keep All My Letters: The Civil War Letters of Richard Henry Brooks, 51st Georgia Infantry.* Macon, Ga.: Mercer University Press, 2003.

Houck, Peter W., ed. *Confederate Surgeon: The Personal Recollections of E.A. Craighill.* Lynchburg, Va.: H.E. Howard, 1989.

Houts, Joseph Kinyoun, Jr., ed. *A Darkness Ablaze: The Civil War Medical Diary and Wartime Experiences of Dr. John Hendricks Kinyoun, Sixty-Sixth North Carolina Infantry Regiment.* St. Joseph, Mo.: Platte Purchase, 2005.

An Impressed New Yorker, Thirteen Months in the Rebel Army Being a Narrative of Personal Adventures in the Infantry, Ordnance, Cavalry, Courier and Hospital Services. New York: A.S. Barnes and Burr, 1862.

Jones, Homer T. *Census of Confederate Veterans Residing in Southeast Alabama in 1907.* Carrollton, Miss.: Pioneer, 1998.

Keen, William Williams. *Addresses and Other Papers.* Philadelphia: W.B. Saunders, 1905.

King, Spencer Bedwill, Jr. *The War Time Journal of a Georgia Girl, 1864–1865 by Eliza Frances Andres.* Macon, Ga.: Ardivan Press, 1960.

Koonce, Donald B., ed. *Doctor to the Front: The Recollections of Confederate Surgeon Thomas Fanning Wood, 1861–1865.* Knoxville: University of Tennessee Press, 2000.

Letterman, Jonathan. *Medical Recollections of the Army of the Potomac.* New York: Appleton, 1866.

Lowe, Jeffrey C., and Sam Hodges, eds. *Letters to Amanda: The Civil War Letters of Marion Hill Fitzpatrick, Army of Northern Virginia.* Macon, Ga.: Mercer University Press, 1998.

Mays, Thomas D. *Let Us Meet in Heaven: The Civil War Letters of James Michael Barr, 5th South Carolina Cavalry.* Abilene, Tex.: McWhiney Foundation Press, 2001.

McCaw, James B. *Confederate Sates Medical and Surgical Journal.* San Francisco: Norman, 1992.

McMullen, Glenn L., ed. *A Surgeon with Stonewall Jackson: The Civil War Letters of Dr. Harvey Black.* Baltimore, Md.: Butternut and Blue, 1995.

The Medical and Surgical History of the War of the Rebellion. Washington, D.C.: Government Printing Office, 1883.

Meriwether, Elizabeth Avery. *The Ku Klux Klan; or, The Carpet-Bagger in New Orleans.* Memphis, Tenn.: Southern Baptist Publication Society, 1877.

Moore, Samuel Preston. *A Manual of Military Surgery, Prepared for the Use of the Confederate States Army.* Richmond: Ayres and Wade, 1863.

Pfanz, Donald C., ed. *The Letters of General Richard S. Ewell: Stonewall's Successor.* Knoxville: University of Tennessee Press, 2012.

Pitcock, Cynthia Dehaven, and Bill J. Gurley, eds. *I Acted from Principle: The Civil War Diary of Dr. William M. McPheeters, Confederate Surgeon in the Trans-Mississippi.* Fayetteville: University of Arkansas Press, 2002.

Reid, Whitelaw. *After the War: A Southern Tour, May 1, 1865–May 1, 1866.* London: Sampson Low, Son and Marston, 1866.

Report of the Joint Committee on the Conduct of the War: Rebel Barbarities. Vol. 3. Washington, D.C.: Government Printing Office, 1863.

Robson, John S. *How a One-Legged Rebel Lives: Reminiscences of the Civil War.* Durham, N.C.: Educator Company, 1898.

Roper, John Herbert, ed. *Repairing the "March of Mars": The Civil War Diaries of John Samuel Apperson, Hospital Steward in the Stonewall Brigade, 1861–1865.* Macon, Ga.: Mercer University Press, 2001.

Schuppert, Moritz. *A Treatise on Gun-Shot Wounds: Written for and Dedicated to the Surgeons of the Confederate States Army.* New Orleans: Bulletin Book and Job Office, 1861.

Smith, John David, and William J. Cooper, Jr., eds. *Window on the War: Frances Dallam Peter's Lexington Civil War Diary.* Lexington, Ky.: Lexington-Fayette County Historical Commission, 1976.

South Carolina Women in the Confederacy: Records Collected by Committee from South Carolina State Division, United Daughters of the Confederacy. Vol. 2. Columbia, S.C.: State Company, 1907.

Straubling, Harold Elk, ed. *In Hospital and Camp: The Civil War through the Eyes of Its Doctors and Nurses.* Harrisburg, Pa.: Stackpole, 1993.

Stromeyer, Louis. *Gunshot Fractures.* Philadelphia: J. B. Lippincott, 1862.

Styple, William B., ed. *Writing and Fighting the Confederate War: The Letters of Peter Wellington Alexander Confederate War Correspondent.* Kearney, N.J.: Belle Grove, 2002.

Sutherland, Daniel E., ed. *A Very Violent Rebel: The Civil War Diary of Ellen Renshaw House.* Knoxville: University of Tennessee Press, 1996.

Swank, Walbrook D., ed. *Confederate Letters and Diaries, 1861–1865.* Shippensburg, Pa.: Burd Street Press, 1988.

Tapp, Hambleton, and James C. Klotter, eds. *The Union, the Civil War and John W. Tuttle: A Kentucky Captain's Account.* Frankfort: Kentucky Historical Society, 1980.

Toalson, Jeff, ed. *No Soap, No Pay, Diarrhea, Dysentery and Desertion: A Composite Diary of the Last Sixteen Months of the Confederacy from 1864 to 1865.* New York: iUniverse, 2006.

Tripler, Charles S., and George C. Blackman. *Handbook for the Military Surgeon.* Cincinnati: Robert C. Clarke, 1861.

Underwood, J. L. *The Women of the Confederacy.* New York: Neale, 1906.

U.S. War Department. *The War of the Rebellion: A Compilation of the Official Records of the Union and Confederate Armies.* 127 vols. Washington, D.C.: GPO, 1880–1901.

Warren, Edward. *An Epitome of Practical Surgery for Field and Hospital.* Richmond: West and Johnston, 1863.

Watkins, Sam. *Co. Aytch: A Side Show of the Big Show.* Wilmington, N.C.: Broadfoot, 1994.

Wiley, Bell Irvin Wiley, ed. *A Southern Woman's Story: Life in Confederate Richmond by Phoebe Yates Pember.* Jackson, Tenn.: McCowat-Mercer Press, 1959.

Wilson, Sadye Tune, Nancy Tune Fitzgerald, and Richard Warwick, eds. *Letters to Laura: A Confederate Surgeon's Impressions of Four Years of War.* Nashville: Tunstede, 1996.

Wilson, Thomas L. *A Brief History of the Cruelties and Atrocities of the Rebellion.* Washington, D.C.: McGill and Witherow, 1864.

Woodward, C. Vann, ed. *Mary Chesnut's Civil War.* New Haven: Yale University Press, 1981.

Yeary, Mamie, ed. *Reminiscences of the Boys in Gray, 1861–1865.* Dallas, Tex.: Smith and Lamar, 1912.

Periodicals

Arkansas Gazette
Atlanta Constitution
Baltimore Sun
British Medical News
Charleston News and Courier
Columbia (Mo.) Herald
Confederate States Medical and Surgical Journal
Confederate Veteran Magazine
Harper's Weekly
Houston Telegraph
Jackson Mississippi Weekly Clarion
The Lost Cause
Macon (Ga.) Daily Telegraph
Memphis Press-Scimitar
Nashville Daily American
New Orleans Daily Picayune
New Orleans Times
New York Times

New York Tribune
Pittsburgh Evening Chronicle
Raleigh Daily North Carolina Standard
Southern Bivouac
Southern Historical Society Papers
Washington Post

Secondary Sources

BOOKS

Abruzzo, Margaret. *Polemical Pain: Slavery, Cruelty and the Rise of Humanitarianism.* Baltimore: Johns Hopkins University Press, 2011.

Adams, George Washington. *Doctors in Blue: The Medical History of the Union Army in the Civil War.* Baton Rouge: Louisiana State University Press, 1952.

Adams, Michael C. C. *Living Hell: The Dark Side of the Civil War.* Baltimore: Johns Hopkins University Press, 2014.

Ayers, Edward L. *The Promise of the New South: Life after Reconstruction.* New York: Oxford University Press, 1992.

——. *Vengeance and Justice: Crime and Punishment in the Nineteenth Century South.* New York: Oxford University Press, 1984.

Bailey, Fred A. *Class and Tennessee's Confederate Generation.* Chapel Hill: University of North Carolina Press, 1987.

Bederman, Gail. *Manliness and Civilization: A Cultural History of Gender and Race in the United States, 1880–1917.* Chicago: University of Chicago Press, 1995.

Bell, Andrew McIlwaine. *Mosquito Soldiers: Malaria, Yellow Fever, and the Course of the American Civil War.* Baton Rouge: Louisiana State University Press, 2010.

Berkin, Carol. *Civil War Wives: The Lives and Times of Angelina Grimké Weld, Varina Howell Davis and Julia Dent Grant.* New York: Knopf, 2009.

Berry, Stephen W. *All That Makes a Man: Love and Ambition in the Civil War South.* New York: Oxford University Press, 2003.

——, ed. *Weirding the War: Stories from the Civil War's Ragged Edges.* Athens: University of Georgia Press, 2011.

Blair, William A. *Cities of the Dead: Contesting the Memory of the Civil War in the South, 1865–1914.* Chapel Hill: University of North Carolina Press, 2004.

Blanton, Wyndham B. *Medicine in Virginia in the Nineteenth Century.* Richmond: Garrett and Massie, 1933.

Blight, David W. *Race and Reunion: The Civil War in American Memory.* Cambridge, Mass.: Harvard University Press, 2001.

Bollet, Alfred J. *Civil War Medicine: Challenges and Triumphs.* Tucson, Ariz.: Galen Press, 2002.

Bowman, John S., ed. *The Civil War Almanac.* New York: World Almanac, 1983.

Brady, Lisa. *War upon the Land: Military Strategy and the Transformation of Southern Landscapes during the American Civil War.* Athens: University of Georgia Press, 2012.

Breeden, James O. *Joseph Jones, M.D.: Scientist of the Old South.* Frankfort: University Press of Kentucky, 1975.

Brinsfield, John Wesley, Jr. *The Spirit Divided: Memoirs of Civil War Chaplains, the Confederacy.* Mercer, Ga.: Mercer University Press, 2006.

Brown, Kathleen M. *Good Wives, Nasty Wenches and Anxious Patriarchs: Gender, Race and Power in Colonial Virginia*. Chapel Hill: University of North Carolina Press, 1996.

Brundage, W. Fitzhugh. *The Southern Past: A Clash of Race and Memory*. Cambridge, Mass.: Harvard University Press, 2005.

Buell, Thomas B. *The Warrior Generals: Combat Leadership in the Civil War*. New York: Three Rivers Press, 1997.

Bynum, Victoria. *Unruly Women: The Politics of Social and Sexual Control in the Old South*. Chapel Hill: University of North Carolina Press, 1992.

Carmichael, Peter S. *The Last Generation: Young Virginians in Peace, War, and Reunion*. Chapel Hill: University of North Carolina Press, 2005.

Carnes, Mark C., and Clyde Griffen, eds. *Meanings for Manhood: Constructions of Masculinity in Victorian America*. Chicago: University of Chicago Press, 1990.

Carter, Hodding. *The Angry Scar: The Story of Reconstruction*. New York: Doubleday, 1959.

Cash, W. J. *The Mind of the South*. New York: Vintage, 1991.

Catton, Bruce. *The American Heritage Picture History of the Civil War*. Avenel, N.J.: Wings Books, 1982.

Censer, Jane Turner. *The Reconstruction of White Southern Womanhood, 1865–1890*. Baton Rouge: Louisiana State University Press, 2003.

Cimbala, Paul A. *Soldiers North and South: The Everyday Experiences of the Men Who Fought America's Civil War*. New York: Fordham University Press, 2010.

Cimbala, Paul A., and Randall M. Miller, eds. *Union Soldiers and the Northern Home Front: Wartime Experiences, Postwar Adjustments*. New York: Fordham University Press, 2002.

Clark, Thomas D., and Albert D. Kirwan. *The South since Appomattox: A Century of Regional Change*. New York: Oxford University Press, 1967.

Clinton, Catherine, and Nina Silber, eds. *Battle Scars: Gender and Sexuality in the American Civil War*. Oxford: Oxford University Press, 2006.

——, eds. *Divided Houses: Gender and the Civil War*. New York: Oxford University Press, 1992.

Connelly, Thomas L., and Barbara Bellows. *God and General Longstreet: The Lost Cause and the Southern Mind*. Baton Rouge: Louisiana State University Press, 1982.

Coulter, E. Merton. *The Civil War and Readjustment in Kentucky*. Chapel Hill: University of North Carolina Press, 1926.

Cox, Karen L. *Dixie's Daughters: The United Daughters of the Confederacy and the Preservation of Confederate Culture*. Gainesville: University Press of Florida, 2003.

Cunningham, H. H. *Doctors in Gray: The Confederate Medical Service*. Baton Rouge: Louisiana State University Press, 1958.

Dabney, R. L. *Life and Campaign of Lieutenant General Thomas J. Jackson*. New York: Blelock, 1866.

Dailey, Jane. *Before Jim Crow: The Politics of Race in Postemancipation Virginia*. Chapel Hill: University of North Carolina Press, 2000.

Daniel, Larry J. *Shiloh: The Battle That Changed the Civil War*. New York: Simon & Schuster, 1997.

——. *Soldiering in the Army of Tennessee: A Portrait of Life in a Confederate Army*. Chapel Hill: University of North Carolina Press, 1991.

Daviess, Maria T. *History of Mercer and Boyle Counties.* Vol. 1. Harrodsburg, Ky.: Harrodsburg Herald, 1924.

Davis, William C. *Battle at Bull Run: A History of the First Major Campaign of the Civil War.* Baton Rouge: Louisiana State University Press, 1977.

Dean, Eric. *Shook over Hell: Post-Traumatic Stress, Vietnam, and the Civil War.* Cambridge, Mass.: Harvard University Press, 1999.

Devine, Shauna. *Learning from the Wounded: The Civil War and the Rise of American Medical Science.* Chapel Hill: University of North Carolina Press, 2014.

Donald, David Herbert, Jean Harvey Baker, and Michael F. Holt. *The Civil War and Reconstruction.* New York: Norton, 2001.

Downs, Jim. *Sick from Freedom: African-American Illness and Suffering during the Civil War and Reconstruction.* New York: Oxford University Press, 2012.

Drago, Edmund L. *Confederate Phoenix: Rebel Children and Their Families in South Carolina.* New York: Fordham University Press, 2008.

Duffy, John, ed. *The Rudolph Matas History of Medicine in Louisiana.* Vol. 2. Baton Rouge: Louisiana State University Press, 1962.

Edwards, Laura F. *Gendered Strife and Confusion: The Political Culture of Reconstruction.* Urbana: University of Illinois Press, 1997.

———. *Scarlett Doesn't Live Here Anymore: Women in the Civil War Era.* Urbana: University of Illinois Press, 2000.

Eicher, David J. *The Longest Night: A Military History of the Civil War.* New York: Simon & Schuster, 2001.

Fahs, Alice. *The Imagined Civil War: Popular Literature of the North and South, 1861–1865.* Chapel Hill: University of North Carolina Press, 2001.

Farman, Christie Anne, ed. *Women of the American South: A Multicultural Reader.* New York: New York University Press, 1997.

Faust, Drew Gilpin. *Mothers of Invention: Women of the Slaveholding South in the American Civil War.* New York: Vintage, 1996.

———. *This Republic of Suffering: Death and the Civil War.* New York: Knopf, 2008.

Foner, Eric. *Reconstruction: America's Unfinished Revolution, 1863–1877.* New York: Harper and Row, 1988.

Foote, Shelby. *The Civil War: A Narrative, Red River to Appomattox.* New York: Vintage, 1974.

Foster, Gaines M. *Ghosts of the Confederacy: Defeat, the Lost Cause, and the Emergence of the New South, 1865 to 1913.* New York: Oxford University Press, 1987.

Freeman, Joanne B. *Affairs of Honor: National Politics in the New Republic.* New Haven: Yale University Press, 2001.

Freemon, Frank R. *Gangrene and Glory: Medical Care during the American Civil War.* Cranbury, N.J.: Associated University Presses, 1998.

Friedmann, Lawrence W. *The Psychological Rehabilitation of the Amputee.* Springfield, Ill.: Charles C Thomas, 1978.

Friend, Craig Thompson, and Lorri Glover, eds. *Southern Manhood: Perspectives on Masculinity in the Old South.* Athens: University of Georgia Press, 2004.

Gallagher, Gary W., and Alan T. Nolan, eds. *The Myth of the Lost Cause and Civil War History.* Bloomington: Indiana University Press, 2000.

Gammage, W. L. *The Camp, the Bivouac, and the Battlefield.* Little Rock: Arkansas Southern Press, 1958.

Gerber, David A., ed. *Disabled Veterans in History*. Ann Arbor: University of Michigan Press, 2000.

Gillespie, Shirley E. *The Lady with the Milk White Hands: A Biography of Captain Sally Louisa Tompkins*. Chandler, Ariz.: Two Dogs, 2006.

Glover, Lorri. *Southern Sons: Becoming Men in the New Nation*. Baltimore: Johns Hopkins University Press, 2007.

Goldfield, David. *America Aflame: How the Civil War Created a Nation*. New York: Bloomsbury Press, 2011.

——. *Still Fighting the Civil War: The American South and Southern History*. Baton Rouge: Louisiana State University Press, 2002.

Green, Elna C., ed. *Before the New Deal: Social Welfare in the South, 1830–1930*. Athens: University of Georgia Press, 1999.

Greenberg, Kenneth S. *Honor and Slavery: Lies, Duels, Noses, Masks, Dressing as a Woman, Gifts, Strangers, Humanitarianism, Death, Slave Rebellions, the Proslavery Argument, Baseball, Hunting, and Gambling in the Old South*. Princeton, N.J.: Princeton University Press, 1996.

——. *Masters and Statesmen: The Political Culture of Slavery*. Baltimore: Johns Hopkins University Press, 1985.

Guelzo, Allen C. *Fateful Lightning: A New History of the Civil War and Reconstruction*. New York: Oxford University Press, 2012.

Hagerman, Keppel. *Dearest of Captains: A Biography of Sally Louisa Tompkins*. White Stone, Va.: Brandylane, 1996.

Haller, John S., Jr. *Battlefield Medicine: A History of the Military Ambulance from the Napoleonic Wars through World War I*. Carbondale: Southern Illinois University Press, 1992.

Harris, William C. *Presidential Reconstruction in Mississippi*. Baton Rouge: Louisiana State University Press, 1967.

Hartman, David, and David Coles. *Biographical Rosters of Florida's Confederate and Union Soldiers, 1861–65*. Vols. 1–4. Wilmington, N.C.: Broadfoot, 1995.

Hasegawa, Guy R. *Mending Broken Soldiers: The Union and Confederate Programs to Supply Artificial Limbs*. Carbondale: Southern Illinois University Press, 2012.

Hettle, Wallace. *Inventing Stonewall Jackson: A Civil War Hero in History and Memory*. Baton Rouge: Louisiana State University Press, 2011.

Hilde, Libra R. *Worth a Dozen Men: Women and Nursing in the Civil War South*. Charlottesville: University of Virginia Press, 2012.

Hogue, James K. *Uncivil War: Five New Orleans Street Battles and the Rise and Fall of Radical Reconstruction*. Baton Rouge: Louisiana State University Press, 2006.

Humphrey, David C. *Peg Leg: The Improbable Life of a Texas Hero, Thomas William Ward, 1807–1872*. Denton, Tex.: Texas State Historical Association, 2009.

Humphreys, Margaret. *Intensely Human: The Health of the Black Soldier in the American Civil War*. Baltimore: Johns Hopkins University Press, 2008.

——. *Marrow of Tragedy: The Health Crisis of the American Civil War*. Baltimore, Md.: Johns Hopkins University Press, 2013.

Jabour, Anya. *Scarlett's Sisters: Young Women in the Old South*. Chapel Hill: University of North Carolina Press, 2007.

Janney, Caroline E. *Remembering the Civil War: Reunion and the Limits of Reconciliation*. Chapel Hill: University of North Carolina Press, 2013.

Jarvis, Christina S. *The Male Body at War: American Masculinity during World War II.* DeKalb: Northern Illinois University Press, 2004.

Johnson, Charles Beneulyn, M.D. *Muskets and Medicine; or, Army Life in the Sixties.* Philadelphia: F.A. Davis, 1917.

Jones, Terry L. *The American Civil War.* New York: McGraw-Hill, 2010.

Labhé, Ronald M., and Jonathan Lurie. *The Slaughterhouse Cases: Regulation, Reconstruction and the Fourteenth Amendment.* Lawrence: University Press of Kansas, 2003.

Linderman, Gerald F. *Embattled Courage: The Experience of Combat in the American Civil War.* New York: Free Press, 1987.

Lindsey, Linda. *Gender Roles: A Sociological Perspective.* Upper Saddle River, N.J.: Prentice Hall, 1997.

Linker, Beth. *War's Waste: Rehabilitation in World War I America.* Chicago: University of Chicago Press, 2011.

Logue, Larry M., and Michael Barton, eds. *The Civil War Veteran: A Historical Reader.* New York: New York University Press, 2007.

Long, Alecia P. *The Great Southern Babylon: Sex, Race and Respectability in New Orleans, 1865–1920.* Baton Rouge: Louisiana State University Press, 2004.

Long, Clarence D. *Wages and Earnings in the United States, 1860–1890.* Princeton, N.J.: Princeton University Press, 1960.

Long, Lisa A. *Rehabilitating Bodies: Health, History, and the American Civil War.* Philadelphia: University of Pennsylvania Press, 2003.

Marlow, Clayton Charles. *Matt W. Ransom: Confederate General from North Carolina.* Jefferson, N.C.: McFarland, 1996.

Marshall, Anne E. *Creating a Confederate Kentucky: The Lost Cause and Civil War Memory in a Border State.* Chapel Hill: University of North Carolina Press, 2010.

Marshall, Park. *A Life of William B. Bate: Citizen, Soldier and Statesman.* Nashville: Cumberland Press, 1908.

Marten, James. *America's Corporal: James Tanner in War and Peace.* Athens: University of Georgia Press, 2014.

——. *Sing not War: The Lives of Union and Confederate Veterans in Gilded Age America.* Chapel Hill: University of North Carolina Press, 2011.

Martin, Samuel J. *Southern Hero Matthew Galbraith Butler: Confederate General, Hampton Red Shirt and U.S. Senator.* Mechanicsburg, PA: Stackpole Books, 2001.

McCawley, Patrick J. *Artificial Limbs for Confederate Soldiers.* Columbia: South Carolina Department of Archives and History, 1992.

McClurken, Jeffrey W. *Take Care of the Living: Reconstructing Confederate Veteran Families in Virginia.* Charlottesville: University of Virginia Press, 2009.

McCurry, Stephanie. *Confederate Reckoning: Power and Politics in the Civil War South.* Cambridge, Mass.: Harvard University Press, 2010.

——. *Masters of Small Worlds: Yeoman Households, Gender Relations and the Political Culture of the Antebellum South Carolina Low Country.* New York: Oxford University Press, 1995.

McPherson, James M. *Battle Cry of Freedom: The Civil War Era.* New York: Oxford University Press, 1988.

——. *For Cause and Comrades: Why Men Fought in the Civil War.* New York: Oxford University Press, 1997.

——. *Ordeal by Fire: The Civil War*. Vol. 2. New York: McGraw-Hill, 2001.

McWhiney, Grady, and Perry D. Jamieson., *Attack and Die: Civil War Military Tactics and the Southern Heritage*. Tuscaloosa: University of Alabama Press, 1982.

Meier, Kathryn Shively. *Nature's Civil War: Common Soldiers and the Environment in 1862 Virginia*. Chapel Hill: University of North Carolina Press, 2013.

Miller, Brian Craig. *John Bell Hood and the Fight for Civil War Memory*. Knoxville: University of Tennessee Press, 2010.

Neff, John R. *Honoring the Civil War Dead: Commemoration and the Problem of Reconciliation*. Lawrence: University Press of Kansas, 2005.

Nelson, Megan Kate. *Ruin Nation: Destruction and the American Civil War*. Athens: University of Georgia Press, 2012.

Nielsen, Kim E. *A Disability History of the United States*. Boston: Beacon, 2012.

Ott, Katherine, David Serlin, and Stephen Mihm, eds. *Artificial Parts, Practical Lives: Modern Histories of Prosthetics*. New York: New York University Press, 2002.

Ott, Victoria E. *Confederate Daughters: Coming of Age during the Civil War*. Carbondale: Southern Illinois University Press, 2008.

Owen, Thomas McAdory. *History of Alabama and Dictionary of Alabama Biography*. Vols. 1, 3, and 4. Chicago: S.J. Clarke, 1921.

Parish, Peter J. *The American Civil War*. New York: Holmes and Meier, 1975.

Pfanz, Donald C. *Richard S. Ewell: A Soldier's Life*. Chapel Hill: University of North Carolina Press, 1998.

Rable, George C. *God's Almost Chosen Peoples: A Religious History of the American Civil War*. Chapel Hill: University of North Carolina Press, 2010.

Robertson, James I., Jr. *Soldiers Blue and Gray*. New York: Warner Books, 1988.

Roland, Charles P. *An American Iliad: The Story of the Civil War*. New York: McGraw-Hill, 1991.

Rosenberg, R. B. *Living Monuments: Confederate Soldiers' Homes in the New South*. Chapel Hill: University of North Carolina Press, 1993.

Rotundo, E. Anthony. *American Manhood: Transformations in Masculinity from the Revolution to the Modern Era*. New York: Basic Books, 1993.

Rubin, Anne Sarah. *A Shattered Nation: The Rise and Fall of the Confederacy, 1861–1868*. Chapel Hill: University of North Carolina Press, 2005.

Rutkow, Ira M. *Bleeding Blue and Gray: Civil War Surgery and the Evolution of American Medicine*. New York: Random House, 2005.

Schantz, Mark S. *Awaiting the Heavenly Country: The Civil War and America's Culture of Death*. Ithaca, N.Y.: Cornell University Press, 2008.

Schmidt, James M., and Guy R. Hasegawa, eds. *Years of Change and Suffering: Modern Perspectives on Civil War Medicine*. Roseville, Minn.: Edinborough Press, 2009.

Schroeder-Lein, Glenna R. *Confederate Hospitals on the Move: Samuel H. Stout and the Army of Tennessee*. Columbia: University of South Carolina Press, 1994.

Schultz, Jane E. *Women at the Front: Hospital Workers in Civil War America*. Chapel Hill: University of North Carolina Press, 2007.

Schweik, Susan M. *The Ugly Laws: Disability in Public*. New York: New York University Press, 2009.

Sears, Stephen W. *Chancellorsville*. New York: Houghton Mifflin, 1996.

Sheehan, Tanya. *Doctored: The Medicine of Photography in Nineteenth-Century America*. University Park: Pennsylvania State University Press, 2011.

Siebers, Tobin. *Disability Aesthetics.* Ann Arbor: University of Michigan Press, 2010.

Silber, Nina. *Gender and the Sectional Conflict.* Chapel Hill: University of North Carolina Press, 2008.

———. *The Romance of Reunion: Northerners and the South, 1865–1900.* Chapel Hill: University of North Carolina Press, 1993.

Simpson, Alicia. *Index of Confederate Pension Applications, Commonwealth of Kentucky.* Frankfort, Ky.: Division of Archives and Records Management, Department of Library and Archives, 1978.

Smith, John David. *Black Judas: William Hannibal Thomas and the American Negro.* Athens: University of Georgia Press, 2000.

Stowe, Steven M. *Doctoring the South: Southern Physicians and Everyday Medicine in the Mid-Nineteenth Century.* Chapel Hill: University of North Carolina Press, 2004.

———. *Intimacy and Power in the Old South.* Baltimore: Johns Hopkins University Press, 1987.

Taylor, Amy Murrell. *The Divided Family in Civil War America.* Chapel Hill: University of North Carolina Press, 2005.

Thompson, Edwin Porter. *History of the First Kentucky Brigade.* Cincinnati: Caxton, 1868.

———. *History of the Orphan Brigade.* Louisville: Lewis N. Thompson, 1898.

Thompson, Rosemarie Garland. *Extraordinary Bodies: Figuring Physical Disability in American Culture and Literature.* New York: Columbia University Press, 1997.

Travis, Jennifer. *Wounded Hearts: Masculinity, Law, and Literature in American Culture.* Chapel Hill: University of North Carolina Press, 2005.

Webb, Ross A. *Kentucky in the Reconstruction Era.* Lexington: University Press of Kentucky, 1979.

Wecter, Dixon. *When Johnny Comes Marching Home.* Cambridge: Houghton Mifflin, 1944.

Wegner, Ansley Herring. *Phantom Pain: North Carolina's Artificial-Limbs Program for Confederate Veterans.* Raleigh: Office of Archives and History, North Carolina Department of Cultural Resources, 2004.

Wells, Jonathan Daniel. *A House Divided: The Civil War and Nineteenth Century America.* New York: Routledge, 2012.

Welsh, Jack D. *Medical Histories of Confederate Generals.* Kent, Ohio: Kent State University Press, 1995.

———. *Two Confederate Hospitals and Their Patients: Atlanta to Opelika.* Macon, Ga.: Mercer University Press, 2005.

Wetherington, Mark V. *Plain Folk's Fight: The Civil War and Reconstruction in Piney Woods Georgia.* Chapel Hill: University of North Carolina Press, 2005.

Whites, LeeAnn. *The Civil War as a Crisis in Gender: Augusta, Georgia, 1860–1890.* Athens: University of Georgia Press, 2000.

———. *Gender Matters: Civil War, Reconstruction and the Making of the New South.* New York: Palgrave Macmillan, 2005.

Whites, LeeAnn, and Alecia P. Long, eds. *Occupied Women: Gender, Military Occupation and the American Civil War.* Baton Rouge: Louisiana State University Press, 2009.

Wiggins, David N. *Georgia's Confederate Sons.* Vol. 1. Carrollton: University of West Georgia Press, 2007.

———. *Remembering Georgia's Confederates.* Charleston, S.C.: Arcadia, 2005.

Wiley, Bell Irvin. *The Life of Johnny Reb: The Common Soldier of the Confederacy.* Baton Rouge: Louisiana State University Press, 1943.

Wilkinson, Warren, and Steven E. Woodworth. *A Scythe of Fire: A Civil War Story of the Eighth Georgia Infantry Regiment.* New York: William Morrow, 2002.

Williams, David. *A People's History of the Civil War: Struggles for the Meaning of Freedom.* New York: New Press, 2005.

Williams, Rusty. *My Old Confederate Home: A Respectable Place for Civil War Veterans.* Lexington: University Press of Kentucky, 2010.

Wilson, Charles Reagan. *Baptized in Blood: The Religion of the Lost Cause.* Athens: University of Georgia Press, 1980.

Wisner, Elizabeth. *Social Welfare in the South: From Colonial Times to World War I.* Baton Rouge: Louisiana State University Press, 1970.

Woodworth, Steven E. *Jefferson Davis and His Generals: The Failure of Confederate Command in the West.* Lawrence: University Press of Kansas, 1990.

Wyatt-Brown, Bertram. *The Shaping of Southern Culture: Honor, Grace, and War, 1760s–1880s.* Chapel Hill: University of North Carolina Press, 2001.

———. *Southern Honor: Ethics and Behavior in the Old South.* New York: Oxford University Press, 1982.

ARTICLES AND PAPERS

Berry, Stephen. "When Metal Meets Mettle: The Hard Realities of Civil War Soldiering." *North and South* 9, no. 4 (August 2006): 12–21.

Brodman, Estelle, and Elizabeth B. Carrick. "American Military Medicine in the Mid-Nineteenth Century: The Experience of Alexander H. Hoff, M.D." *Bulletin of the History of Medicine* 64, no. 1 (Spring 1990): 63–78.

Carroll, Dillon. "'The Living Souls, the Bodies' Tragedies': A Comparative Analysis of Amputation and PTSD in the Civil War." Paper presented at the Southern Association for the History of Medicine and Science meeting, Atlanta, March 3, 2012.

DeBrava, Valerie. "The Offending Hand of War in *Harper's Weekly.*" *American Periodicals* 11(2001): 49–64.

Edwards, Laura F. "The Problem of Dependency: African Americans, Labor Relations and the Law in the Nineteenth-Century South." *Agricultural History* 72, no. 2 (Spring 1998): 313–40.

Escott, Paul. "'The Cry of the Sufferers': The Problem of Welfare in the Confederacy." *Civil War History* 23 (September 1977): 228–40.

Fairclough, Adam. "'Scalawags,' Southern Honor, and the Lost Cause: Explaining the Fatal Encounter of James H. Cosgrove and Edward L. Pierson." *Journal of Southern History* 77 (November 2011): 1–28.

Figg, Laurann, and Jane Farrell-Beck. "Amputation in the Civil War: Physical and Social Dimensions." *Journal of History of Medicine and Allied Sciences* 48, no. 4 (1993): 454–75.

Frick, Daphne Frick. "Soldiers with Empty Sleeves: The Minie Ball and Civil War Medicine." *Proceedings and Papers of the Georgia Association of Historians* 14 (1993): 46–53.

Gold, Susanna W. "'Fighting It Over Again': The Battle of Gettysburg at the 1876 Centennial Exhibition." *Civil War History* 54, no. 3 (September 2008): 277–310.

Gorn, Elliot J. "'Gouge and Bite, Pull Hair and Scratch': The Social Significance of Fighting in the Southern Backcountry." *American Historical Review* 90, no. 1 (supplement) (February 1985): 18–43.

Graber, John W. "One Man's Civil War." *Minnesota History* 52, no. 4 (1990): 144–45.

Grant, Susan-Mary. "The Lost Boys: Citizen-Soldiers, Disabled Veterans, and Confederate Nationalism in the Age of People's War." *Journal of the Civil War Era* 2, no. 2 (June 2012): 233–59.

Hacker, J. David. "A Census-Based Count of the Civil War Dead." *Civil War History* 57, no. 4 (December 2011): 307–48.

Hacker, J. David, Libra Hilde, and James Holland Jones. "The Effect of the Civil War on Southern Marriage Patterns." *Journal of Southern History* 76, no. 1 (February 2010): 39–72.

Jabour, Anya. "Male Friendship and Masculinity in the Early National South: William Wirt and His Friends." *Journal of the Early Republic* 20, no. 1 (Spring 2000): 83–111.

Jones, Charles T., Jr. "Five Confederates." *Alabama Historical Quarterly* 24, no. 2 (1962): 133–221.

Jordan, Brian Matthew. "Living Monuments: Union Veteran Amputees and the Embodied Memory of the Civil War." *Civil War History* 57, no. 2 (June 2011): 121–52.

Koven, Seth. "Remembering and Dismemberment: Crippled Children, Wounded Soldiers, and the Great War in Great Britain." *American Historical Review* 99, no. 4 (October 1994): 1167–1202.

Lewellen, Faye. "Limbs Made and Unmade by War." *America's Civil War*, September 1995, 38–45.

Lindman, Janet Moore. "Acting the Manly Christian: White Evangelical Masculinity in Revolutionary Virginia." *William and Mary Quarterly* 57, no. 2 (April 2000): 393–416.

Mayfield, John. "'The Soul of a Man!': William Gilmore Simms and the Myths of Southern Manhood." *Journal of the Early Republic* 15, no. 3 (Fall 1995): 477–500.

McClintock, Megan. "Civil War Pensions and the Reconstruction of Union Families." *Journal of American History* 83 (September 1996): 456–80.

McDaid, Jennifer Davis. "With Lame Legs and No Money: Virginia's Disabled Confederate Veterans." *Virginia Cavalcade* 47 (Winter 1998): 14–25.

Meier, Kathryn S. "'No Place for the Sick': Nature's War on Civil War Soldier Mental and Physical Health in the 1862 Peninsula and Shenandoah Valley Campaigns." *Journal of the Civil War Era* 1, no. 2 (June 2011): 176–206.

Nelson, Megan Kate. "A Worthy Substitute for Nature: Prosthetics and the Problem of Authenticity in Civil War America." Paper presented at the American Historical Association meeting, New Orleans, La., January 3, 2013.

Parsons, Elaine Frantz. "Midnight Rangers: Costume and Performance in the Reconstruction-Era Ku Klux Klan." *Journal of American History* 92, no. 3 (December 2005): 811–36.

Schurr, Nancy. "It Is Heart-Breaking to Hear Them Groan: Female Workers in Confederate General Hospitals." Paper presented at the Society of Civil War Historians meeting, Richmond, June 18, 2010.

Scribner, R. L. "A Short History of Brewton." *Alabama Historical Quarterly* 11, no. 1 (1949): 7–131.

Short, Joanna. "Confederate Veteran Pensions, Occupation, and Men's Retirement in the New South." *Social Science History* 30 (Spring 2006): 75–101.

Vinovskis, Maris A. "Have Social Historians Lost the Civil War? Some Preliminary Demographic Speculations." *Journal of American History* 76, no. 1 (June 1989): 34–58.

Zornow, William Frank. "State Aid for Indigent Soldiers and Their Families in Louisiana, 1861–1865." *Louisiana Historical Quarterly* 39, no. 3 (July 1956): 375–80.

DISSERTATIONS

Gross, Jennifer L. "'Good Angels': Confederate Widowhood and the Reassurance of Patriarchy in the Postbellum South." Ph.D. diss., Emory University, 2001.

Herschbach, Lisa Marie. "Fragmentation and Reunion: Medicine, Memory and Body in the American Civil War." Ph.D. diss., Harvard University, 1997.

FILMS

Gone with the Wind. Los Angeles: Metro Goldwyn Mayer, 1939.

The Horse Soldiers. Los Angeles: Metro Goldwyn Mayer, 1959.

Lincoln. Los Angeles: DreamWorks, 2012.

WEBSITES

http://www.collectorsweekly.com/articles/war-and-prosthetics

http://dartmed.dartmouth.edu/summer11/html/years_of_change.php

http://www.history-sites.com/cgi-bin/bbs62x/nccwmb/webbs_config.pl?md=read;id=2472

http://www.huffingtonpost.com/2012/07/26/ied-afghanistan-war-veterans_n_1705397.html

http://http://ncgenweb.us/cumberland/cumberland.htm

http://www.tshaonline.org/handbook/online/articles/ynt05

http://unitproj.library.ucla.edu/biomed/his/painexhibit/panel4.htm

http://usatoday30.usatoday.com/news/nation/2005-04-28-female-amputees-combat_x.htm

INDEX

Adam, Nicholas, 187n11
Adams, James, 80
Adams, John, 59–60
Afghanistan, 174–75
African Americans, 4, 9, 89, 121, 126–27,
    132, 146; and bodies, 6, 188n21; and
    interaction with Confederates, 87
Agnew, Samuel A., 25
Alabama, 23, 36, 88, 124, 131, 137, 149,
    197n21; anger over artificial limbs, 149,
    155; and artificial limb expenditures,
    150–51, 180, 212n18, 216n24, 216n26;
    hospitals in, 41; and pensions, 164,
    204n46, 221n39
Albany, Georgia, 124
alcohol, 29, 70, 84, 212n17
Alexander, Peter Wellington, 47–48
Alexandria, Louisiana, 88–89
Allen, B. W., 70
Allen, George, 53
Allen, Henry Watkins, 58–59
almshouses, 132, 135, 145, 158
amputation, 116, 119, 122, 126, 128,
    136, 139, 154, 160, 161, 177–78; from
    accidents, 52, 146; arms, 20–22, 39–48,
    50–51, 53, 58–68, 70, 72, 75–76, 79–80,
    87–90, 93–95; chloroform, 20, 23, 28–
    31, 48, 52, 59–60, 75, 84, 116; civilian
    views of, 107–9, 121–26; data pertaining
    to, 39–42, 177–79; dreams about, 91, 175;
    emotional reaction to, 52, 53, 72–76, 120,
    122; fatality rates, 39–42, 177–79, 192n47,
    193n49, 194n51; fingers, 48, 50, 52, 67,
    70, 72, 75, 79, 88, 120, 160; hands, 20–
    22, 31, 39, 42, 48, 50, 63, 70, 72, 75, 79–
    80, 88; hips, 11, 39, 41–42, 66, 79, 83,
    171; legs, 38–48, 64–68, 70–72, 74–77,
    79–81, 83–87, 89–90; legs (prewar), 6;
    limited sources, 12; memory of, 1, 2, 4–6,
    9–14; numbers of in the Confederacy,
39–42, 177–79, 192n47, 193n49, 194n51;
    numbers of in the United States, 39;
    organs, 72; perception of in South before
    Civil War, 6–7; piles of limbs, 20–22;
    primary, 28, 31; resistance to, 50, 54–55,
    58–60; results in death, 28, 44–45, 65,
    76, 79, 83–84, 95, 97–99; secondary, 28,
    42, 97; surgeons and, 17–20, 22–25, 27–
    31, 33–35, 37, 39–46, 50–61; toes and
    feet, 21, 29, 41–42, 45, 54–55, 70, 72, 75,
    84, 89, 120; tools, 27
amputees, 6–15, 140, 156–57, 159;
    acceptance from women, 101–5, 107–
    15; and accepting amputation, 63–68;
    accepting death, 58–59; begging, 118,
    133–35; benevolence and, 138–39; burial
    of limbs, 22, 63, 65, 89; and captivity,
    44, 61, 86–88, 170; care from nurses,
    43–46, 56, 76, 86, 93–100; cowardice,
    72, 79, 84, 119; depression, 52–53, 75–
    76; difficulty with prosthetic devices,
    7, 119, 127, 129, 136, 154–55, 175;
    disillusionment, 76–77; education, 127–
    28; employment of, 127–35; farming,
    127; fear of rejection from women, 104–
    7; historians and, 18; humor, 55, 75, 79,
    99, 122; and manhood, 54–90, 91–115;
    manual labor, 127, 132–33; mobility,
    4, 50, 68, 144, 151, 154, 172; modern
    perceptions of, 173–76; patriotism, 72,
    79–80, 84, 120–21, 136, 162; phantom
    limbs, 118–20; politics and, 129–32;
    prosthetic devices and, 144–46, 148–
    55; and race, 87; resisting amputation,
    54–58, 84–86; return home, 121–27;
    returning to the battlefield, 59–63, 65–
    67; seeking pensions, 143, 160–70; and
    southern oaks, 5–6, 103; suicide, 116–17;
    surgeons and, 39, 42, 72, 75; symbols of
    Lost Cause, 117–18, 137–39; teaching,

Polk, John D., 160
Polk, Leonidas, 88
Pollard, Edward, 123–24
Portis, John C., 89
poverty, 111–12, 152, 160–61, 163, 172
Power, J. L., 150
Preston, Sally Buchannan, 106–7
Price, George W., 146
primary amputation, 28, 31
prosthetic devices, 120, 133, 141, 159, 161,
    172–76; and benevolent groups, 135–39;
    and industry, 129, 147–50; pain and, 118–
    19, 127–28, 143; soldiers and, 52, 65–66,
    81, 90; and state programs, 150–57, 180–
    82, 211n14, 211n16, 211n18, 213nn19–20,
    213n21, 214n22, 215nn23–24, 216n26;
    usage before the Civil War, 7
Purple Heart, 173

Quaile, Lizzie, 109, 130

Rable, George, 53
Rainwater, Charles, 122
Raleigh Daily Standard, 150
Raleigh Sentinel, 151
Ransom, Matthew Whitaker, 58
Rawls, Samuel B., 113
Read, John, 127
Readjusters, 131–32
Ready, Alice, 102
reconciliation, 15, 121, 125–26, 131, 167–
    68, 172
Redding, John, 107
redemption, 145, 152, 160
Reid, Whitelaw, 108, 123
religion, 13, 23, 51; and amputation, 53,
    75, 125
Republican Party, 130, 152, 158
resections, 24, 68, 150, 193n47, 194nn50–51
Richardson, John Manly, 128
Richardson, T. G., 28, 66
Richmond, Virginia, 11, 24, 64, 67, 83,
    106–7, 146; battles around, 86; benevolent
    groups in, 100, 135–36; hospitals in,
    30, 36–37, 40, 46, 61, 97, 99–100, 114;
    postwar, 124–25, 133; women in, 53

Ride with the Devil (Lee), 2
Robarts, Henrietta, 113–14
Robarts, James, 113
Robinson, John, 151
Robson, John, 30, 127
Roden, James B., 25
Rothermel, Peter, 141–42
Rowland, Kim, 122
Rudd, W. Z., 170
Rush, Columbus J., 78, 81–82
Russell, William A., 70

Samples, John Bunyon, 127
San Antonio, Tex., 6
Savannah, Ga., 108, 123
Sayers, Joseph D., 164
Scales, Cordelia, 93
Schuppert, Moritz, 17
Second Alabama Cavalry, 75
secondary amputation, 28, 42, 97–98
Second Florida, 68
Second Manassas, 21, 44, 57, 70, 178
Second Tennessee, 54
sensory hallucination, 119
Seven Days, 21, 40, 179
Seven Pines, 20, 60, 67, 75, 113
Seventh Kentucky, 170
Seventh Louisiana, 25
Shakespeare Alms House, 135
Sharpsburg, 48, 60, 172. *See also* Antietam
Sheppard, Deacon Elliott, 158
Sherman, William T., 2, 123
Shiloh, 1, 3, 7, 53–54, 59, 61, 75, 98, 160,
    170; and high number of amputations, 38
Shivers, Jesse B., 68, 216n26
Sick Soldiers Relief Society, 100
Sisters of Charity, 55
Sixteenth Mississippi, 119
Sixteenth Tennessee, 79
Sixth Florida, 75
Sixty-Second Georgia, 52
slavery, 5, 57–58, 92, 121, 125, 143
Sloan, John Mather, 67, 98
smallpox, 34
Smith, Janie, 94
Smith, John David, 117

UnCivil Wars

CPSIA information can be obtained at www.ICGtesting.com
Printed in the USA
LVOW08s0254140416

483523LV00002B/9/P